THEORY AND PRACTICE IN
AMERICAN MEDICINE

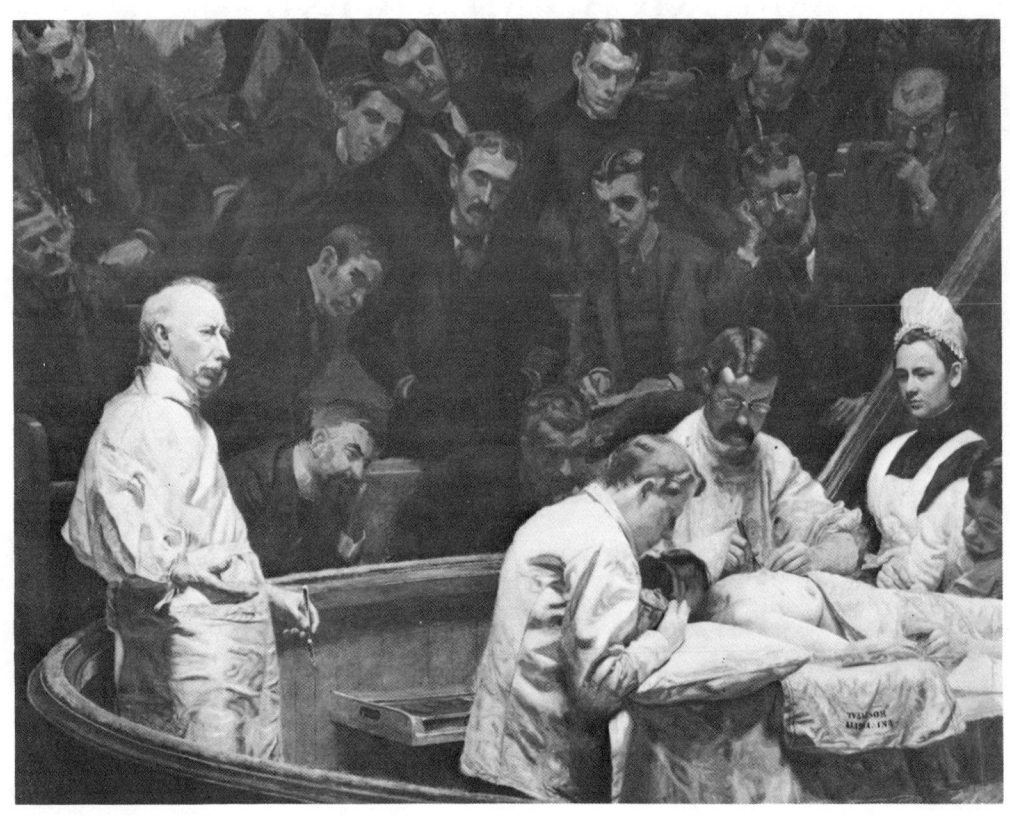

Agnew Clinic by Thomas Eakins. Courtesy the *School of Medicine of the University of Pennsylvania.*

Theory and Practice in American Medicine

Historical Studies from the Journal of the History of Medicine & Allied Sciences

GERT H. BRIEGER

Editor

SCIENCE HISTORY PUBLICATIONS
NEW YORK
1976

Science History Publications
a division of
Neale Watson Academic Publications, Inc.
156 Fifth Avenue
New York, New York 10010
© 1976 The Journal of the History of Medicine and Allied Sciences
Designed and manufactured in the U.S.A.
First Edition 1976

Publisher's Note: We would like to express our appreciation to the Journal for granting permission to reprint the articles in this volume. If the publishers have unwittingly infringed the copyright on any illustration reproduced, they will gladly pay an appropriate fee on being satisfied as to the owner's title.

Contents

Introduction
    GERT H. BRIEGER ... vii

Medical Education

Dr. Thomas Bond's Essay on the Utility of Clinical
Lectures (1947, 2: 10-19)
    CARL BRIDENBAUGH ... 1

The Study of Medicine at the Vermont Academy of Medicine
(1827-1829) as Revealed in the Journal of Asa Fitch
(1969, 24: 416-429)
    SAMUEL REZNECK ... 11

The New England Journal of Medicine, 1812-1968
(1969, 24: 125-139)
    JOSEPH GARLAND ... 25

Medical Theory and Medical Research

William Beaumont, Robley Dunglison, and the
"Philadelphia Physiologists" (1970, 25: 3-21)
    JEROME J. BYLEBYL ... 39

American Attitudes toward the Germ Theory
of Disease, 1860-1880 (1954, 9: 428-454)
    PHYLLIS ALLEN RICHMOND ... 58

Poliomyelitis and the Rockefeller Institute
(1974, 29: 74-92)
    SAUL BENISON ... 85

Medical Practice

Glossary of Historical Fever Terminology
(1961, 16: 76-77)
    PHYLLIS ALLEN RICHMOND ... 104

Smallpox Inoculation in Colonial Boston
(1953, 8: 284-300)
    JOHN B. BLAKE ... 107

The Medical and Surgical Practice of the Lewis
and Clark Expedition (1959, 14: 273-279)
    DRAKE W. WILL ... 124

Neo-Thomsonianism in the United States
(1956, *11*: 133-155)
    ALEX BERMAN   149

The Medical History of the Fredericksburg Campaign
(1963, *18*: 241-256)
    GORDON W. JONES   173

Surgery

Surgical Anesthesia, 1846-1946
(1946, *1*: 505-514)
    JOSIAH C. TRENT   193

Development and Use of the Rubber Glove in Surgery
and Gynecology (1958, *13*: 373-381)
    CURT PROSKAUER   203

Evarts A. Graham, The American College of Surgeons,
and The American Board of Surgery (1972, *27*: 247-261)
    PETER D. OLCH   212

Medical Care

Class, Ethnicity, and Race in American Mental
Hospitals, 1830-1875 (1973, *28*: 207-229)
    GERALD N. GROB   227

Social Class and Medical Care in 19th-Century America:
The Rise and Fall of the Dispensary (1974, *29*: 32-54)
    CHARLES E. ROSENBERG   250

Introduction

IN this, America's bicentennial year, it seems fitting to publish a collection of essays about the nation's medical history. We celebrate also the thirtieth year of *The Journal of the History of Medicine* which has so enriched students of the history of science and medicine for these last three decades. In his introductory statement to volume one of the *Journal*, the first editor, George Rosen, said he hoped to present historical papers "... that can be of interest to as large a section of the medical profession as possible." He and his distinguished board of editors that included Erwin H. Ackerknecht, Max H. Fisch, John F. Fulton, and Josiah C. Trent, did "... not want to cultivate medical history as a mere search for antiquities, as a kind of hunt for curios, but rather as a vital integral part of medicine. We believe this can be done." Now thirty volumes later, owing to the scholarship and dedication of several succeeding editors, the judgment must be that the original goals have been amply fulfilled.

One benefit for an editor of a volume such as this selection represents is that he must go back to the beginning in 1946 and look through each issue. What an enjoyable task! I come away with awe, for the *Journal* has published a remarkable set of papers. The breadth in both subject and time is great.

Because this volume of selections is intended to contain only papers dealing with the history of medicine in America, a number of others that have an important bearing on that subject must be left out. One cannot properly comprehend American developments and practices without taking into account previous or simultaneous European events. A persistent thread in American medical history is the continuing dependence upon our overseas forebears and contemporaries coupled with a perceptible tension produced by the efforts to free ourselves intellectually as well as politically. These tensions are readily apparent in the medical literature until the early decades of the present century, when American medicine began its real rise to world preeminence. Prior to half a century or so ago, it is really not correct to speak of American medicine. With the exception of a few remarkable developments such as the work of Cotton Mather and Zabdiel Boylston on small pox inoculation, the surgical triumphs of Ephraim McDowell and J. Marion Sims, the physiological studies of William Beaumont, and the discovery of anesthesia, there were not a great number of American contributions. But the articles in this volume, as indeed is true for our entire medical story, should not be viewed as a series of isolated discoveries or events nor as the saga of a few major figures about whom we seem to hear over and over again. Much of the recent criticism from within our ranks and from sociologists and general historians has stressed the undue attention given to great men and their great discoveries. It is true, I am afraid, that far too often medicine has used its own history merely as a means of self-glorification. All of the editors of the *Journal* have tried to avoid this approach.

One criticism of medical historiography was published in the *Journal* by Erwin Ackerknecht in 1967. Only three and a half pages long, it is a statement of great force. Ackerknecht argued for a behaviorist approach in writing the history of medicine. "We must admit to ourselves," he pointed out, "that we often do not know the most elementary facts of either medical practices or of social aspects of medical practice even for periods not very far removed at all." Quoting his own teacher Henry Sigerist's statement that, "the history of medicine is infinitely more than the history of the great doctors and their books," Ackerknecht called for more medical history that provides not just anecdotal data about the day to day conditions of medical practice, but a much fuller understanding of what the average patient in a given place at a particular time in the past actually experienced at the hands of the physicians.

Unfortunately, far too few of us have seriously heeded this call. A few of the papers in this volume do qualify, however, and one may hope that more will follow. One of Ackerknecht's own students, Charles Rosenberg, has shown us the way. In an article published in the *Bulletin of the History of Medicine* in 1967, he detailed the practice of medicine in New York City a century before. In the article on the dispensary included here, Rosenberg again demonstrates the importance and the usefulness of focussing on an institution that was at the heart of the urban medical care system of the latter nineteenth century. What we need now is similar treatment of the hospital and it s role as the focus of medical treatment. George Rosen and others have written about the sociological aspects of the use of hospitals, but we need further study of hospital clinics, of the hospital as a teacher of physicians, and of the medical and surgical care received by hospital patients, along the lines suggested by Ackerknecht and Rosenberg. That Gerald Grob has begun to do this for mental hospitals is nicely illustrated by a number of his recent writings, including the article in this volume.

One of the most potent forces in the history of medical literature has been the medical journal. Far too little has been written about its impact on advancing medical science, its role in teaching, its function as the repository of medical knowledge. Most historians make extensive use of the periodical literature in their own researches, just one indication of its great importance. Yet we know little about the actual circulation of journals. How many physicians subscribed to what journals? How many actually read those they purchased, and so on?

Joseph Garland, one of our most successful medical editors of recent decades, does not directly address such questions, but his account of the *New England Journal of Medicine* deserves reprinting, I believe, for it calls to our attention the place of this one influential journal in our medical heritage. The *Boston Medical and Surgical Journal,* founded as the *New England Journal of Medicine and Surgery and the Collateral Branches of Science,* in 1812 (and now again known as the *New England Journal of Medicine*) was one of very few American medical journals that survived for any length of time. Only in the twentieth century have numerous titles been in continuous publication, now to the point of saturating library shelves and most readers' patience.

Hospitals, dispensaries, and medical literature, are but a few of the many themes reappearing in the history of medicine in America. In the beginning, the intellectual baggage brought to America by the early colonists included the current seventeenth-century theories and practices of the British and Continental physicians. One need only recall that both Jamestown and Plymouth were settled before the publication of William Harvey's *De motu cordis*. Edward Eggleston, in his *The Transit of Civilization* published in 1900, devoted a long chapter to the medical notions at the time of settlement. Subsequent historians of colonial America, including Carl Bridenbaugh, Daniel Boorstin, and Perry Miller, among others, have continued to discuss the medical-historical aspects of the period. Medical historians such as Richard Shryock, John Duffy, Whitfield Bell, and John Blake, have all written extensively about colonial physicians and the diseases they and their patients had to face. Dr. Shryock's little book, *Medicine and Society in America,* is readily available. The *Journal* is rich in articles about colonial medicine. One of the virtues of Dr. Blake's article about small pox inoculation is that it also contains a discussion of the disease as it affected Colonial Boston.

Perhaps no single theme in nineteenth-century medicine in America is as important as the rise of the medical sects, their practices, and their relationships to the so-called regular physicians. The homeopaths have in recent years come in for scrutiny and discussion in several books. The activities of botanical practitioners, especially the followers of Samuel Thomson, were extensively described by Alex Berman in his 1954 doctoral dissertation at the University of Wisconsin, *The Impact of the Nineteenth Century Botanico-Medical Movement on American Pharmacy and Medicine.* As noted in the first page of the article on the Neo-Thomsonians in this book, Berman published much of his dissertation in his two 1951 *Bulletin* articles. The extension of the old Thomsonian practices by the Neo-Thomsonians, as Berman described it, was partly a matter of survival in an age of slowly increasing scientific respectability for regular medicine. One of the therapeutic tensions prevalent in the middle of the nineteenth century may be seen in the tradition of Rational Medicine as espoused by eminent regular practitioners such as Jacob Bigelow and Worthington Hooker. Doctors could use purges and sedatives, sudorifics and anodynes, but still they had to rely most heavily upon the healing power of nature.

The middle years of the last century witnessed not only the rise of the medical sects, but the growth of many of the institutions we have come to associate with the medical profession, such as medical schools, medical societies, medical literature, and later in the century, hospitals. At the time of the centennial celebrations in 1876 there were only about 200 general hospitals in the United States. A century later there are over 7000, and building seems to proceed apace. While hospitals are not sufficiently represented in this volume, medical education does receive its share of space. Dr. Bond's ideas about clinical teaching are frequently mentioned, but his essay is not often read any more. Asa Fitch, on the other hand, was not a well-known physician, which makes the notes about his experiences while learning to become a physician a useful primary source.

Two major topics of interest to general historians of nineteenth-century America are the westward migration of the frontier settlements and the advent of the bloody Civil War in the middle of the century. Health and disease on the frontier and the life and work of the early western physicians is of inherent interest to many. Drake Will's chronicle of the medical conditions confronting the early explorers of the West is a vivid portrait of an heroic time. Not only was this the age of so-called heroic therapy, but the trials of migration and settlement of the later followers of Lewis and Clark are written in much blood, not all of it let by physicians, as well as sweat and tears. The disease burden was often heavy, and retreat to a comfortable bed was rarely an economic possibility.

The middle years of the century were a time of medical advance as well as a time of turmoil. The single greatest American gift to the world, many believed, was anesthesia. No volume on American medical history would be complete without some mention of it. The final issue of the inaugural year of the *Journal* was an anesthesia centennial number, and it contained a number of eminently reprintable articles. The article by Josiah Trent in the present volume speaks for itself.

I have deliberately refrained from adding biographical information about the authors represented in this volume, many of whom I know personally and admire. One whom, unfortunately, I did not know, but to whom I have been drawn by personal association is Josiah C. Trent. Dr. Trent died tragically of a lymphoma at the age of thirty-four. Prior to his death in 1948, he collected a major library, now at Duke University, wrote extensively in the history of surgery, was one of the founding editorial board of this *Journal*, and has left an important legacy to those of us attempting to work in the same vineyards.

The most important American contributions to medicine are often said to have been in surgery. Such accomplishments as Ephriam McDowell's ovarian operations and J. Marion Sims's repair of vesico-vaginal fistulae were grand indeed. To the list one might add Reginald Fitz's proper description of appendicitis and William Stewart Halsted's introduction of rubber gloves, as well as a host of other examples. Certainly the Civil War was a proving ground for many surgeons. The conditions described by Gordon Jones for Fredericksburg were true of many other battle sites. After the war surgical training improved, yet surgery was just beginning to emerge as a definable medical specialty. Samuel D. Gross, one of the country's leading surgical teachers, wrote in 1876 that, "there are, strange to say, as a separate and distinct class [of surgeon], no such persons among us. It is safe to affirm that there is not a medical man on this continent who devotes himself exclusively to the practice of surgery." While frequently quoted, this statement should be read in connection with his welcome to the delegates to the first American Surgical Association meeting in Philadelphia in 1882. Here, in his presidential address, Gross noted that

> we have in the United States, according to a reasonable estimate, not fewer than 60,000 medical men. Among these are large numbers of surgeons, who, in point of culture, practical skill, and reputation as writers and teachers, would be an honor to any country, however its standards of excellence.

In the organizational context as well, surgeons have come to wield much power in American medicine. Surgeons played a leading role in the pioneer teaching of anatomy and bacteriology. The early schools of nursing were frequently supported by the surgical staffs of hospitals for the surgeons saw the need for skilled nursing very clearly. The American College of Surgeons took the lead in raising hospital standards. In short, much of the practice of medicine today, its hospital-centered locus especially, is owing to the field of surgery and the surgical subspecialties. In this context Peter Olch's article about the certification of surgeons assumes importance.

Scientific medicine, a term we tend to use rather loosely, is generally associated with our present century. Early physiology as described by Jerome Bylebyl and discussions about the germ theory of disease detailed by Phyllis

Richmond clearly reveal the scientific roots. In the writing of the history of medicine in America, as is evidenced by the articles in the *Journal* for instance, the emphasis has been on the years up to about 1870. The medical story of the last hundred years is yet to be written, though important segments are beginning to appear. Saul Benison's article is one such example. Only when we come to grips with the changing patterns of medical organization and research as influenced by such things as the changing disease picture will we have a better understanding of the history of more recent medicine. The role of philanthropy, of the federal government, of medical education in relation to higher education as a whole, are all parts of the story.

Since medicine, as it is taught in medical schools today, and as the patient-public has come to view it also, is so distinctly science-oriented, it is regrettable that public health could not be better represented in these selections. The reason certainly is not that there are insufficient articles from which to choose. The *Journal* is, in fact, particularly rich in this area. Some of the articles appeared in two parts. So far as American medical subjects are concerned, public health and Colonial medicine are probably the best represented throughout the thirty volumes. Whitfield Bell's recent collection of essays on Colonial medicine will provide readily accessible materials. For the classroom, George Rosen's recently published collection, *From Medical Police to Social Medicine*, should serve the need in part at least, to turn students' attention toward the development of an all important attitude that is social medicine. In addition, a book of Charles Rosenberg's essays soon to be published by the Johns Hopkins Press will also provide readily accessible materials about the social dimensions of health and disease.

I have chosen sixteen papers from a group of sixty-nine good candidates. Obviously many fine articles have found no room, and other editors would certainly have chosen differently. My purpose has been to present as wide a range as possible. Biographical articles, even though some, such as George Rosen's 1965 study of Noah Webster, won prizes, generally tend to be more narrow in focus than most of those included. I have also avoided including two articles by the same author with the one exception of Phyllis Richmond. Her very short glossary of fever terminology is so useful that I hoped hereby to call to it the attention that it deserves. It should be especially helpful in the classroom.

Since I hope this collection will be of particular interest to teachers and students of the history of medicine, one issue of the *Journal* deserves particular mention. The January, 1968 number was dedicated to Richard H. Shryock. All of us who have followed him have been in his continuing debt, both for ideas in his writing, published as well as personal, and from his encouragement to all younger scholars. On pages eight to fifteen of volume 23 of the *Journal* is a bibliography of his published work through 1967. It will be useful to all students of medical thought and medical practice in America. For those wishing to learn more about Dr. Shryock, Whitfield Bell's fine tribute in the January 1974 issue of the *Journal* is highly recommended.

I hope, then, that this collection will find some use in the increasing number of courses in medical history being taught in universities and medical schools. The articles, while representing many themes in the development of medicine in America, raise as many questions as they answer. I shall leave it to students to pose these questions for themselves and wish them well in their search for the answers.

Gert H. Brieger, M.D.

A Short List of Useful References
(*have appeared in paperback editions)

Erwin H. Ackerknecht, *Malaria in the Upper Mississippi Valley 1760-1900,* 1945.
*George W. Adams, *Doctors in Blue,* 1952.
*Whitfield J. Bell, *The Colonial Physician and Other Essays,* 1975.
John B. Blake, *Public Health in the Town of Boston, 1630-1822,* 1959.
Thomas N. Bonner, *American Doctors and German Universities,* 1963.
Gert H. Brieger, *Medical America in the Nineteenth Century,* 1972.
James G. Burrow, *AMA, Voice of American Medicine,* 1963.
George W. Corner, *A History of the Rockefeller Institute,* 1964.
Harris L. Coulter, *Divided Legacy,* vol. III., *Science and Ethics in American Medicine: 1800-1914,* 1973.
John D. Davies, *Phrenology, Fad and Science,* 1955.
*John Duffy, *Epidemics in Colonial America,* 1953.
*Richard Dunlop, *Doctors of the American Frontier,* 1962.
Elizabeth Etheridge, *The Butterfly Caste, The Social History of Pellagra in the South,* 1972.
Donald Fleming, *William H. Welch and the Rise of Modern Medicine,* 1954.
*James T. Flexner, *Doctors on Horseback,* 1937.
Martin Kaufman, *Homeopathy in America,* 1971.
Joseph F. Kett, *The Formation of the American Medical Profession,* 1968.
Monroe Lerner and Odin Anderson, *Health Progress in the United States: 1900-1960,* 1963.
Vernon W. Lippard, *A Half Century of American Medical Education, 1920-1970,* 1974.
William F. Norwood, *Medical Education in the United States Before the Civil War,* 1944.
Madge E. Pickard and R. Caryle Buley, *The Midwest Pioneer: His Ills, Cures, and Doctors,* 1945.
George Rosen, *Fees and Fee Bills: Some Economic Aspects of Medical Practice in 19th Century America,* 1946.
   *—*From Medical Police to Social Medicine: Essays on the History of Health Care,* 1974.
*Charles E. Rosenberg, *The Cholera Years,* 1962.
Barbara Rosenkrantz, *Public Health and the State, Changing Views in Massachusetts, 1842-1936,* 1972.
William Rothstein, *American Physicians in the 19th Century,* 1972.
Henry B. Shafer, *The American Medical Profession, 1783-1850,* 1936.

Richard H. Shryock, *American Medical Research*, 1946.
  *—*Medicine and Society in America, 1620-1860*, 1960.
  —*Medicine in America*, 1966.
  —*Medical Licensing in America, 1650-1965*, 1967.
*Herman and Ann Somers, *Doctors, Patients, and Health Insurance*, 1961.
Rosemary Stevens, *American Medicine and the Public Interest*, 1971.
Stephen P. Strickland, *Politics, Science, and Dread Disease*, 1972.
Greer Williams, *Virus Hunters*, 1960.
*James Harvey Young, *The Toadstool Millionaires, A Social History of Patent Medicines in American before Federal Regulation*, 1961.
  *—*The Medical Messiahs, A Social History of Health Quackery in Twentieth Century America*, 1968.

Dr. Thomas Bond's Essay on the Utility of Clinical Lectures

CARL BRIDENBAUGH*

AMONG many sociologists and historians it has become an accepted axiom that Eighteenth-Century America suffered from the "cultural lag" which is commonly observed in all colonies when their achievements are compared with those of older, established societies. Upon close examination, however, there appears considerable doubt of the validity of this sweeping generalization. For example, the cultural flowering of Philadelphia, 1740–1776, placed it not on the periphery but squarely in the center of the Enlightenment.[1] In this second city of the British Empire there was often no "lag" at all, for in such activities as electrical research, organized philanthropy, prison reform, and scientific publications, Philadelphians set the pace for Europeans to follow — and were recognized by European savants as so doing.

By 1750, Philadelphia medical men, with ideas of their own and thoroughly cognizant of current European developments, began energetically to provide their community with the best possible facilities for the prevention and cure of disease by promoting legislation for the cleaning and paving of streets and the draining of swamps, by founding the Pennsylvania Hospital (1751), by establishing a Medical School at the College (1765), and by founding a Medical Society (1766). The towering figure in this noteworthy advance was Dr. Thomas Bond, who as philanthropist, physician, surgeon, and organizer of medical and scientific activities proved himself the outstanding member of the faculty in the thirteen colonies.

Although Giovanni Battista Morgagni of Padua had published his *Seats and Causes of Disease,* which established the study of pathological anatomy, as recently as 1761, Dr. Bond was ready by 1766 to add lectures at the Pennsylvania Hospital on this new and fundamental subject to the theoretical instruction provided by Doctors Morgan and Shippen at the

---

* Institute of Early American History and Culture, Williamsburg, Virginia.
[1] This thesis is developed in detail by Carl and Jessica Bridenbaugh in *Rebels and Gentlemen: Philadelphia in the Age of Franklin* (New York 1942).

1

Medical School.[2] To the Sitting Managers of the Hospital Dr. Bond addressed a letter in which he proposed that "they would give Liberty and Encouragement for the Reading Clinical Lectures, to the Students in Physic, on the Nature, Cause and Cure of Diseases, and to put up a Meteorological Apparatus in the Picture Room, for observation of the Weather, and keeping an Exact Account of the Epidemic Diseases thereby caused." The Board was agreeable and designated December 11, 1766, as the day upon which it would assemble to listen to "the plan intended to be prosecuted by the Physicians of the Hospital."

This lecture, delivered at Dr. Bond's home before an enthusiastic audience composed of the Managers of the Hospital, professors of the College, leading physicians of the city and "near thirty Students," ranks with Dr. Morgan's *Discourse upon the Institution of Medical Schools in America* (1765) as one of the early classics of American medical literature. It sets forth a point of view which was ignored between the Revolution and the Civil War, but which today is recognized as valid.[3] Largely overlooked by students of our medical history, it has been twice printed in publications now generally inaccessible: the *North American Medical and Surgical Journal* 4 (1827) 264-75; and in the appendix of T. G. Morton and F. Woodbury, *The History of the Pennsylvania Hospital* (Philadelphia 1897). The text here produced is taken from the Minutes of the Managers of the Pennsylvania Hospital (pp. 277-289), from whom, through the good offices of Miss Florence Greim, permission has been generously granted for publication. In the interest of clarity a few minor changes have been made in punctuation and spelling.

DOCTOR THOMAS BOND'S INTRODUCTORY LECTURE TO A COURSE OF CLINICAL OBSERVATIONS IN THE PENNSYLVANIA HOSPITAL, DELIVERED THERE DECEMBER THE 3RD 1766

When I consider the unskilful hands the Practice of Physic and Surgery has of necessity been Committed to, in many Parts of America, it gives me pleasure to behold so many Worthy Young Men, training up in those professions, which, from the nature of their Objects, are the most interesting to the Community, and yet a greater pleasure in foreseeing, that the unparalled public Spirit, of the Good

---

[2] Dr. John Morgan, founder of the Medical School, had met Morgagni and had been presented with an autographed set of his works (which is now in the Library of the College of Physicians, Philadelphia). He does not, however, appear to have conceived of the need for clinical lectures in connection with his school.

[3] See Richard H. Shryock, "Factors Affecting Medical Research in the United States, 1800-1900," *Bulletin of the Society of Medical History of Chicago* 5(1943) 1-5. For the medical scene in Philadelphia at the time of the delivery of Dr. Bond's lecture, consult Bridenbaugh, *Rebels and Gentlemen*, Chapter VIII.

People of this Province, will shortly make Philadelphia the Athens of America, and Render the Sons of Pennsylvania, reputable amongst the most celebrated Europeans, in all the liberal Arts and Sciences. This I am at present Certain of, that the institutions of Literature and Charity,[4] already founded, and the School of Physic lately open'd in this City[5] afford sufficient Foundation for the students of Physic to acquire all the Knowledge necessary for their practising every Branch of their professions, reputably, and Judiciously.

The great Expence in going from America, to England, and thence from Country to Country, and Colledge to Colledge, in Quest of Medical Qualifications, is often a Barr to the cultivation of the Brightest Geniuses amongst us, who might otherwise be Morning Stars in their professions, and most useful Members of Society.[6] Besides every Climate produces Diseases peculiar to itself, which require experience to understand and cure; and even the Diseases of the several Seasons in the Same Country, are found to differ so much some Years, from what they were in others, that Sydenham, the most Sagacious Physician that ever lived, acknowledges that he was often difficulted and much mistaken in the treatment of Epidemic's for some time after their appearance.

No Country then can be so proper for the instruction of Youth in the knowledge of Physic, as that in which 'tis to be practised; where the precepts of never failing Experience are handed down from Father to Son, from Tutor to Pupil.

That this is not a Speculative opinion, but real Matter of Fact, may be proven from the Savages of America, who without the assistance of Literature have been found possessed of Skill in the cure of Diseases incident to their climate, Superior to the Regular bred, and most learned Physicians, and that from their discoveries the present practice of Physic has been enrich'd with some of the most valuable Medicines now in use.

Therefore from Principles of Patriotism and Humanity, the Physic school here, should meet all the protection and Encouragement, the Friends of their Country, and Well Wishers of Mankind can possibly give it. Though 'tis yet in its Infancy from the Judicious Treatment of it's Guardians, it is already become A forward Child, and has the promising appearance of soon arriving to a Vigorous and Healthful Maturity. The professors in it at present are few; but their departments include the most Essential parts of Education; Another, whose distinguish'd Abilities will do honour to his Country and the Institution, is Expected to join them in

[4] Dr. Bond doubtless had in mind the Library Company and the College of Philadelphia in which he, personally, had taken an active part. The cultural life of Philadelphia is discussed against its provincial and European backgrounds in Bridenbaugh, *Rebels and Gentlemen.*

[5] During commencement, May 30-31, 1765, Dr. John Morgan delivered before the College audience, in two parts, his notable *Discourse upon the Institution of Medical Schools in America* (Philadelphia 1765; reprinted in *Bibliotheca Medica Americana* 2 [Baltimore 1937]), and in September came the joint announcement of Dr. Morgan's lectures on Materia Medica and those of Dr. William Shippen on anatomy and surgery. *Pennsylvania Gazette,* Sept. 26, 1765.

[6] Not only did the cost of a European education confine medical training to the upper class, it was dangerous. At least two young medical students lost their lives in the Atlantic crossing. Bridenbaugh, *op. cit.* 276-78.

the Spring,[7] And I think he has little Faith who can doubt that so good an undertaking will ever fail of Additional Strength, and a Providential Blessing. And I am certain nothing woud give me so much pleasure, as to have it in my Power to contribute the least mite towards it's perfect Establishment.

The Professor of anatomy and Physiology,[8] is well qualified for the Task; his Dissections are accurate and Elegant, and his Lectures, Learned, Judicious, and Clear.

The Professor of the Theory and Practice of Physic,[9] has had the best opportunities of improvement, join'd to Genious and application, and cannot fail of giving Necessary and instructive Lessons to the Pupils.

The Field this gentleman undertakes is very Extensive, and has many difficulties which may mislead the Footsteps of an uncautioned Traveller, therefore Lectures, in which the different parts of the Theory and Practice of Physic are Judiciously Classed and Systematically explain'd, will prevent many Perplexities the student would otherwise be Embarrassed with, will unfold the Doors of Knowledge, and be of great use in directing and abridging his future Studies, Yet there is something further wanting, he must Join Examples with Study, before he can be sufficiently qualified to prescribe for the Sick; for Language and Books alone, can never give him Adequate Ideas of Diseases, and the best methods of Treating them. For which reasons Infirmaries are Justly reputed the Grand Theatres of Medical Knowledge.

There the Clinical professor[10] comes into the Aid of Speculation and demonstrates the Truth of Theory by Facts: he meets his Pupils at stated times in the Hospital, and when a case presents adapted to his purpose, he asks all those Questions which lead to a certain knowledge of the Disease, and parts affected; this he does in the most exact and particular manner, to convince the Students how many, and what minute circumstances are often necessary to form a judgment of the curative indications, on which, the safety and Life of the Patient depend, from all which Circumstances and the present Symptoms, he pronounces what the Disease is, whether it is curable or Incurable, in what manner it ought to be treated, and gives his reasons from Authority or Experience for all he says on the occasion; and if the Disease baffles the power of Art, and the Patient falls a sacrifice to it, he then brings his knowledge to the Test, and fixes Honour or discredit on his Reputation by exposing all the Morbid parts to view,

---

[7] Dr. Adam Kuhn, armed with an Edinburgh degree, returned from botanical study with Linnaeus to become Professor of Materia Medica in January, 1768. Bridenbaugh, *op. cit.* 291; *Pennsylvania Journal*, May 5, 1768.

[8] Dr. William Shippen, also an Edinburgh graduate with additional training in surgery at London under Dr. William Hewson and the Hunters, began his courses in anatomy under the sponsorship of the Pennsylvania Hospital in 1762 and continued them until 1765, when he became a professor in the Medical School. *Pennsylvania Gazette*, Nov. 11, 1762.

[9] Dr. John Morgan "graduated at Edinburgh with an éclat almost unknown before," and came home after the Grand Tour "flushed with honors"— Fellow of the Royal Society, Corresponding Member of the Royal Academy of Surgery at Paris, Licentiate of the Royal College of Physicians in London as well as in that of Edinburgh. *Pennsylvania Magazine of History and Biography*, 18 (1894) 37, 40; *Pennsylvania Gazette*, Oct. 3, 1765; Dec. 8, 1766.

[10] Here Dr. Bond refers to the clinical lectures he proposes to give.

and Demonstrates by what means it produced Death; and if perchance he finds something unsuspected, which betrays an Error in Judgment, he like a great and good Man, immediately acknowledges the mistake, and for the benefit of survivors points out other methods by which it might have been more hapily Treated. The latter part of this field of Tuition is the surest method of obtaining just Ideas of Diseases. The great Booerhave[11] was so attentive to it, that he was not only present at the opening of Human Bodies, but frequently attended the Slaughter Houses in Leyden, to examine the Carcases of Beasts; and being asked by a learn'd Friend, by what means he had acquired such uncommon certainty in the Diagnostic's and Prognostic's of Diseases, answered by examining dead Bodies, studying Sydenhams observations, and Bonetus's *Sepulchretum Anatomicum,* both which he had read ten times, and each time with greater pleasure, and improvement.[12]

But to give you more familiar instances of the utility of this practice, let me remind several of You, who were present last Fall at the opening two Bodies,[13] One of which died of Astmatic complaints, the other of a Phrenzy succeeded by a Palsey, and ask you whether any thing short of occular demonstration, cou'd have given you just Ideas of the causes of the Patients Death, in one we saw a Dropsy in the left side of the Thorax, and a curious Polypus with its growing Fimbriae of 14 Inches in length (now in the Hospital) extending from the left Ventricle of the Heart, far beyond the Bifurcation of the pulmonary Artery, in the other we found the Brain partly superated and the Ventricle on the opposite side to that affected, with the Paralysis, distended by a large Quantity of Limpid Serum; and you must Remember, that the state of all the Morbid parts were predicted, before they were exposed to View: which may have a further advantage, by rousing in you an industrious pursuit after the most hidden causes of all the affections of the Human Body; and convince you what injury they do to the living, who oppose a decent, painless, and well timed examination of the Dead.

Thus all the professors in the best European Colledges,[14] go hand in hand, and co-operate with each other by regular chains of Reasoning and occasional demonstrations, to the satisfaction and improvement of the Students.

But more is required of us in this late settled world, where new Diseases often occurr, and others common to many parts of Europe visit us too frequently, which it behoves the Guardians of Health, to be very watchful of, that they may know them well, and by an hearty union, and Brotherly communication of observations investigate their causes, and check their progress. The Task is Arduous, but 'tis a Debt we owe to our Friends and our Country. The Atmosphere that Surrounds

---

[11] Herman Boerhaave of Leyden, under whom several Philadelphians had studied. His influence was strong in Edinburgh too. See Richard H. Shryock, *The Development of Modern Medicine* (Philadelphia 1936) 67-68.

[12] For Thomas Sydenham, the great English clinician, see David Riesman, *Thomas Sydenham* (New York 1926); and on the somewhat uncritical pathological observations of Théophile Bonet, consult Shryock, *op. cit.* 63-64.

[13] Probably the bodies of patients who died either at the Pennsylvania Hospital or at the Bettering House. In 1764 Dr. Shippen had dissected the body of a Negro suicide before students in his "theatre." *Pennsylvania Gazette,* Apr. 12, 1764.

[14] This was true of Continental medical schools, rather than of those in the British Isles.

us is fine, and the Air we breath, free, pure, and Naturally healthy, and I am fully perswaded we shall find on strict enquiry, when it becomes otherwise, 'tis mostly from contagion imported, or neglected Sources of Putrifaction, amongst ourselves, and therefore when ever we are able to Demonstrate the Causes, they may be removed and the Effects prevented.

Our Fathers after insuring to us the full enjoyment of the inestimable blessings of Religious and Civil Liberty, have settled us in a Country that affords all the real comforts of life, and given us the prospect of becoming one Day, a great and happy People, and I know only one Objection to a prudent Mans giving North America the preference to any other part of the British Dominions for the place of his residence, which is, that the climate is sometimes productive to severe Epidemic Diseases in the Summer and Fall:[15] the Country is otherwise free from those tedious and dangerous Fevers which frequently infest most parts of Europe. The last wet Summer and a short space of hot dry Weather in Autumn, caused so many Intermittents from the Southern Suburbs of this City all the way to Georgia, that I may venture to assert two thirds of the inhabitants were not able to do the least Business for many Weeks, and some families and even Townships were so distress'd that they had not well persons sufficient to attend the Sick, during which time this City was unusually Healthy. How respectable then wou'd be the Characters of those Men, who shou'd wipe this Stain out of the American Escutcheon and rescue their Country from such frequent calamaties.

Sufficient encouragement to make the attempt is found both in History, the Books of Physic, and our own Experience. Several instances are recorded of places that were so sickly, as to be uninhabitable, until Princes have ordered their Physicians to search into the causes of their Unhealthiness, and having discover'd and removed them, made thereby valuable additions to their Kingdoms. Was not our Antient and Great Master, Hippocrates, so knowing in the cause of Pestilential Contagion, as to foresee an approaching Plague, and send his pupils into the cities to take care of the Sick, and has not *He,* and Sydenham the English Hippocrates, done infinite Service to the healing Art, and gained immortal Honours to themselves, by their Essays on Epidemic's in which they not only accurately describe the Diseases of their Respective Countries, but shew the depraved constitution of the Air which produced each of them. Our own Experience also affords much Encouragement, when I first came into this City the Dock[16] was the common Sewer of Filth, and was such a Nuisance to the inhabitants about it, every Fall, that they were obliged to us more pounds of Bark,[17] than they have Ounces since

---

[15] Physicians of Philadelphia and of the Southern Colonies spent much time in the study of the causes and cure of "Fevers." The most significant work on this subject was *An Essay on Fevers,* by Dr. Lionel Chalmers of Charleston, S. C., which ran serially in the *Pennsylvania Chronicle* (Dec. 19, 1768-Jan. 2, 1769) through the good offices of Dr. Morgan and the American Society for Promoting Useful Knowledge. It was published in book form in Philadelphia in 1769 and at London in 1776.

[16] For years the "Dock" had been a receptacle for dead dogs, carrion and filth — "a publick nuisance injurious to health." In 1763 the authorities ordered it filled in to form the present Dock Street. *Statutes at Large of Pennsylvania* (Vols. 2-13 Harrisburg 1896–1908) 5. 234-836.

[17] In colonial days quinine was commonly called Jesuit Bark or Catholic Bark.

it has been raised, and levell'd. Another striking instance of the Advantage of Cleanliness for the preservation of Health, affords me an Opportunity of paying a Tribute, justly due, to the Wisdom of the Legislature of this Province, in framing the salutary Laws for paving and regulating the Streets of this City,[18] and to the indefatigable industry and Skill of the Commissioners in excuting them, whereby they have contributed so much to the Healthiness of the Inhabitants, that I am confident the whole Expence will be repair'd in ten Years, by the lessening of Physic Bills alone. A Farm within A few miles of this city was remarkably healthy for Fifty Years, whilst the Tide overflow'd the Low Lands, near the dwelling House, but after they were Bank'd in by Ditches so ill contrived that they often did not discharge the Water that fell into them for considerable time, and until it became putrid, and thereby rendered the place as remarkably Sickly, as it had before been healthy, I was told by a Gentleman of Veracity that he saw the Corps of One of Nine tenants that had been carried from it in a few Years.

The Yellow Fever, which I take to be exactly the same distemper as the Plague of Athens, described by Thucydides, has been five different times in this City since my residence in it, the causes of three of them I was luckily able to Trace, and am certain they were the same, which produced a Goal Fever in other Places, and am of opinion the difference betwixt the appearance of these Fevers, arises from the Climate, and the different state the Bodies are in when they Imbibe the Contagion; if so, the Same methods which are taken to prevent a Goal Fever, will equally prevent a Yellow Fever; 'Twas in the Year Forty One,[19] I first saw that horrid Disease which was then imported by a Number of Convicts from the Dublin Goal. (The second time it prevailed it was indigenous from Evident causes, and was principally confined to One Square of the City.) The third time it was generated on Board of Crowded Ships in the Port, which brought in their Passengers in Health, but soon after became very Sickly. I here saw the appearance of Contagion like a Dim Spark which gradually encreased to a Blaze, and soon after burst out into a terrible Flame, carrying Devastation with it, and after continuing two Months was extinguish'd by the profuse Sweats of Tertian Fevers, but this is not the ordinary course of the Contagion, 'tis usually check'd by the cool Evenings in September and dies on the Appearance of an October Frost.

I lately visited an Irish Passenger Vessel, which brought the People perfectly healthy untill they came in our River. I found five of them Ill, and others Unwell, and saw that the Fomes[20] of infection was spreading among them, I therefore ordered the Ship to lay Quarantine, to be well purified with the Steams of Sulphur,

---

[18] As a result of an aroused public opinion, agitated for years by the pressure of such citizens as Dr. Bond and Benjamin Franklin, the Assembly finally passed a law in 1762 providing for the paving and cleansing of Philadelphia's streets, and appointed Commissioners to carry out the program. The Commissioners' Minutes, 1762–1768, are in the Historical Society of Pennsylvania. 1750/1; Apr. 15, 1762; *Statutes at Large of Pennsylvania* 6. 196-214; 230-846.

[19] So many Palatines arrived with malignant fevers in 1741 that their plight aroused public interest and resulted in 1743 in the establishment of an isolation hospital on a 342 acre tract on Province Island. *Statutes at Large of Pennsylvania* 4. 382.

[20] Foams. Dr. Bond was one of the Port Physicians at this time who were employed by the Province to examine immigrant vessels. See his report on sick Palatines made with Dr. Thomas Graeme in 1754. *Pennsylvania Magazine of History and Biography* 36(1912) 476.

and with Vinegar, directed the Bedding and Cloathing of the People to be well wash'd and Air'd, before any person should be permitted to Land out of her, after which I advised separating the Sick from the Healthy. This was done by putting twelve in different Rooms in one House, and fourteen in another, out of the City, the conveniences of the two Houses were much the same, in one of them little care was taken of the Sick, who were laid upon the same foul beds, they (contrary to orders) brought on Shore with them; the consequence was, that all the Family catch'd the distemper, and the Landlord Died. In the other my directions were Strictly observed, the Sick had clean Cloaths, and clean Bedding, were well attended and soon Recovered, without doing the least Injury to any person that visited them; which confirms Observations I had often made before, that the Contagion of Malignant Fevers, lies in the Air confined and corrupted, by a neglect of Rags and other filth about the Helpless Sick, and not from their Bodies.

As each of these heads, shall be a Subject of a future Lecture, I shall at present only mention to you further, a few of those Methods which have preserved Individuals from prevailing diseases.

The inhabitants of Hispaniola have found the wearing Flannel Shirts to be a preservative against Intermitting Fevers in that sickly Island, and as that Disease is known to arise principally from inhaling a great Quantity of the Humidity of the Air, I make no doubt 'twould also be of use in preventing them in our low, moist, level Countries.

We know that the Bark of Sassafras contains many Excellent Medicinal Virtues, my Worthy Friend Mr. Peter Franklin[21] told me that he being in the Fall of the Year, in the River Nantikoke in Maryland, and on seeing the People on Shore much afflicted with Intermitting Fevers, advised the Marriners of the Ship to drink freely, by way of prevention, of that Aromatic and Antiseptic Medicine, but cou'd not prevail on more than half the company to do it, and that he and all the others who took it, enjoy'd perfect Health, whilst not a single Person of the rest, escaped a severe attack of the Epedemic Disease, I have known other similar Instances, which 'tis needless to mention, since this is remarkably pertinent.

But I have many reasons to expect that a more agreeable, and equally certain preventative against our Autumnal Fevers, will be found in Sulphures Chalybeate Waters, which may readily be procured in most parts of America, especially where those Diseases are most prevalent, A Spring of this Kind at Gloucester[22] within a few Miles of this Place has been much used of late, and has been so very serviceable to Invalids, it has the appearance of being a valuable conveniency to the City, Persons under various Diseases took Lodgings in the Village the

[21] Peter Franklin, post-master of Philadelphia and brother of Benjamin Franklin, had died several months before Dr. Bond's lecture, in July, 1766. Carl Van Doren, *Franklin* (New York 1938) 212, 261, 358.

[22] Each of Philadelphia's physicians appears to have had his favorite mineral spring. Water from the Gloucester spring was bottled over in New Jersey for sale in the city. Carl Bridenbaugh, "The Baths and Watering Places of Colonial America," *William and Mary Quarterly*, 3rd. ser., 3 (1946) 173-74, 177.

last Season, for the advantage of drinking the Waters at the Fountain head, and though the Fall was more sickly than has been known in the Memory of Man, not one, who went there for health, nor any one of the Inhabitants near the Spaw, who drank it freely, had a touch of the prevailing Disease, whilst a Major part of those that did not, had more the appearance of Ghosts, than living Creatures, there were two Houses, the Habitations of Father and Son, within twenty Feet of each other, the Family of the Father had suffered greatly from Intermitting Fevers the preceding Fall, and some of them continued Invalids 'till the middle of Summer, when they were prevailed on, to take the Waters, after which they daily recovered Health, Bloom, and Vigour, and pass'd the sickly Season without a Complaint, whilst scarcely a person in that of the Son, who did not take them, escaped a severe Illness; 'Tis well known from experience that Mineral Waters are not only the most Palatable, but the most Salutary parts of the Materia Medica, and that the Effect of those which are pure and properly impregnated with chalybeate Principles, Strengthen digestion, brace and counteract the Summers Sun, dilute a thick putrid Bile, (the instrument of Mischief in all Hot Climates) and immediately wash away putrification through the Emuntaries of the Bowels, Skin, or Kidneys, and therefore appear to be natural preservatives against the Effect of an hot, moist, and putrid atmosphere. Whether these Waters will answer my sanguine Expectations or not, must be left to the Decision of Time. If they should be found wanting, that ought not discourage our further pursuit, for since providence has furnish'd every Country with defences for the Human Bodies, against the inclemencies of Heat and Cold, why shou'd we Question whether infinite wisdom and Goodness has made equal Provision against all other natural injuries of our Constitutions; Experience and Reason, encourages us to believe it has, and that the means might be discovered by diligent investigation were our researches equal to the Task, the above instances are therefore related to convince you, that the prevention of some of the Epedemic diseases of America is not only a laudable and rational Pursuit, but is more within the limits of human precaution than has generally been imagined, and to excite your particular attention to the improvement of this Humane and interesting part of your profession, in which, and all other useful undertakings, I most sincerely wish you Success.

I am now to inform you, Gentlemen, that the Managers and Physicians of the Pennsylvania Hospital, on seeing the great number of you attending the School of Physic in this City, are of opinion, this excellent institution likewise affords a favourable opportunity of farther improvement to you in the practical part of your Profession, and being desirous it should answer all the good purposes intended by the generous Contributors to it, have allotted to me the Task of giving a course of Clinical, and Meteriological Observations in it, which I chearfully undertake (though the season of my Life points out relaxation and retirement, rather than new Incumbrances.[23]) in hopes, that remarks on the many curious Cases that must daily occurr, amongst an Hundred and thirty Sick persons, collected together at one time, may be very instructive to You. I therefore purpose

[23] Dr. Bond was at this time fifty-four years of age.

to meet you at stated times here, and give you the best information in my Power of the nature and treatment of Chronical Diseases, and of the proper management of Ulcers, Wounds and Fractures. I shall shew you all the Opperations of Surgery, and endeavour, from the Experience of Thirty Years, to introduce you to a Familiar acquaintance with the acute Diseases of your own Country, in order to which, I shall put up a compleat Meteriological Apparatus, and endeavour to inform you of all the known Properties of the atmosphere which surrounds us, and the effects it's frequent variations produce on Animal Bodies, and confirm the Doctrine, by an Exact register of the Weather, and of the prevailing Diseases, both here, and in the Neighbouring Provinces, to which I shall add, all the interesting observations which may occurr in private practice, and sincerely wish it may be in my power to do them to your Satisfaction.

I likewise have the Pleasure to inform you, that Doctor Smith,[24] has promised to go through a course of experimental Philosophy in the Colledge, for your instruction in Pneumatic's, Hydraulic's, and Mechanic's, which will be of the greatest advantage to a ready comprehension of the Meteriological Lectures, and other parts of your Medicinal Studies, and lay you under the highest obligations to that learned Professor.

---

[24] The Reverend William Smith, D.D., Provost of the College of Philadelphia. For his lectures, see *Pennsylvania Gazette*, Dec. 11, 1766; Aug. 24, 1769.

The Study of Medicine at the Vermont Academy of Medicine (1827–29) as Revealed in the *Journal of Asa Fitch*

SAMUEL REZNECK

HE special distinction of Asa Fitch as a student of medicine at the Vermont Medical Academy in Castleton lay in the fact that he was already a graduate of the Rensselaer School in Troy, New York, as were a number of his fellow students. Rensselaer was then the only school of its kind in the country exclusively dedicated to the teaching of natural science and its applications by student experimentation and demonstration. Founded in 1824 by Stephen Van Rensselaer, the principal landlord of the Upper Hudson Valley, it was actually the creation of Amos Eaton, its first head, for the 'application of science to the common purposes of life.'[1] In a sense, medicine was then already an established study of a similar character, and there was a natural affinity between the two types of schools. Both faculty and students moved freely between them, as in the case of Amos Eaton, Dr. Lewis Beck, and Asa Fitch, and many physicians played a prominent role in the early history of American science.[2]

Asa Fitch was one of those whose career combined both medicine and science, especially entomology. He was graduated from the Rensselaer School in 1827 and from the Castleton Medical School in 1829.[3] Born in 1809 in Salem, New York, scion of an old and distinguished Connecticut family and son of a physician of the same name, Fitch kept the diary, which he began at twelve, during most of his life. Still preserved in manuscript at

---

1. A biography of Asa Fitch, the author of the diary and the subject of this article, is in the *Dictionary of American Biography*, VI, 424. For the history of the Rensselaer School and its graduates, see H. B. Nason, *Biographical record . . . of Rensselaer Polytechnic Institute, 1824–86* (Troy, 1887); Ethel M. McAllister, *Amos Eaton, scientist and educator* (New York, 1941); and Samuel Rezneck, *Education for a technological society: A sesquicentennial history of Rensselaer Polytechnic Institute* (Troy, 1968).

2. For Fitch and other Rensselaer students and professors at the Medical Academy in Castleton, see F. C. Waite, *The first Medical College in Castleton* (Montpelier, Vermont, 1949), pp. 72ff., 177, 185, 196, 209. There is an interesting account of the Vermont Academy of Medicine in the *Troy Sentinel*, 23 Dec. 1823.

3. Of the ten men in the Rensselaer second class of 1827, four became physicians including Fitch. Three of them apparently were at Castleton.

11

the Yale University Library, it provides an informative and intimate account of a young man's life and inner thoughts in early America. Particularly does it portray with remarkable felicity and detail a student's experience in the then still new (in America) fields of science and medicine. To the account was subsequently added the record of a young doctor's life in western Illinois, at Greenville, where he spent an unhappy winter unsuccessfully trying to adjust himself to the crudities of life and practice on the frontier. This was in 1830–31, at precisely the time when young Abraham Lincoln, also born in February 1809, arrived at nearby New Salem to begin his career in storekeeping.

This introduction is not intended to provide a sketch, however fragmentary, of Fitch's life, but to set the stage and offer perspective for his study at the Vermont Medical Academy as revealed in his extensive and illuminating journal. His education was novel but quite thorough, although somewhat haphazard and peripatetic. It began at the Salem Academy and at Bennington, Vermont. In May 1826 he entered the recently established Rensselaer School at Troy, the youngest member of a kind of experimental traveling school of science on the newly opened Erie Canal. He spent a whole year at Rensselaer and received its degree (A.B.) in 1827.

Returning to Salem, he followed the family tradition of medicine, although he had already acquired a deep and lifelong interest in entomology which was ultimately to become his principal preoccupation. He was apprenticed according to the fashion of the day to a Dr. Freeman, who was apparently an uncle, with whom he pursued the study of medicine more or less continuously for several years. His first scheduled program was strenuous—'to get up with the sun and to attend to Natural History until breakfast.' Then he spent most of the day at the 'shop,' and six hours on anatomy.[4] For more formal instruction Fitch attended a variety of institutions which gave the relatively brief courses of lectures then usual, each lasting approximately four months. He spent two such terms at Castleton, in 1827 and 1829, the intervening winter at the Rutgers Medical College in New York City, and a short time privately at Albany with Dr. Alden March, who was a professor at Castleton and who was later to found the Albany Medical College, still in existence. Altogether, he studied medicine for some three years following the year at the Rensselaer School.

---

4. Fitch's Journal, E, pp. 120ff. This journal, in many volumes both lettered (A–G) and numbered (1–15), is preserved in the Historical Manuscripts Division at the Yale University Library and is used here with the permission of its officials, for which I am grateful. Further references will be made hereafter, by volume and page, in parentheses immediately following the quotation in the text.

The principal concern of this article is Fitch's life and study at Castleton, as described in his journal, but it must be viewed in relation to his whole life and career. According to his record he arrived at Castleton from Salem on 3 September 1827, and his first impressions were agreeable if not overwhelming: 'It is a pleasant place, but does not contain near the number of buildings that I had expected, and these are scattered along so that it would be difficult to tell the precise spot which is village.' He found lodging and board at $1.50 per week. There were only four boarders, and thus the house would not be crowded. One of his roommates was Frederick Header from Alstead, New Hampshire, which perhaps indicated the range of Castleton's drawing power. Two of Fitch's classmates at the Rensselaer School were also at Castleton. One, Jonathan Chandler, also from Alstead, New Hampshire, was already a practicing physician; the other, Orlin Oatman, from Middletown, Vermont, was a fellow student at the Academy (F, 23ff.).

Fitch opened the account of this term by unexpectedly noting: 'I do not anticipate much if any hard study the present winter and therefore expect to pass the time away agreeably.' This apparently meant he anticipated the continued pursuit of scientific interests acquired at Rensselaer. He early went out into the country to collect insects, his primary avocation, and also to 'geologize' some crystallized feldspar discovered there by Dr. Ebenezer Emmons, another graduate of the Rensselaer School, who was in medicine (F, 28). On 5 September 1827 Fitch attended the introductory lecture of the term. It was delivered by a figure familiar to him, Dr. Lewis C. Beck, one of three Albany medical brothers, who was also Junior Professor at the Rensselaer School. Delivered to a 'motley collection' of persons in a well-filled room, the lecture was, not surprisingly, on the importance of natural history to medicine (F, 30).

Thus began the season's program, which consisted usually of five lectures daily. Beck began at 8:30 a.m. and he ended the day with a second lecture of the afternoon on botany. Drs. Theodore Woodward and William Tully filled in the rest of the day. Dr. Woodward lectured very fast on Inflammation, and Fitch could hardly understand him. Dr. Tully was especially voluble, 'though not equal in constancy to Professor Eaton. I sat mum for about two hours.'[5] The rest of the time, day and evening, he busied himself

---

5. Dr. William Tully was a graduate of Yale College, with an honorary M.D. also from Yale. He taught Materia Medica at both Castleton and Yale and was the author of a work on the subject. He was highly regarded as one of the most learned and scientific physicians in New England. Dr. Theodore Woodward was one of the founders of the Castleton Medical Academy in 1818 and served it as both registrar and professor of surgery and obstetrics for twenty years. He studied medicine at Dartmouth College, but his M.D. was honorary, from both Middlebury and Harvard Colleges. Dr. Alden

transcribing his lecture notes. He probably used a system of 'steneography,' since he reports learning this method in preparation for note-taking while still in Salem (F, 6, 31).

Very early in the term Fitch gave an account of an excursion to nearby Hubbardton, notorious subsequently as the site of a grave robbery charged to students at Castleton. Several wagonloads of students set out to witness an amputation on a woman shot in the knee joint. On arrival, however, they discovered that it was only some 'partridge shot' in the calf and not serious enough for amputation. There was almost a tone of disappointment in this report. A few weeks later, with some trepidation, Fitch recorded the beginning of his work in dissection: 'For the first time I took the knife and laid open the integuments of the thigh. I no longer fear on going into the room, though I should not dare to attempt it alone' (F, 35, 38).[6]

The concentrated character of the Castleton course of medical instruction was well illustrated when, toward the end of October, Fitch made note of changes of lecturers. Dr. Allen took the place of Dr. Beck, and Professor Eaton of the Rensselaer School and Dr. March of Albany arrived for their lectures: 'Now is the busiest part of the course. I take down and transcribe pretty full notes from Eaton's lectures, and have scarcely time to read Bell's *Anatomy* as fast as March progresses in his lecture' (F, 39ff.). Nevertheless, Fitch found time to collect and report gossip that Dr. Tully, who was the President, would resign from the institution and would be hard to replace. Drs. Beck and March might join him. These were the best lecturers; their plan was to establish a private medical school at Albany, with degrees granted by Union College. This development, foreseen thus early in 1827, did not, however, materialize until 1839, and the association with Union College not until 1873 (F, 36).

As is often the way with diaries, routine activities are disregarded, such as the daily lectures to which Fitch had become accustomed, or in which he perhaps lacked interest. The record of this first term is here abbreviated in order to permit a more complete treatment of the second term when Fitch was more experienced and better able to profit by it and to report it more

---

March was a graduate in medicine from Brown University who settled in Albany. He was a visiting professor of anatomy at Castleton. His distinguished career was, however, principally in New York state, where he became successively president of the Albany County and New York State Medical Societies, as well as president of the American Medical Association. He was a vigorous advocate and ultimately the founder of the Albany Medical College in 1839, still in existence. (Sylvester Willard, *Annals of the Medical Society of the County of Albany* [Albany, 1864]; Waite [n. 2]).

6. The 'Hubbardton Raid' of 1830 was celebrated half a century later in poetry, which is reproduced in *J. Amer. med. Ass.*, 1968, *204*, 678. Cf. article on 'The Castleton Medical College,' by Dr. M. Therese Southgate (*Ibid.*, pp. 699–701).

fully. His account for the remainder of the term of 1827 tended to be limited to more unusual events, such as a case of 'hydrocele' in a Mr. Parker, who was to be operated on before the class by Dr. Woodward (F, 42). Almost equally noteworthy was Thanksgiving Day, celebrated on Thursday, 6 December, both with church services and a Thanksgiving dinner consisting of 'roasted turkey and chicken, pickles, bread, butter, applesauce, pudding, and pie. Thanksgiving does not come every day'—which perhaps accounts for the full report (F, 43).

On 10 December Fitch prepared to leave Castleton for home: 'I think most probably never to see it again.' He said farewell to the professors and noted that 'it is contemplated to raise the standing of the Medical School.' Tuition was to be increased a few dollars above the current forty-three dollars, and each professor was to stay for the whole term. He was not content with his own performance: 'I regret I have not learned more. I have often been too inattentive, and have heard whole lectures, without remembering scarcely an idea which they contained. It is now, however, too late to repent, and I must make amends in my future application' (F, 44, 50ff.). He, nevertheless, lauded 'the high advantages for medical instruction which the institution established in this village affords,' and concluded, notwithstanding his own deficiencies, that 'the doctrines here inculcated have been carried by numerous graduates into various parts of the country . . . It is no wonder that this institution has become the resort of students, not merely from the immediate section of the country, but also from distant and remote parts of the Union' (F, n. p.).

At the beginning of 1828 Fitch was back home in Salem, New York, determined 'to commence studying and keep at it the rest of the winter more regularly than I have yet done. Altogether then six hours of each day shall be spent in reading Cullen (on Practice).' He also reported reading Bell's *Anatomy*. Later on he estimated that he must average fifteen pages a day to get through the book by August. He was now reading about the heart, in the second volume, and was drawing a plan of the arteries (F, 58, 88ff.).

Thus did the course of self-instruction continue, with occasional references to actual visits to sick patients. He also engaged in crudely inept and painful mutual bleeding procedures with a fellow-student, William Savage. Equally pointless seemed to be an experiment which appeared to be more a self-indulgent lark than a serious venture in self-instruction. The two young men went out into a field with a supply of 'nitrous oxyd,' which they breathed in, with the result that they broke out 'laughing most heartily . . .

The sensations which it produced were of the most agreeable nature, nay ecstatic' (F, 92ff.). Later, at Castleton, this type of practice went on with other drugs as well.

Life at home during 1828 offered numerous distractions, and despite his studious intentions the time and effort that went into medical study were neither continuous nor intensive. There was seasonal work to be done on the farm, beside which Fitch had considerable interest in reading general literature, and a preoccupation with his botanical collection and particularly with entomology. Occasionally he made visits to nearby Troy and renewed acquaintances at the Rensselaer School. All of these activities, added to the social events typical of youth in a small town like Salem, left little time or opportunity for consecutive medical study or practice. The journal for the winter of 1828 spent in New York when Fitch was attending the lectures at Rutgers Medical College is extensive but must be omitted here. He was back in Salem early in 1829 for further practice under Dr. Freeman's tutelage. He did not care much for Dr. Freeman, who never took his 'students out to see sufficient practice.' Freeman's method was quite permissive, for example, in one case when he knew Fitch was very busy, 'he said he should like to have me go down, if I wished, to see a young man at McLean's Mills having a lumbar abscess. It is the only time he has made a similar proposition, except in the case of Mr. Culver's child last spring' (F, 117ff.).

On 26 August 1829 Fitch again packed his bags and other belongings, as well as his instruments, said his farewells, and departed for Castleton, not to return to Salem as his home 'till after I finish my studies, and perhaps not then' (2, 84). Still only twenty years old, he had had a considerable variety of educational experience, which included both Castleton and New York City. Now back at Castleton, though as an advanced student, he attended the same program of lectures as in his previous course. His father accompanied him, and advised him 'to stick closely to my studies, and let other things, as politics, antimasonry alone' (2, 86).

Fitch actively joined the other second-term students in arranging a ceremony for the opening day. They printed and distributed a circular, and on the appointed day, 27 August, at least sixty students gathered, and more than a hundred persons joined in the procession to the College. These included the students, the President and Chaplain, professors, corporation, practicing physicians, citizens, and strangers. At the ringing of a bell the procession marched to the Old College, where the students opened rank to right and left and raised their hats, allowing the others to march in. After prayer, Dr. William Tully, President of the College and Professor of the Theory and Practice of Materia Medica, delivered an excellent lecture on its history, 'and its present state among the various inhabitants of the savage and civilized world. The subject was novel and one which has seldom received the attention of writers, and then only superficially.' All listened with close attention and evident gratification, and 'the Junior students were confirmed in their high opinion of Dr. Tully' (F, n. p.; 2, 88ff.).

Fitch's lecture schedule was long, although not arduous, from 8 a.m. to 12 noon daily, and on several afternoons as well. Indeed, Drs. Beck and Tully lectured twice each day. Relations with the professors were apparently close and intimate, whether because of Fitch's medical family or his acquaintance with some of the faculty, such as Beck and Eaton, from his Rensselaer days. Dr. Woodward gave him Bégin's *Therapeutics* to read, and was greatly pleased with his progress in it. On taking Dr. Tully's ticket, he discussed other medical schools with him as well as his future destination, and 'he told of all very cheerfully.' On another occasion he took a visiting physician from Salem, Dr. Abram Allen, to see Dr. Tully, and they had a long conversation, 'chiefly on medicine, the illiberality and enmity of physicians, and particular cases to illustrate it' (2, 91ff., 112).

Fitch turned to writing, and his account of the opening day's lecture appeared in the *Vermont Statesman*. He was greatly pleased with this first venture in publication, as he put it: 'I have often had an itching for this .... The ice is broken ....' With the novice's vanity he sent copies of this to his family and friends. Nevertheless, he early became homesick and somewhat melancholy: 'Impatient of study, I want to see home ... But I must conquer such reveries. Still they cling to me and will not be driven away' (2, 95, 98).

Castleton's resources for diversion were limited. There was, of course, church, and Fitch was pious and conventional enough to attend services, often twice on Sunday, reporting the subjects of the sermons in his journal. There was the debating society, in which he participated actively by contributing compositions and discussion, and whose meetings offered opportunity for association with young ladies. Of a very special nature was the arrival of a 'caravan of animals,' which attracted a great crowd. It included 'an elephant very large and one of the finest I have ever seen, which, moreover, performed tricks. There was also a camel with two humps, a tiger, a leopard, a kangaroo, llama, and several monkeys, one of which rode a pony.' This account is significant for its revelation of the naive character and the occasions for diversion available in a small American community in the early nineteenth century (2, 99).

Most revealing, however, were the uses to which drugs were then put for the edification or, more likely, the entertainment of medical students. Perhaps it was a crude kind of experimentation. One evening, early in September, Fitch saw several students in Dr. Woodward's yard. They were 'taking ether, by inhalation, to receive the effect similar to that of exhilerating (*sic*) gas. I had not much faith in it, and it was not heightened by seeing others take it. At the close of the scene, however, I tried it myself, and found the effect, if not identical, the next best thing to the gas,' thus referring to his earlier experimentation with nitrous oxide in Salem. Suggesting more modern drug experimentation, he now described the effects: 'I flew about as though on eagle's wings vanquishing whoever happened in my way' (2, 100).

A few days later a breakfast conversation on a Sunday turned to Dr. Tully's statement that 75 grains of opium might be taken in twenty-four hours without detriment. It was doubted, and Fitch undertook to try the experiment. Beginning at 9 a.m. and continuing until 6 p.m., he took a dose every twenty minutes, a total of thirty-five or forty grains. The effects were severe, as he described them to a friend, 'turns of nausea, retching, and eructation of air were common through the night. I was glad to see the morning.' The next day brought further consequences: 'My countenance marked the state of my health. My breath is sore and offensive .... A diarrhea has existed all day,' but he felt better by Tuesday (2, 100).

As Fitch noted, 'the evening is about the only part of the day that furnished ought of interest for my diary.' Apparently the medical lectures did not. Despite his frequent comments about his shyness and lack of sociability, Fitch found ample opportunity for association with the fair sex, which seemed to preoccupy his public actions as well as private thoughts. One young lady, who lived in the same house, a Miss Angelica Parmenter, especially engaged his interest. They went on walks together and he found her charming. When he learned that 'she was worth her thousands,' he became even more speculative about her: 'That is a fact of which I did not dream before. What will become of my poor heart, when these ponderable—those "solid charms" are added to the former attractions .... Heigho, well, I am quite indifferent.' When she left for home in Brandon, Fitch promised to visit her, 'for her company had become quite pleasing. Long will the hours I spent with her live in my memory' (2, 117ff., 123).

With a characteristic sense of student values, Fitch occasionally skipped his medical lectures for other activities. One time he stayed away from Dr. Beck's lecture in order to transcribe his composition for the debating society. It was on antimasonry, then a lively public subject. It was well received, and Fitch accepted the role of 'composist' for the next writing (2, 116ff.). He also found occasion to add to his practical experience in medicine. Thus he stayed up all night with a Mr. Munroe, 'who is dangerously ill of a typhus fever.' Dr. Tully came in about ten o'clock: 'Notwithstanding the opium I dozed some before morning, but read all that I cared about in the *Wreath*,' which was an English 'Annual' volume (2, 115).

Fitch combined a remarkable sensitivity for nature and love of literature with his knowledge and appreciation of science, particularly natural history. Thus, on a long walk in the Castleton countryside one October Saturday during Indian summer, he waxed eloquent about nature's beauties. His interest in entomology shone through prophetically as he addressed a wasp: 'Lovely insect! May I yet contribute to bring thy species to the knowledge of the world! I have almost declared: "I will—I will do it!"' (2, 126ff.).

This kind of restful appreciation of the beauties of nature alternated with a wild, almost orgiastic, experience, as he joined a group of students in again 'taking ether on the green, this side of the church.' Ether was, as he described it, 'as free as water.' He took dose after dose, five altogether, and subsequently described his reactions: 'At first I fought, and scuffled, especially with Beech. We both appeared to have quite an antipathy toward each other.' Another fellow became 'quite oratorical and began to speak in flowing style. I opposed him, standing behind him, with whimsical gesticulation, etc., etc., ridiculing or denying whatever he said. He got mad and chased me.' This tired Fitch so much that 'it seemed as though I must sink to the ground' (2, 130ff.).

A few days later, this experience was repeated in the presence of Dr. Tully. At first Fitch stayed out, saving himself for a ball the next night. But apparently he eventually submitted to the pressure and inhaled the ether. He got into a fight with another ether-taker, who tried to trip him up. Fitch jumped over Ferry, catching his foot in his forehead: 'A gash was cut, entirely down to the bone, even separating the periostium.' The next day, the day of the ball, Fitch felt languid, but he rested and 'about noon commenced stimulating with opium.' He went to the ball and danced until three in the morning, until he 'was weary enough.' He paid his bill of $1.80 at the tavern and escorted a young lady home in the lovely night (2, 134ff.).

On another occasion a group of students decided to attend the performance of a visiting theatrical company at East Poultney. They hired a carriage and drove off at breakneck speed, racing a stage, and were nearly upset. On the way they were a noisy band, 'singing all the villainous songs ever heard of.' The comedy was only 'indifferently acted,' but the farce, 'Animal Magnetics, was quite ludicrous.' Fitch did not get to bed until 2 a.m. (2, 119). A few days later, on a Saturday night, his roommate, a Mr. Mazuzan, 'tried the effect of opium in large doses, and the room is in a pretty pickle. He has vomited upon the floor and lies here, half dead, taking one grain every half hour, and I am sitting up to take down the symptoms.' This was apparently an experiment applied by Mazuzan toward his thesis on the effects of opium on health, and Fitch was helping him with it (2, 121). The next night he again sat up all night with Mr. Munroe, the typhus patient, and read the *North American Review* (2, 122).

Fitch varied such activities with the more homely one of 'paring quinces with Mr. Hamilton for Mrs. Kellogg, who was their landlady' (2, 133). The following Friday, Dr. Beck gave a public lecture, 'a sketch of the history of chemistry, and several experiments.... The laboratory was crowded as full nearly as it could be.' Somewhat later Fitch reported a reduced schedule of lectures, only three daily and two on Saturday, 'hardly enough to pay for staying here, but the dancing school, ah yes, I will stay ... for what more do I want ...' (2, 137, 139, 140). Dr. Beck completed his course at this time, and Dr. March began his.

At the same time Fitch bade farewell to a fellow-student, a Mr. Hamilton, who left for home in South Carolina. One wonders at how he got up to Vermont. Fitch added to the mystery by writing of him as 'a young man so favored by fortune, that he spends his time and money to suit himself and cannot content himself with study. Otherwise he is a fine fellow. His father is a nephew of General Alexander Hamilton' (2, 138).

Fitch, as a member of the second-year or senior class, became involved in a 'warm quarreling' over the form of the catalogue. As chairman of a student committee, Fitch compiled a list of students, with the assistance of Dr. Woodward, which finally contained 102 names. There were two subscription lists, and Fitch was accused of 'wishing to rule the whole class.' In addition, he had minor troubles with his roommates and with the landlady. Two students left because of 'dissatisfaction with the victuals,' but particularly because 'Mrs. Kellog's tongue is certainly too limber and she is too inquisitive with the affairs of others which do not concern her in the least.' His roommate, Mazuzan, 'is sans exception the most miserable shirk of a roommate that I ever yet had ... he never brings a pitcher of water or thinks of doing his share of our little choars (*sic*)' (2, 141f., 148, 152ff.).

Dr. March lectured on anatomy and lost no opportunity to agitate for a medical college at Albany. Once he said to Fitch: 'Come, Mr. Fitch, I must electioneer some. It may as well come out first as last. We must get a Medical School chartered in Albany. It will be opposed here, but I cannot help that. Who are some of the most influential men in your county?' The bell then rang for the lecture, and Fitch helped carry the anatomical subject from the dissecting room to the lecture room (2, 160).[7]

By 27 November, with the end of term still several weeks away, Fitch recorded that he was wearying of the lectures, reporting that the thought of another lecture gave him the 'hyp.' They had become 'an old story, inconceivably tedious, and the lecture room looks awfully sad and gloomy.' He was not alone in this feeling; student drop-outs seemed common, for there was 'scarcely half the class there a month ago' (3, 4). The question of completing the course for a degree now came up, and Fitch told the registrar, Dr. Woodward, that his time was not up until next July. It could, however, be completed earlier 'if I count six months of the Rensselaer degree, which is here allowed' (3, 5). So Fitch at once entered his application as a candidate for a degree.

Now began a race to finish his work. Fitch was deficient in many fields. He had never read on surgery or midwifery and could not do so now, but he began to review Dr. Tully's notes on the treatment of diseases. The lectures ended on 1 December, and Fitch turned to his dissertation, which was to be on 'Natural Sciences and Their Importance to Medicine' (3, 6). In the meantime he waited his turn for the examination, which took place quite informally. On Friday, 4 December 1829, he was called up for oral examination before the professors, and he gave a vivid account of what went on in that examination. Dr. Beck was easy on him, announcing he had known Fitch for several years, back in his Rensselaer days, and was satisfied with his qualifications. Then came Dr. Woodward, who was 'a tough one.' He began with inflammation in its many manifestations: 'I was woefully puzzled. I was even angry at the minuteness of thrust of his questions.' Next was Dr. March, who was very easy. Tully came last, 'on opium and its effects, Tone, Atomy, Eutomy, Nervines, Narcotics, etc.' The examination lasted nearly three hours (3, 6ff.).

Fitch handed in his dissertation and started immediately for home 'to get certificates of my time.' In the absence of Dr. Freeman, his father wrote out a certificate testifying to his studies of medicine since 2 July 1827. Fitch re-

---

7. Early in the following year, 1829, Fitch attended Dr. March's private medical class in Albany and became the assistant to him (*Journal*, 3, *passim*).

turned to Castleton, assured that his 'passports for the M.D. were pretty fair' (*3*, 8ff.). In a few days came the reading of dissertations. His thesis proved longer than was necessary and passed easily. His roommate, Mazuzan's paper sounded flat; he might have been ashamed of it, since 'I wrote the whole of it.' One thesis Fitch singled out for particular comment was on Fecundation: 'A nastier and more disgusting piece could scarcely have been composed. Every motion and appearance in the act of copulation was minutely described, and professors and students were convulsed with laughter' (*3*, 12).

In the evening Fitch paid Dr. Woodward the $16 fee for graduation, and all was finished. The notable day of commencement finally arrived: 'It dawned bright and clear ... our big business was drawing rapidly to a consummation.' The graduates advanced and lined up in two rows before the President's chair. Dr. Tully read the list of those qualified and asked the corporation if they had any objections. None being made, the diplomas were handed out, 'and we were invested, by power granted from the supreme authority of the State of Vermont, with the title of Doctor of Medicine, and with all the rights, honors, and privileges which law and custom has bestowed on Doctors in Medicine.' The newly invested doctors then seated themselves: 'old Tully looked as dignified as a high priest, while performing these ceremonies. His appearance was noble.' He then delivered an excellent address 'on the duties of patients and nurses, and on those of physicians. It was a masterpiece.' Everybody adjourned to Moulton's hotel, where they partook of 'a public dinner at the expense of the graduates' (*3*, 13ff.).

Fitch did not attend the dinner for want of funds, but instead exchanged cards with a number of fellow students and went to his room to pack for departure. As a final sad mission, he went to see the body of his friend and fellow student, Norton, who had been sick but died that morning. Later that day a number of them departed on a special stage for Poultney: 'a jolly, jolly load of young puces,' singing, whistling, hallooing, and talking. One of the songs was apparently a kind of alma mater: 'So fare thee well, old Castleton, I ne'er shall see you more' (*3*, 15).

Strangely enough, even with his M.D. from Castleton, Fitch's medical education was not yet completed, but continued for several months longer. He returned to Salem, where he was soon embroiled in a controversy with the local church, and with his family, over his dancing. Young Fitch took a firm position on the subject, explaining that it was part of his quest for poise and maturity: 'I am not prepared to renounce it, nor do I think I shall be ... my determination at the outset was to shake off, rid myself of the extreme diffidence, timidity, and tongue-tiedness ... which I had two years ago. This would never do for me when I became a doctor.... I was resolved to cure myself of it, and in order to do so I must go into company.' He elaborated an extensive apology for his behavior: 'Better success never followed an undertaking. I can now go into company, yes, and polite company, and feel myself at home.... I have danced. I have played. I have kissed rosy cheeks. I have won maidens' smiles. Yet I do not think I have gone astray, or opened the wounds of my Saviour ... or sinned against my God. I have not caroused ...' (3, 18ff.).

In the meantime, Dr. Freeman apparently tried to atone for his previous neglect and offered Fitch wider opportunity for sharing in medical practice. The cases ranged from a woman with dyspepsia and sympathetic tooth- and-headache to a twelve-year-old boy who had had his leg amputated halfway up the thigh, and to ulcers, 'catarrhal' consumption, and syphilis. Salem obviously had a substantial and varied incidence of illness, whatever was done for it. Fitch had most difficulty with the Goodale boy who had lost a leg. In dressing the wound he reported: 'I trembled slightly ... the first pin I stuck in the bandage went through and the boy screamed.' Nevertheless the boy did well, and the ligatures of the arteries were soon removed (3, 21ff.).

Fitch acquired a license to practice, which completed his education, and he broached a plan to migrate to the Illinois frontier. In the summer of 1830 he accompanied the Rensselaer traveling school of science on the Erie Canal as an assistant professor and continued on westward to Greenville, Illinois. There he spent an unhappy winter in an attempt to establish himself in practice.[8] He returned to Salem in 1831 and never again ventured far afield from the paternal farm. Subsequently he abandoned the practice of medicine and dedicated himself to the pursuit of entomology. He was designated as state entomologist of New York and became known as the 'Bug Catcher of Salem,' but his fame in entomology was nationwide and even international.

Thus did Fitch fulfill his aspirations in the field of science, perhaps distinguishing himself far more than he would have as a rural practitioner. In his customary New Year's speculations, Fitch recorded on the last night of 1829 that he had attained 'the summit of my wishes, the degree of M.D.,' adding the uncertain question: 'where and how will I be situated on the last day of December, 1839!' Actually he was then back on the family farm, having

---

8. Fitch's western experiences are recorded in several volumes of his journal (4–6) and in Samuel Rezneck, 'Diary of a New York doctor in Illinois, 1830–31,' *J. Illinois hist. Soc.*, 1961, *14*, 25ff.

put medicine aside, and was combining farming with scientific observation and the study of 'noxious and beneficial insects' for the state of New York (*3*, 38).[9]

---

9. Cf. D. L. Collins, 'The bug catcher of Salem,' *N. Y. St. Bull.*, March, 1954; Asa Fitch, 'Reports on the noxious, beneficial, and other insects of the state of New York,' *Trans. N.Y. St. agric. Soc.*, 1855–72, vols. 14–30, in addition to various other miscellaneous publications.

The New England Journal of Medicine, 1812-1968

JOSEPH GARLAND

NEARLY forty-five years ago, impressed with the journalistic prolificity of our own unique region, I prepared for the *Boston Medical and Surgical Journal* an account of medical journalism in New England.[1] Approximately eighty titles were included, of various types of medical publications, and others may have been omitted. The list began with the single volume of *Cases and Observations* produced in 1788 by the Medical Society of New Haven County in the State of Connecticut. Not to be considered a medical journal, it nevertheless had the distinction of including Hezekiah Beardsley's original description of congenital pyloric stenosis.

Two years later the first of the *Medical Papers Communicated to the Massachusetts Medical Society* appeared. These transactions, also hardly journalistic in nature, were published until 1914, when their function was taken over by the *Boston Medical and Surgical Journal*.

Meanwhile Connecticut was carrying on with its customary zeal. The *Proceedings of the Connecticut State Medical Society* were published at intervals from 1805 for the next eighty-five years, first in Hartford and then in New Haven; the *Communications of the Medical Society of Connecticut* appeared in New Haven five years after the *Proceedings* were initiated. The *Monthly Journal of Medicine* began publication in Hartford in 1823 but continued for two years only. The *Quarterly Journal of Inebriety* pursued its righteous course, also in Hartford, from 1876 until 1906, when it was consolidated with the *Archives of Physiological Therapy* of Boston and continued as the *Journal of Inebriety* for seven years. It then gave up what must have seemed a losing battle, although prohibition was not far over the horizon.

1. Joseph Garland, 'Medical journalism in New England, 1788-1924,' *Boston med. surg. J.*, 1924, *190*, 865-879.

The Annual Beaumont Lecture on the William H. Carmalt Foundation delivered before the Beaumont Medical Club at their meeting on 3 May 1968 in New Haven, Connecticut.

land *Journal of Medicine and Surgery and the Collateral Branches of Science* (Conducted by a Number of Physicians), the first quarterly issue of which appeared that January.

The founders associated with themselves in their journalistic enterprise other leading Boston physicians: John Gorham, Jacob Bigelow, and Walter Channing, later adding Drs. George Hayward, John Ware, and John W. Webster, the eight meeting each month 'to sup and read the papers submitted.' The first issue had as its lead article 'Remarks on Angina Pectoris' by John Warren, father of the editor; 'Remarks on the Morbid Effects of Dentition' by James Jackson; 'Case of Apoplexy with Dissections' by John C. Warren; 'Treatment of Injuries Occasioned by Fire' by Jacob Bigelow, and 'Remarks on Diseases Resembling Syphilis' by Walter Channing.

In accordance with the promise that the Journal would also represent the 'Collateral Branches of Science,' various issues contained such communications as 'On the Vegetation of High Mountains, with Reference to the Pyrenees, translated from the French,' a 'History of the Forest Trees of North America, Considered Primarily with Regard to their Use in the Arts and their Introduction into Commerce.' Later one may find 'Some Account of the Grand Monadnock' and 'Some Account of the White Mountains of New Hampshire,' preceded by 'Some Account of Harvard University in Cambridge' and closely followed by 'Some Account of Iodine,' as well as 'Observations on the Utility of Blood-letting and Purgatives, in a Fever which Prevailed in the Russian Fleet.'

Volume VII contains a report from the Dutch that eight grains of freshly gathered and cleaned cobwebs made up into seven pills with mucilage of gum arabic, two being taken shortly before a paroxysm of ague, three during it, and two shortly after it, will generally have the effect of preventing the next attack.

Two articles of considerably greater importance, if less picturesque, appeared during these early years. In the last quarterly issue of 1822 James Jackson published a paper 'On a Peculiar Disease Resulting from the Use of Ardent Spirits'—a careful description of peripheral neuritis; and two years later M. F. Cogswell of Hartford gave an 'Account of Operation for Extirpation of Tumour, in which a Ligature was Applied to the Carotid Artery.' The operation was reported nineteen years after it had been performed!

Volume XVI, for 1827, appeared under the title *The New England Medical Review and Journal*, and was conducted by Walter Channing and John

Ware. Channing, a graduate of Harvard College, took his medical degree at the University of Pennsylvania in 1809. He was Harvard's first Professor of Obstetrics and Medical Jurisprudence and held the deanship for twenty-eight years. John Ware was graduated from Harvard Medical School in 1816 and practiced first in Duxbury, then in Boston. A president of the Massachusetts Medical Society for four years, he succeeded James Jackson as Hersey Professor of Theory and Practice in 1856.

Meanwhile, in 1823, the year in which Thomas Wakley founded the *Lancet*, the first issue of the weekly Boston *Medical Intelligencer* appeared. The subscription rate was $2.00 per annum and it consisted of a four-page, three-column folio, designed to present, according to its title page, 'Extracts from Foreign and American Medical Journals, a Variety of Local Intelligence on Subjects Connected with Medicine; Biographical Sketches of Distinguished Surgeons and Physicians; Descriptions of the Principal Hospitals in Europe; Original Articles on Various Diseases; with Concise Views of the Improvements and Discoveries in the Medico-Chirurgical Sciences. Conducted by Jerome V. C. Smith, M.D.'

Volume III was conducted by James Wilson, M.D., 'Assisted by an Association of Physicians' who, alarmed at the deterioration of their profession, warned that the name of Physician had come 'to be associated with every species of speculation, and almost every pursuit, that it is nearly synonymous with politician, farmer, merchant, stockjobber, and in some instances horse jockey and gambler.'

John G. Coffin edited the last two volumes, announcing in January, 1828, that on 19 February the first number of the *Boston Medical and Surgical Journal* would appear as a continuation of the *New England Medical Journal* and of the *Boston Medical Intelligencer*. . . . 'Its object will be to present, in as condensed a form as possible, the Medical and Surgical intelligence of the day, both domestic and foreign. For this purpose arrangements have been made for publishing in it all the most interesting practices of the Massachusetts General Hospital' and so forth. The purchase of the *Intelligencer* had been made by Drs. Warren, Ware, and Channing for $600.00, and the two journals were united, Dr. Warren commencing the editorship.

Dr. Warren was then fifty years old, and according to Edward Warren, his biographer, 'At this period he rose in winter and breakfasted by candle-light and went directly out to visit his patients until one; except during the lectures, when he passed usually two hours at the Medical College. From one to two he received patients at his home. He devoted about twenty minutes to his dinner; after which, he retired to his room for an hour. In the latter part of the afternoon, he visited such patients as required a second visit, and then took a cup of tea in his study at seven; after which he wrote and worked upon the subjects before mentioned, often, if not generally, until two in the morning.'

The first issue of the *Boston Medical and Surgical Journal*, under which title the periodical was to continue in weekly publication for a hundred years, contained as its first article 'Cases of Neuralgia or Painful Affections of Nerves,' by John Collins Warren. Dr. Channing submitted reports from the medical department of the Massachusetts General Hospital, and Dr. John Gorham contributed a 'Medical Report of the Weather and Prevalent Diseases for the Last Three Months.'

Mingled with the erudite communications that appeared in the first volume of the *Journal* a few may be found which, if less erudite, are certainly more imaginative. I may mention in particular an 'Account of the Blowing Snake,' as narrated in a letter from Dr. H. Conant, of Maumee. It appeared that on the tenth of May in 1828 Dr. Conant had been called to visit a lad of fifteen whom he found 'much swollen in his countenance, much affected with nausea and giddiness,' violent pain in the limbs, pulse weak, and finally a universal prostration. The treatment was palliative, consisting of an emetic-cathartic. Two miles further on the doctor visited a forty-year-old man with identical symptoms to whom the same therapy was administered. The next day he was called to see a girl of fourteen with similar symptoms, but more severe. Under the same treatment, but with the addition of olive oil, her recovery was more rapid.

It transpired that three days before these patients were seen 'they had all been exposed to the effluvia of the blowing snake. The man had killed two and the boy and girl had each passed one, at the distance of a yard or so to the leeward. According to a native Frenchman of the region something must have gone amiss, for persons blown upon always swell and burst open and invariably die.' Dr. Conant honestly concludes in respect to the snake: 'It is said, that during its expiration, a yellowish steam is visible issuing from its mouth to the distance of several inches, but I know nothing of it, having never seen a living snake of the kind.'

In September 1833 a letter to the editor from Thomas Sewall of Washington describes a demonstration by William Beaumont, of his not invariably co-operative patient, Alexis St. Martin. A longer account appears in January of the following year and in April a short note that 'the faculty of this city have been very highly gratified the present week by a visit from Dr. Beaumont . . . who demonstrated his patient on this occasion.'

Dr. Jerome V. C. Smith, originator of the *Medical Intelligencer*, assumed the editorship of the *Journal* in 1835 and carried on for twenty-two years, when, having been health officer of Boston, he became its mayor and disappeared from the medical journalistic scene. He was succeeded by W. W. Morland and Francis Minot.

During Dr. Smith's editorship a number of interesting and sometimes important events were chronicled. In 1841 Dorothea Dix discovered the conditions under which the insane of the Commonwealth were confined in many of its institutions—'wretched in our prisons and more wretched in our Alms-Houses.' The career that was to occupy the rest of this indomitable woman's life began with an investigation and a report to the General Court that appeared in the *Journal* of 3 March 1843. 'I proceed, Gentlemen, briefly to call your attention to the state of Insane Persons confined within this Commonwealth, in cages, closets, stalls, pens: Chained, naked, beaten with rods, and lashed into obedience!' Her disclosures had the desired effect, resulting in an enlargement of the state hospital at Worcester, the building of the Butler Hospital in Providence, and the establishment of the Trenton State Hospital in New Jersey. Before she was through, she had visited every state east of the Rocky Mountains and was instrumental in the creation of thirty hospitals before turning her attention to Great Britain! The controversial documentary film *Titicut Follies*, aside from the legal and moral questions that have been raised regarding its propriety, is a sad reminder that reforms may be neither complete nor permanent.

In the same issue with Miss Dix's inspired battle cry is a note that the Duke of Marlboro had mesmerized a dog in Ireland. 'American dogs continue to resist the magnetic influence.'

Certainly the most significant papers to be published in the long history of the *Boston Medical and Surgical Journal* were those announcing the first public demonstration, in the operating theater of the Massachusetts General Hospital, of the administration of ether as a general anesthetic agent. No one would today fail to recognize the prior claim of Crawford W. Long of Georgia as a result of his own bold experiments made five years previously, but to John Collins Warren must go the credit for having performed the now famous operation on 16 October 1846. He was then sixty-nine years of age. It was perhaps an act of generosity, the operation having proved successful, for him to permit the young Henry Jacob Bigelow, one of the spectators, to publish 'Insensibility During Surgical Operations Produced by Inhalation' in the *Journal* of 18 November of the same year. Dr. Warren's own cautiously optimistic paper, 'Inhalation of Ethereal Vapor, for the Prevention of Pain in Surgical Operations' appeared three weeks later.

The trial in the case of the famous Harvard Medical School murder on 23 November 1849 of Dr. George Parkman by John W. Webster, Professor of Chemistry and a member of the original group of editors, was amply covered in the *Journal*, detail by detail, including the eventual confession, the conviction, the sentencing, and the public hanging on 30 August 1850, tickets for which were in great demand.

It is salutary after this grim recital, to note in the *Journal* of 19 March 1851, that within the past week the editor had had an opportunity of examining an artificial leg made by Mr. B. F. Palmer of Springfield. 'It is made of a light wood [he wrote], covered with an enamel that is impervious to liquids, has flexible joints, and is as complete a substitute for the natural limb as we can conceive of . . . so well did it correspond in movements with the natural one that it was difficult to say which was the artificial leg.' Those who have read *Dr. Dogbody's Leg*, by James Norman Hall, will be reminded of the automatic self-propelled limb reported as having been designed and constructed by Benjamin Franklin for that incorrigibly imaginative ship's surgeon and veteran of the Napoleonic Wars.

Four years later, in Volume 52, Gilman Kimball of Lowell reported another bold and successful pioneering effort under the title 'Successful Case of Extirpation of the Uterus.'

The *Journal* experienced a rapid succession of editors after Smith's retirement, with a 'New Series' starting in 1868 under David W. Cheever and Oliver F. Wadsworth. According to an announcement at that time its nobler size and double columns conformed in 'shape and appearance to the best modern specimens of hebdomadal literature.'

Perhaps the *Journal*'s greatest crisis is related in a handwritten note headed 'Collapse to Survival' enclosed in the Boston Medical Library's bound Volume 87 for the latter half of 1872. Francis H. Brown, the editor, was seriously ill and his assistant, F. W. Draper, unprepared to cope with the situation. The cupboard was bare except for one manuscript. Benjamin E. Cotting, having been appealed to, threw into the breach an address he had delivered to the Norfolk District Society, entitled 'My First Question as a Medical Student.' A footnote cited the pertinent retort made to an 'upbraiding professor' by John Homans when a medical student: 'I prefer to be called a fool for asking the question, rather than to remain in ignorance.' This paper, and the interest of six physicians in subscribing $100 each for three years, saved the day; before the time elapsed they had purchased the *Journal* outright, J. Collins Warren, grandson of the original founder, assuming the editorship with Thomas Dwight.

Warren continued as editor until 1881, during which time (in 1877) the *Journal* was instrumental in effecting the abolishment in Massachusetts of the old, largely political and often corrupt, system of lay coroners and their replacement by professionally trained physicians as medical examiners. He was succeeded by George Brune Shattuck, who occupied the editorial chair for a record thirty-one years. During this period, in 1882 and 1883, the *Journal* published three of Oliver Wendell Holmes's most felicitous essays: 'Medical Highways and Byways,' 'Farewell Address to the Harvard Medical School,' and 'The New Century and the New Building of the Medical School of Harvard University.' On 14 February 1889 Reginald H. Fitz's original paper on 'Acute Pancreatitis' appeared.

Dr. Shattuck retired in 1912 and was succeeded by E. Wyllys Taylor, with Robert M. Green as his assistant. In 1914 the *Journal* became the official publication of the Massachusetts Medical Society, Dr. Green, master of English prose and verse, surgeon, obstetrician, anatomist, Latin scholar and teacher of Greek, assuming the editorship in 1915 and carrying on until the actual purchase of the *Journal* by the Society in 1921. The price agreed on was $1.00, which, according to a persistent rumor, was never paid. Dr. Walter P. Bowers—'Uncle Walter' to his younger associates—had been instrumental in persuading the Council to approve the purchase, and, as a form of penance perhaps, he was pressed into service as editor, aided by an editorial board that met each month to discuss the papers submitted, following the pattern established in 1812. In the following year George Gilbert Smith, William B. Breed, and I became associate editors, and a year later the publication of the Case Records of the Massachusetts General Hospital was assumed. Each new subscriber was asked whether the inclusion of the Case Records had been responsible for his investment. If the answer was in the affirmative, under an interesting fiscal arrangement which continued for some time a percentage of his subscription was allocated to the Hospital, which may account for that Institution's continued prosperity.

Occasional noteworthy papers have been published over the years, a score of which were listed by Henry R. Viets in the *Journal*'s sesquicentennial issue of 4 January 1962.[2] Certain of these have already been mentioned;

2. H. R. Viets, 'A score of significant papers published in the *Journal* during the last hundred and fifty years,' *N. Engl. J. Med.*, 1962, 266, 23-28.

among others were J. Homer Wright's 'Origin and Nature of Blood Plates,' Legg's description of an 'Obscure Affection of the Hip-joint,' Tracy Putnam's 'Treatment of Hydrocephalus by Endoscopic Coagulation of the Choroid Plexus,' and the report by Albright, Butler, Hampton, and Smith of a 'Syndrome Characterized by Osteitis Fibrosa Disseminata, Areas of Pigmentation and Endocrine Dysfunction, with Precocious Puberty in Females.' And certainly Donald Munro's papers on rehabilitation of paralyzed veterans, with special emphasis on tidal drainage of the atonic bladder, represent an important contribution.

On 18 February 1928 a dinner was held to celebrate a century of publication as the *Boston Medical and Surgical Journal* and the change of name to the present title. Only seven minor orations were delivered before Morris Fishbein, the speaker of the evening, was given the floor. He prefaced his remarks by quoting from Oliver Wendell Holmes' dedicatory address at the opening of the Boston Medical Library in 1878 in respect to the growth of periodical literature: 'We must have the latest thought in its latest expression; the page must be newly turned like the morning bannock; the pamphlet must be newly opened like the anteprandial oyster.'

During the 1920s the *Journal* made its only attempt at empire building by gradually acquiring a group of organizations for which it served as the official publication. These included the New England Surgical Society, the Boston Surgical Society, the New Hampshire and Vermont Medical Societies, the New England Pediatric Society, and the New Hampshire Surgical Club. There is no evidence that the state societies of Maine, Rhode Island, or Connecticut were ever tempted to enter the fold. The course of empire having long since moved westward, the *Journal*, essentially conservative, returned to its geographical traditions, and the empire gradually fell away.

Dr. Bowers retired at the close of 1936, being then eighty, and was succeeded by my contemporary, Robert N. Nye, who carried on with distinction until his untimely death in 1947, when I was asked to take his place. Robert Green had put on the *Journal* the stamp of his own superior literary acumen; Dr. Bowers and Dr. Nye, in their twenty-six consecutive years of editorship for the Society, stabilized its position as a uniquely acceptable general medical journal.

Within the last two decades, continuing under the impetus that it had acquired, the *Journal* has gradually grown in size from an average of fifty-eight pages per issue in 1947 to approximately twice that number in 1967. Three hundred and six original articles were submitted in 1947, of which about half were accepted, and over five times that number in 1967, of which fewer than a fifth were published. The medical progress articles, mostly solicited, have continued in regular publication and have become immeasurably more sophisticated, being now so comprehensive that they usually require serialization. The century-old department of Medical Intelligence has been revived, at least in title, to serve as the repository of brief miscellaneous material, technical or otherwise, including such features as the short biographical Doctors Afield sketches, John Lister's Monthly London Post, which has missed only one deadline in over fifteen years, Law-Medicine Notes, and so-called Current Concepts.

Special articles on a variety of subjects have increased in number and importance. They included, in the last issue of May 1962, a four-part symposium on the 'Medical Consequences of Thermonuclear War,' the following year 22 papers on the social and organizational aspects of medical care, and in 1964 the 27 papers that made up the Boston City Hospital's centennial symposium. A year and a half ago the *Journal* presented a series of eight articles on Environmental Hazards, ranging from hearing loss resulting from community noise, to electromagnetic and ionizing radiation, and urban solid waste management.

In a different and apparently controversial class was a paper in the same year by Henry K. Beecher on 'Ethics and Clinical Research,' dealing unequivocally with the problems of experimentation on human beings and attempting to define informed consent. Also, within the last two years the publication of the monthly Seminars in Medicine of the Beth Israel Hospital of Boston has been instituted, and more recently the Physiology for Physicians papers, prepared by the American Physiological Society.

Our real year of decision for these two decades was 1952, when a professional appraisal of the *Journal*'s organization and operation was made. The most important advice resulting from this study was that a business manager be obtained, and this was done, with remarkable success. Since the resulting reorganization went into effect, the publication has remained in the black, and the circulation has risen by steady increments from around 25,000 to well over 100,000 subscribers.

It has been the conviction of the editors, occasionally challenged by an ultraconservative reader, that editorials in a medical journal need not necessarily be confined strictly to medical or even paramedical subjects. Doctors, they assume, are intelligent and educated persons with wide interests. Consequently, with a good stable of editorial writers, the number of editorials per issue has been increased to an average of four, with considerable license in the choice of subjects, to include whatever might interest, inform, persuade, inspire, or even, sometimes, entertain the physician.

Thus a cursory inspection of volume indexes shows editorial titles ranging from 'Abdominal Pain during Intravenous Infusion' to 'Zymoses of 1857,' and sage discussions of many important scientific subjects are to be found. One may read also a description of the 'Old Farmer's Almanac,' a comment on the British New Year's Honours, and a congratulatory note on the appointment of Paul Beeson of Yale to the Nuffield Professorship of Clinical Medicine at Oxford, the establishment at Yale of the Beeson Visiting Professorship, and the summoning of Dr. Beeson as the first Beeson Professor.

Sometimes the sequence of these titles as indexed conveys a sort of message, i.e., 'Gerontocracy, Perhaps,' 'Grandfather Complex,' and 'Great Expectations.' On another occasion, 'Problems of Alcoholism' followed immediately by 'Problems of Internal Combustion.' In the same volume, in 1954, an editorial note appears on the dedication at Mackinac Island of a Beaumont Memorial consisting of the reconstruction, on the original site and foundation, of the American Fur Company store in which St. Martin's accident occurred. It seems impossible to escape a certain preoccupation with the gastric juices.

I cannot resist reference to a quasi-clinical or pseudo-scientific discussion of 'Famous First Words' relative to the supposed utterance of audible and possibly meaningful cries by an infant several hours before birth. 'From the evidence submitted' the comment continues, 'it must be concluded that intrauterine voices are simulated by the shrill winds in the pregnant abdomen. There may be music in the air, as the familiar song insists, "when the infant dawn is nigh," but unborn-infant voices are suspect.'

Rarely has verse of a sort intruded, as in the case of a sonnet submitted by an anonymous contributor—after its rejection, we discovered, by the *Atlantic*. Entitled 'A Gaggle of Mother Geese,' it seems to have been inspired by the success of the Russians in putting the little dog Laika into orbit:

> Like fleas of which each higher tries to leap
> Than any other flea, on souped-up feet,
> So we, committed to our cosmic 'beep'
> For place in space seem destined to compete.
> Hey diddle diddle! Puss, with horsehair laid
> Across her gut in tuneful masochism,

>Salutes each effort with a serenade
>Of paradoxical ventriloquism.
>What satellites are in their orbits now!
>A flying saucer fleeing with its spoon
>While Mother Goose's space-commuting cow
>Bounds on her milky way from earth to moon.
>The twinkling stars look down in gay rapport
>And ghostly Laika laughs to see such sport.

In 1962, without pomp but with some circumstance, the *Journal* celebrated its 150th anniversary with Wilder Penfield as guest speaker.

In the development of medical journalism, the general or all-purpose journal, like the general or all-purpose practitioner, was first on the scene, and both, I assume, will persist as the cornerstone of the services that they represent. 'Experience,' it has been said, 'still has its uses, even in relation to experiment, and a devotion to the latter still needs to be tempered with the wisdom born of the former if knowledge gained is to be translated into service rendered.' I might quote from Dr. Holmes's valedictory address to the graduating class of the Bellevue Hospital College in 1871, in which he suggested that 'the young man knows the rules, but the old man knows the exceptions.'

Sir Theodore Fox, then editor of the *Lancet*, expanded on this general theme in his University of London Heath Clark Lectures on 'Crisis in Communication,' delivered five years ago.[3] Recognizing that communication in the aggregate passes through many channels toward a multitude of objectives, he simplifies the problem for medicine by dividing its journals into two main categories—the 'recorders' and the 'newspapers,' 'The former reserve their pages for new observations, experiments, and techniques; the latter have as their function "to inform, interpret, criticize, and stimulate," ' and many of those that were primarily of the newspaper type have taken on a hybrid quality.

Concerned with the increasing potential of the physician for the improvement of human health, and yet, too frequently, his loss of touch with the vital aims of his calling, the *Journal* three years ago questioned a considerable number of its subscribers, whose professional classification was already part of the record, regarding their interest in the *Journal*'s content. The results were summarized at an assembly of the World Medical Association in London that fall. Reports of medical progress led the list in

---

3. Sir Theodore Fox, *Crisis in communication* (University of London Heath Clark Lectures 1963, delivered at the London School of Hygiene and Tropical Medicine) (London, 1965).

popularity, then came the original articles, the Case Records of the Massachusetts General Hospital and the special articles on a variety of usually nontechnical subjects.

Classified according to their various professional pursuits, approximately 19 per cent of our readers were internists, over 11 per cent general practitioners, and 8 per cent surgeons. It is gratifying that 35 per cent, or then about 35,000, were interns, residents, and students.

In continuing to unfold his concept of a crisis in communication, Dr. Fox draws a comparison between the recording and the newspaper functions of a hybrid journal, which may be stated simply as knowledge versus information, fact versus opinion, depth versus breadth. The real function of the first division is to be published; of the second, to be read. Whereas expert advice is desirable in selecting scientific material for publication, it must be remembered that the risk inherent in expertness lies in resistance to new ideas. Group decisions are admittedly safer than those made by one person alone, but they ensure justice to honest work only as it falls 'within the framework of established ideas,' and they lessen the chance of acceptance of original but unorthodox views.

The 'recorder' pages of a journal must be exact; the newspaper section must be critical, and the editor must have freedom to express his opinions. In respect to the function of putting on record the revelations of research (often, unfortunately, in little understood language), the former editor of the *Lancet* does not claim that editing of a paper makes it more readable, but only less unreadable, and I confess that many of us would agree with this comment.

However, all that is possible must be done to interpret the results of scientific investigation, for any of these records may be or may become important, like Mendel's law, the exposition of which lay for thirty-five years forgotten in the pages of an obscure journal. So far as any crisis in communication is concerned, there will be better communication, clearer communication, and possibly even less journalistic competition as time goes on. The printed word will no more be replaced by the spoken word or the moving picture on a screen than was the spoken word replaced when the Sumerians invented their cuneiform chirography. One need not fear a twilight of the printed word—a *Wörterdämmerung*—as has been suggested, especially so long as a journal retains its invaluable capacity of staying quiet until one is ready to consult it, and is then on hand with its original content unchanged.

Crises, after all, are of the essence of progress, and even if progress itself is a sort of *folie circulaire*, as may sometimes be suspected, it goes forward to meet its other end by a succession of crises, encountered and overcome or successfully bypassed.

In attempting briefly to outline the history and development of the *New England Journal of Medicine*, at least as I have viewed them, I have touched on what I have believed its functions to be and can now express the hope that in some degree the worthier of these objectives are being attained. Its future course will be determined by the expanding needs of mankind. The struggle against inhumanity in its efforts to destroy humanity, against the ills of great poverty and those of great prosperity, against the littleness of man in competition with his greatness, must be unremitting if it is to meet with any degree of success—and any permanent victory is hardly to be expected.

Scientific achievement, which may, perhaps fancifully, be called a product of the brain, will continue to advance, and it must be matched by a continually expanding social consciousness, which is a product, according to a long-cherished sentiment, of the heart. The virtue of an all-purpose journal is that it must give space to both.

The future of any of the works of man depends on their continued usefulness to man, and the future course of medicine will depend on the exploration of new horizons, faithfully recorded and intelligently interpreted, in which its periodical literature must be an important factor. The strictly interpersonal traditional doctor-patient relation, whereas it must be nurtured and strengthened, must itself welcome and be included in a greater appreciation of the broader needs that medicine must help to fulfill, as in planning to meet the health requirements of the community.

These new horizons, in the development of which the schools and the whole profession are involved, will include the better adaptation of scientific advances to the real needs of the patient and of society, studies in the economics of medical care, the shaping of teaching curricula to the vast amount of available knowledge and to social needs, where the students themselves are already pressing the issue.

The schools are taking an increasingly active interest in the continuing education of the physician as intern, resident, and beyond, inculcating an understanding of the subtle nuances of the true ethics of practice, including such sometimes difficult matters as the prolongation of existence, which may mean only the prolongation of the harrowing process of dying, to the point where decisions to permit death to intervene must be made.

Not only must the schools of medicine exert leadership in such progress, but so also must the organized profession of medicine. And so, too, must the responsible medical journals stand ready to 'inform, interpret, criticize, and stimulate,' to follow and to lead in the strengthening of medicine and of human aspirations, if mankind is to have a future.

Finally, I wish to congratulate our Committee on Publications on the selection of Franz J. Ingelfinger as the *Journal*'s present editor. Endowed with medical knowledge, common sense, literary ability, and a sense of humor, fully aware of the problems and purposes of our profession, he is a fitting product of his uniquely superior education. For he is a graduate of Yale College and of the Harvard Medical School. The results would have been the same had the order been reversed.

As the editors announced in the first issue of the *Boston Medical and Surgical Journal* 140 years ago: 'The list of subscribers being now large, it will go forward in some shape or other; and efforts will not be wanting to make it useful.'

Chestnut Hill, Massachusetts

William Beaumont, Robley Dunglison, and the 'Philadelphia Physiologists'

JEROME J. BYLEBYL

BY the late eighteenth century, Reaumur, John Hunter, and, above all, Spallanzani had gone a long way toward establishing the theory that certain fluids which collect in the stomach, generally referred to as 'gastric juice,' have the power of reducing diverse forms of food to chyme.[1] This idea was based primarily on the demonstration that food can be digested out of pierced metal containers in the stomach, and was strongly confirmed by the ability of the gastric fluids to dissolve food outside the stomach, in the technique known as 'artificial digestion.' Sir Michael Foster has stated that by Spallanzani's work, 'the solvent power of gastric juice ... whether within or outside the stomach, became an established fact, a definite addition to our knowledge of digestion, never afterwards taken away.'[2] When one reads Spallanzani's lengthy account of his careful and exhaustive experiments, it seems that Foster's statement ought to have been true.[3] Nevertheless, the gastric juice theory had a stormy history during the fifty years following the publication of Spallanzani's work around 1780.[4] Only against this background of continued controversy and uncertainty can one understand why William Beaumont undertook some of his observations, and why some European physiologists welcomed his demonstration of things that, to the modern observer, might not seem to have needed further demonstration.

One problem was that the gastric juice long remained a hypothetical substance, that is, something known primarily through its effects of dissolving food, preventing or halting putrefaction, and curdling milk, but which had not been chemically identified as a specific secretion.[5] Spallan-

---

I would like to thank Professors Frederic L. Holmes, Lloyd G. Stevenson, and Leonard G. Wilson, and Dr. Samuel X. Radbill for their suggestions and encouragement.

1. Michael Foster, *Lectures on the history of physiology* (Cambridge, 1901), pp. 209–223.
2. *Ibid.*, p. 219.
3. Lazzaro Spallanzani, *Expériences sur la digestion de l'homme et de différentes espèces d'animaux*, Jean Senebier, tr. (Geneva, 1783).
4. For a thorough survey of controversies over digestion during the late eighteenth century, see D. Bates, 'The background to John Young's thesis on digestion,' *Bull. Hist. Med.*, 1962, *36*, 341–361.
5. *Ibid.*, pp. 351–356. For an indictment of Spallanzani's theory on these grounds, see François Chaussier and N. P. A. Adelon, 'Digestion,' *Dictionaire des sciences médicales* (Paris, 1818), IX, 422.

zani had used the term 'gastric juice' simply to refer to the heterogeneous mixture of saliva, esophageal, and gastric secretions which collect in the stomach, though he recognized that the secretions of the stomach proper have the greatest degree of solvent power.[6] He reported that 'pure' gastric juice is clear, colorless, insipid, and slightly salty.[7] He knew that acid is frequently present in the stomach, but he firmly maintained that this acidity is the accidental result of the digestion of vegetable substances rather than a necessary property of the gastric juice.[8] Until the 1820s this view was generally accepted, and, with organic analysis in its infancy, it is not surprising that more detailed studies of the components of the gastric fluids produced widely conflicting results and failed to reveal any other substances which might account for their solvent powers.[9]

But although the failure to identify chemically the specific components of the gastric juice was a serious problem, the chief source of difficulty over the theory seems to have been the underlying assumptions about digestion prevalent in the early nineteenth century which had changed but little since antiquity. Digestion was considered to be part of the process of 'animalization,' by which crude and heterogeneous food was gradually assimilated into a uniform living substance, namely blood, whose final constituents might bear little relationship to those of the food originally consumed. Within this framework, chymification, or gastric digestion proper, was thought to produce the first degree of animalization, and men tended to think of chyme, like blood, as a more or less specific substance, the identifiable product of chymification.[10] Thus if the gastric juice were to be the main agent in gastric digestion, it would have to possess not only the power of dissolving diverse forms of aliment, but also that of converting them all into the same chymous solution. To say that an apparently insipid fluid, once it had been secreted, could accomplish these marvellous changes independently of the living organism was a claim that was not to be taken lightly. During the second and third decades of the nineteenth century, the experiments of Magendie and of Tiedemann and Gmelin began to dispel the idea that the chyme resulting from different forms of aliment is the

6. Spallanzani (n. 3), pp. 45–56, 86–88, 234, 247, 251–252.
7. *Ibid.*, pp. 56, 217, 234.
8. *Ibid.*, pp. 284–296.
9. For a survey of various analyses of gastric juice, see F. Tiedemann and L. Gmelin, *Die Verdauung nach Versuchen* (Heidelberg and Leipzig, 1826–27), 2 vols., I, 146–150.

10. Bates (n. 4), pp. 342–347, where he discusses these problems with respect to the process of chylification. During the early decades of the nineteenth century, physiologists tended to use the term 'chylification' with reference to the stage of digestion occurring in the intestines, while that in the stomach was called 'chymification.'

same,[11] but the nature of the transformation produced in the stomach remained a mystery.

For some men, such as John Hunter, it was sufficient to point out that the gastric juice had, after all, been secreted by a living animal in the first place and to maintain that its effect on food was totally unlike any other natural process.[12] Hunter said that digestion differs from fermentation in that the latter is only a decomposition, whereas digestion is a form of conversion, of animal and vegetable substances into chyle. It is also unlike chemical solution, 'which is only a union of bodies by elective attraction. But digestion is an assimilating process.... It is a species of generation, two substances [gastric juice and food] making a third [chyle]; but the curious circumstance is its converting both vegetable and animal matter into the same kind of substance or compound, which no chemical process can effect.'[13] Thus Hunter incorporated the gastric juice theory into a fundamentally vitalistic physiological system and, due largely to his influence, the theory became well established in Britain.

With the growth of a more thoroughgoing vitalism in France during the late eighteenth and early nineteenth centuries, however, even the sort of gastric juice theory maintained by Hunter was too 'chemical' for some men, who found it impossible to believe that true digestion could take place without the direct and continuous action of the living stomach. Thus they denied that the product of artificial digestion is really the same as natural chyme formed in the stomach.[14]

In 1812 A. Jenin de Montegre reported to the French Institute a series of experiments which gave considerable support to those who doubted the importance of the gastric juice in digestion.[15] Montegre had set out to test the validity of the gastric juice theory by attempting to duplicate Spallanzani's artificial digestions, but nearly all of his experiments resulted only in putrefaction.[16] A series of comparative experiments seemed to show that gastric juice behaves just like saliva, and Montegre suggested that the so-

11. F. Magendie, *Summary of physiology*, John Revere, tr. (Baltimore, 1822), p. 216; Tiedemann and Gmelin (n. 9), I, 162–208.
12. Bates (n. 4), pp. 345–346; John Hunter, *Observations on certain parts of the animal economy* (Philadelphia, 1840), p. 148.
13. Hunter (n. 12), pp. 135–136.
14. E.g., Anthelme Richerand, *Nouveaux élémens de physiologie*, 2nd ed. (Paris, 1802), 2 vols., I, 44, where he generally accepts Spallanzani's gastric juice theory, but states: 'N'assimilons cependant point complètement cette dissolution des alimens par les sucs retirés de l'estomac, à ce qui se passe dans la digestion stomacale. Tout nous prouve qu'il ne doit point être considéré comme un vase chimique....'
15. A. Jenin de Montegre, *Expériences sur la digestion dans l'homme* (Paris, 1814), 55 pp.
16. *Ibid.*, pp. 16–27.

called gastric juice is really little more than saliva that has been swallowed.[17] His main conclusion was that 'one cannot, in consequence, regard this gastric juice as a solvent *sui generis*, whose particular properties enable it to prevent the putrefaction of animal matters, and even less that it can bring about a true digestion independently of the action of the stomach.'[18] Montegre conjectured that the stomach brings about digestion through 'a vital and elective absorption,' carried out by the vessels of the stomach 'by virtue of their particular sensibility.'[19]

In retrospect it is not difficult to see why Montegre obtained these results which confirmed what was probably a predisposition on his part to distrust the gastric juice theory. For his artificial digestions Spallanzani had obtained gastric juice by having birds swallow dry sponges, which would later be disgorged soaked with juice, or by opening the stomachs of dogs and cats which had previously been made to swallow metal tubes containing food, and the abundance of the fluid which he obtained in these ways convinced him that the gastric juice normally collects in the stomach between meals.[20] To ensure that what he had learned from animals would be applicable to humans, Spallanzani thought it desirable to repeat the artificial digestions using human gastric juice.[21] He found, however, that he could obtain the latter only by inducing vomiting in himself in the morning before eating, something which he did only twice because he found it extremely disagreeable. The amount of fluid obtained in this way was not sufficient to carry his artificial digestions to completion, but he maintained that the fluid did begin to dissolve meat which had been cooked and mashed and also prevented putrefaction. Montegre was able to disgorge the contents of his stomach at will with no unpleasantness, and for his artificial digestions he made use of this ability to obtain the pure gastric juice which according to Spallanzani was supposed to collect in the fasting stomach.[22] Thus he probably got little more than mucus and saliva, and the results of his experiments are not surprising.

Montegre also studied digestion within the stomach by bringing up portions of its contents at various intervals after eating.[23] He found that the gastric contents are always acid when digestion is in progress, which seemed to confirm the idea that the acidity is the result of digestion rather than a pre-existing agent of it. He also found that the contents of the fasting stomach are occasionally acid, which he attributed to the action of the

17. *Ibid.*, pp. 22–27, 42–44.
18. *Ibid.*, pp. 43–44.
19. *Ibid.*, pp. 44–45.
20. Spallanzani (n. 3), pp. 52, 56, 83–88, 217, 232.
21. *Ibid.*, pp. 234–235, 246–250.
22. Montegre (n. 15), pp. 3–4.
23. *Ibid.*, pp. 28–34.

digestive process on swallowed saliva.[24] He admitted that on the rare occasions when this acid is very strong, it will naturally have a solvent effect on food outside the stomach, but he denied that this is the same as true chymification. He maintained that artificially acidified saliva has the same effect on food as the acid contents of the stomach, and suggested that Spallanzani had probably observed the corrosive action of stomach acid in his artificial digestions and drawn the erroneous conclusion that it is the same as true chymification.

In an official report prepared for the Institute, Thenard, Berthollet, and Cuvier concluded: 'The observations of M. de Montegre have the merit of dispelling the false notions which we have received concerning the gastric juice from experiments made by men whose names are most imposing.'[25] In his textbook of physiology, Magendie likewise accepted Montegre's results as showing that the so-called artificial digestions are not the same as true chymification.[26] The extreme vitalists Chaussier and Adelon gloated over Montegre's results,[27] and a follower of Chaussier declared in 1821 that, because of Montegre's work, 'Physiologists who are not alien to the progress of biology today reject [Spallanzani's] gastric juice . . . .'[28] Writing in 1825 Leuret and Laissaigne expressed regret that Montegre's experiments had led to widespread doubts concerning the role of the gastric juice in digestion, despite the apparent decisiveness of Spallanzani's demonstrations.[29]

Many of those who accepted the validity of Montegre's results did not, however, go as far as he did in rejecting the gastric juice theory. Chaussier developed his own highly modified version of the gastric juice theory, the key element of which was that the gastric juice is not a specific chemical substance which collects in the fasting stomach, but is a 'vital solvent' created by the stomach after it has received an impression of the ingested aliment, so that digestion cannot take place without the ability of the stomach to perceive what is necessary in each individual case.[30] Magendie said that Montegre's experiments simply demonstrated the impossibility of duplicating outside the stomach the precise conditions needed for the action of the gastric juice, but he also saw some merit in Chaussier's

24. *Ibid.*, pp. 36–42.
25. *Ibid.*, p. 53.
26. Magendie (n. 11), p. 221.
27. Chaussier and Adelon (n. 5), pp. 422–423.
28. [Anonymous], 'Chymose,' *Dictionaire abrégé des sciences médicales* (Paris, 1821), IV, 282.
29. François Leuret and J. L. Laissaigne, *Recherches physiologiques et chimiques pour servir à l'histoire de la digestion* (Paris, 1825), pp. 118–120.
30. Chaussier and Adelon (n. 5), pp. 416–425.

theory.[31] Broussais also emphasized the mysterious and peculiarly vital character of digestion and favored a modified version of the gastric juice theory in which assimilation is 'produced by the action of the mucous membrane, aided by fluids peculiar to the person in whom the process takes place . . . .'[32]

Montegre's work seems to have had little influence in England, where Hunter's version of the gastric juice theory generally persisted. In 1821 a British reviewer gave a fairly long account of Montegre's experiments, which he then refuted on the basis of Spallanzani's conflicting results.[33] In 1824 C. T. Thackrah reported some experiments on the comparative solvent powers of saliva and gastric juice which confirmed Spallanzani's findings against Montegre's attack.[34] In his textbook of physiology John Bostock likewise adhered to the gastric juice theory, though he repeatedly expressed amazement that apparently inert fluids such as those found in the stomach could have so drastic effect on the food, and he emphasized that the whole process of digestion remained essentially a mystery.[35] He noted that these difficulties had led 'many of the most eminent among the modern physiologists' to attribute digestion to a peculiar vital property of the stomach lining rather than to the gastric juice, but he felt that this idea did nothing to dispel the mystery surrounding the process.

The obscurity which had come to surround the subject of digestion since the time of Hunter and Spallanzani was not just the result of experiments such as Montegre's which conflicted with the earlier findings, but was due in large part to the development of new modes of physiological thought which revealed the inadequacies of the older theories. The whole new field of organic analysis had developed in the late eighteenth and early nineteenth centuries,[36] and the more men learned about organic compounds, the less they felt they knew about the nature of digestion, whatever its cause might be. By 1823 the French Academy decided that the techniques of organic analysis had reached a point where it should be possible to overcome some of the ignorance concerning the chemical changes involved in digestion, and so they announced a prize essay contest on this

31. Magendie (n. 11), pp. 221–222.
32. F. J. V. Broussais, *A treatise of physiology applied to pathology*, John Bell and R. La Roche, trs. (Philadelphia, 1826), pp. 283–286, 296–298, 324.
33. [Anonymous], 'The alimentary function and its disorders' [a review article], *Edinb. med. surg. J.*, 1821, *17*, 582–592.
34. C. T. Thackrah, *Lectures on digestion and diet* (London, 1824), pp. 13–14.
35. John Bostock, *An elementary system of physiology* (Boston, 1828), 3 vols., II, 379–388, 407–417.
36. On these developments, see F. L. Holmes, 'Elementary analysis and the origins of physiological chemistry,' *Isis*, 1963, *54*, 50–81.

subject for the year 1825. The contestants were to analyze the various digestive juices and, using simple food substances such as starch, fat, and gelatine, to try to determine the chemical changes which take place at each stage of digestion.

The entries were two large volumes by a German team, Tiedemann and Gmelin, and a slim little volume by two Frenchmen, Leuret and Laissaigne.[37] Though the original scope of the project far exceeded the limits of analytic methods then available, the Germans nevertheless came up with some important results, such as the discovery that starch is converted to sugar in digestion.[38] The immediate impact of their work was, however, blunted by conflicts between their findings and those of the French team. For example, the results of their respective attempts to analyze the gastric juice differed widely, and they did not even agree over whether the main acid in the stomach is muriatic (as the Germans found) or lactic (as the Frenchmen concluded).[39]

The two teams did, however, concur in some non-chemical observations which helped to discredit Montegre's findings.[40] Both showed that the gastric juice does not collect in the fasting stomach but is secreted only after the stomach lining has been mechanically or chemically stimulated.[41] Both also found that the gastric juice is already acid when it is secreted. Both carried out artificial digestions,[42] though to clinch the matter they should have done more than simply repeat Spallanzani's experiments, since the opponents of the gastric juice theory conceded that the gastric fluids have some solvent powers. As a British reviewer complained, 'the question should have been set at rest by subjecting the food [to artificial digestion] ... and then comparing the chemical changes which take place with those produced in the food [by] ... natural chymification.'[43]

Unknown to this reviewer, William Beaumont, an American army surgeon stationed at Fort Niagara in western New York, was already taking advantage of a gastric fistula in his patient Alexis St. Martin to make observations which were to go a long way toward dispelling the uncer-

37. See notes 9 and 29 above.
38. For an appreciation, see Nikolaus Mani, 'Das Werk von Friedrich Tiedemann und Leopold Gmelin: "Die Verdauung nach Versuchen," und seine Bedeutung für die Entwicklung der Ernährungslehre in der ersten Hälfte des 19. Jahrhunderts,' *Gesnerus*, 1956, *13*, 190–214.
39. Tiedemann and Gmelin (n. 9), I, 150; Leuret and Laissaigne (n. 29), pp. 112–117.
40. Tiedemann and Gmelin mention Montegre only in passing (I, 7, 145–147), while Leuret and Laissaigne were much more concerned with specifically discrediting his results (n. 29), pp. 118–123.
41. Tiedemann and Gmelin (n. 9), pp. 91–145; Leuret and Laissaigne (n. 29), pp. 110–114.
42. Tiedemann and Gmelin (n. 9), pp. 209–211, 306; Leuret and Laissaigne (n. 29), pp. 121–123.
43. [Anonymous], *Edinb. med. surg. J.*, 1827, *28*, 368.

tainties about the gastric juice theory of digestion. Beaumont did not use chemical analyses to test the results of his experiments, but from the very beginning of his work he seems to have realized that the effect of the gastric juice on foods outside the stomach was of crucial importance for understanding digestion. One of the first experiments that he did on St. Martin in August 1825 was to draw gastric juice from the stomach through a tube and observe its ability to dissolve meat out of the stomach.[44] Simultaneously he tied a piece of the same meat to a string and inserted it into the stomach through the fistula, then periodically withdrew it to observe the progress of digestion. He concluded: 'The effect of the gastric fluid upon the piece of meat suspended in the stomach was exactly similar to that in the phial, only more rapid. . . .' Altogether, Beaumont reported over seventy examples of artificial digestion in his *Experiments and Observations*, many of which had the explicit purpose of showing that chymification is essentially the same in and out of the stomach. These were not just the obvious things to do, since twenty years before, in making observations on a patient with a similar gastric fistula, Jacob Helm had studied digestion within the stomach but seems to have seen little need for testing the activities of the gastric fluids outside the stomach.[45]

How did Beaumont know what to look for? By late in 1824 he had recognized the possibilities for experimenting on St. Martin, though at this time he seems to have been concerned only with digestion within the stomach.[46] He perhaps wrote to Surgeon General Lovell, his friend and superior, for advice on what to do, but Lovell was obviously not the source of Beaumont's inspiration, for his suggestion was to try to see whether different kinds of food eaten at the same time will be digested simultaneously or in succession.[47] Lovell did, however, promise to send Beaumont 'some book of experiments on the gastric liquor,' and though it is not known what book he sent (if indeed he did send one), a likely choice would have been *A Physiological Essay on Digestion* by Nathan Ryno Smith, which was published in New York early in 1825.

---

44. William Beaumont, 'Further experiments on the case of Alexis San Martin,' *Med. Recorder*, 1826, 9, 95–96. The account of these experiments, slightly reworded, was included in Beaumont's *Experiments and observations on the gastric juice and the physiology of digestion* (Plattsburgh, 1833), pp. 128–129 (hereafter cited as *Experiments*).

45. Bruno Kisch, 'Jacob Anton Helm and William Beaumont. With a translation of the first of Helm's *Zwei Kranken-Geschichten* (1803),' *J. Hist. Med.*, 1967, 22, 54–80. In his Editorial Addendum to this article, Lloyd G. Stevenson calls attention (p. 80) to Beaumont's particular interest in the gastric juice per se in contrast to Helm.

46. J. S. Myer, *Life and letters of Dr. William Beaumont* (St. Louis, 1939), p. 117.

47. *Ibid.*, pp. 119–120, quoting a letter of 9 Nov. 1824 from Lovell to Beaumont.

Smith, a young professor at Jefferson Medical College in Philadelphia and son of the famous Nathan Smith of Yale, was a strong adherent of the vitalism of Bichat. Smith found the gastric juice theory unacceptable on general principles because it presupposed a similarity between chemical solution and the vital process of digestion.[48] Moreover, he claimed that 'the more recent experiments of Montegre and others, performed with more accuracy and precision . . . , show that these results [i.e., those of Spallanzani et al.] were fallacious.'[49] He also argued that even if the gastric fluids do have some solvent effects on food outside the stomach, no one had shown that these are really the same as chymification which occurs in the stomach. Smith maintained that digestion is accomplished primarily by the direct and peculiarly vital action of the gastric villi on the food.[50]

Reading a challenge to the gastric juice theory such as Smith's might have made Beaumont aware of the central importance of artificial digestion and thus stimulated his investigations in that area. In any case, Beaumont was able to perform only a few experiments before St. Martin 'absconded to Canada.'[51] Not until 1829 did St. Martin rejoin Beaumont, who was now at Fort Crawford in Michigan, and over the next two years he carried out a second long series of experiments, many of them to elucidate further the solvent properties of the gastric juice in artificial digestion.[52] He found that heat is necessary for gastric juice to act on food, and that a certain amount of juice will dissolve only a limited amount of food, after which more juice must be added for the process to continue. He compared the action of the gastric juice with that of vinegar and plain water and confirmed the ability of the juice to coagulate milk and egg white. He found that the gastric juice does not collect in the fasting stomach but is secreted only when the stomach lining is stimulated mechanically or by contact with food.

Late in 1832, having apparently decided that he had exhausted his own resources for devising further experiments, Beaumont went to Washington with St. Martin to consult the literature available there and to seek expert assistance.[53] His notes reveal his diligence in reading about digestion, but, as S. X. Radbill has noted, 'of all the reputable scientists to whom

---

48. N. R. Smith, *A physiological essay on digestion* (New York, 1825), pp. 7–15, 30–40.
49. *Ibid.*, p. 30, also pp. 41–43.
50. *Ibid.*, pp. 46–73.
51. Beaumont, 'Further experiments' (n. 44), p. 97.
52. Beaumont, *Experiments*, pp. 131–169. Most of these additional observations had already been made by earlier investigators.
53. Myer (n. 46), pp. 151–152.

Beaumont applied, only [Robley] Dunglison came to his aid....'[54] Dunglison was the young professor of medicine at the University of Virginia who had come from England in 1825 at the invitation of Thomas Jefferson, the founder of the University.[55] He had recently completed his medical education at Edinburgh, London, and Paris and, though not himself actively engaged in research, he was probably more familiar with the latest developments in physiology than anyone else in the United States.

Though Dunglison eventually rose to prominence in Philadelphia medicine as a professor at Jefferson Medical College, his early reception by the physicians of that city, most notably Nathaniel Chapman, was a hostile one since they regarded him as a foreign intruder on the American medical scene.[56] The subject of digestion became one of the points of friction between Dunglison and the Philadelphians. There had been a long tradition of interest in digestion among the students and faculty of the University of Pennsylvania, some of whom rejected a chemical theory of chymification.[57] Early in the nineteenth century, Professor Benjamin Barton propounded a vitalistic view of digestion,[58] and his successor, Nathaniel Chapman, reserved judgment on the question of the identity of artificial and natural chyme.[59] In 1832 Professor Samuel Jackson published a textbook of physiology and medicine containing yet another vitalistic theory of chymification.[60] Basing his opinion largely on Montegre's experiments, he denied the existence of a specific solvent gastric juice.[61] He knew the work of Tiedemann and Gmelin and conceded that the gastric fluids have some solvent effect on food, but he denied that this effect is the same as true chymification. A reviewer of his book in *The American Journal of the Medical Sciences*, which was published in Philadelphia, concurred with Jackson's reliance on Montegre.[62]

Late in 1832, not long before receiving Beaumont's request for assistance, Dunglison published his own textbook of physiology. In discussing

54. S. X. Radbill, in the Introduction to his edition of 'The autobiographical ana of Robley Dunglison, M.D.,' *Trans. Amer. Phil. Soc.*, 1963, n.s.53, part 8, p. 4.
55. Biographical information from *ibid*.
56. *Ibid.*, p. 25.
57. Bates (n. 4), pp. 342, 356–357.
58. *Ibid.*, p. 357.
59. A. Richerand, *Elements of physiology*, G. J. M. De Lys, tr., with notes by N. Chapman (Philadelphia, 1813), p. 116.
60. Samuel Jackson, *The principles of medicine, founded on the structure and functions of the animal organism* (Philadelphia, 1832), pp. 345–355.
61. However, whereas Montegre concluded that gastric juice is little different from saliva and that neither is important for digestion, Jackson particularly stressed the role of swallowed saliva in chymification.
62. 'E.G.' *Amer. J. med. Sci.*, 1832, *10*, 190.

chymification, he relied chiefly on the work of Tiedemann and Gmelin and of Leuret and Laissaigne, who he felt had adequately confirmed Spallanzani's findings against Montegre's attack.[63] Dunglison held that chymification is the chemical dissolution of food by a specific fluid secreted by the stomach. He acknowledged that the widely varying results of analyses of the gastric juice tended to cast doubt on its existence, but he maintained that if the gastric juice had not yet been isolated, it nevertheless exhibited the constant properties of dissolving food, preventing putrefaction, and curdling milk.[64] Dunglison regarded chyme not as a uniform substance but simply as the variable solution of whatever food had been eaten, and he rejected the need for a special vital power to explain its creation.[65] He did not, however, think that the acidity of the gastric juice alone could account for its solvent powers, and he conjectured, 'organic chemistry may hereafter exhibit to us some chemical agent . . . which is capable of rapidly reducing to chyme all substances—animal and vegetable.'[66]

Dunglison was probably aware that his views on digestion would be unpopular among the Philadelphians, and he may even have known that an attack on them was about to appear in the *American Journal of the Medical Sciences*, and so he was quite pleased to be asked to participate in Beaumont's experiments on St. Martin.[67] The invitation was extended early in January 1833 by Surgeon-General Lovell through Nicholas P. Trist, who was President Jackson's private secretary and a friend of Dunglison's.[68] Dunglison could not come to Washington immediately because of the poor condition of the road at that time of year, and so on 12 January he wrote a long letter containing numerous suggestions for experiments.[69] A week later he decided to brave the elements and proceeded to Washington, where he and Beaumont carried out a number of these experiments.[70]

---

63. Robley Dunglison, *Human physiology* (Philadelphia, 1832), 2 vols., I, 476–500, especially pp. 486–490, 494–497.
64. *Ibid.*, pp. 482, 488–493.
65. *Ibid.*, pp. 482, 494–497.
66. *Ibid.*, p. 497.
67. The tone of the letters exchanged by Dunglison and Beaumont on 6 and 10 Feb. seems to imply that they had already discussed the views of the Philadelphians when they met in January.
68. Dunglison, *Ana*, p. 50.
69. Dunglison included this letter, which was addressed to Lovell, in its entirety in his *Ana*, pp. 50–51, and Beaumont's copy was published by Myer (n. 46), pp. 156–158.
70. Dunglison, *Ana*, p. 54. Dunglison described the experiments which he performed with Beaumont in a letter to Isaac Hays, 5 Feb. 1833, which he subsequently published in his *Elements of hygiene* (Philadelphia, 1835), pp. 216–222 (hereafter cited as *Elements*). This letter is discussed further below. Some of these experiments correspond with ones described by Beaumont for the dates 18–20 Jan. in his *Experiments*, pp. 206–208, although, as we shall see, Beaumont did not report all of the experiments described by Dunglison.

Subsequently he sent Beaumont several letters containing additional suggestions, and Beaumont replied to inform him of some of the results.[71]

Dunglison's first suggestion was to compare the action of gastric juice on food with that of saliva in order to verify the distinctness of the two against Montegre.[72] Beaumont's experiments showed that the two fluids differ notably in their ability to dissolve food and resist putrefaction.[73] Dunglison also had him confirm the ability of gastric juice to correct putrefaction and coagulate milk,[74] and Beaumont demonstrated to him that the gastric juice is secreted only after the stomach lining has been stimulated.[75] Dunglison himself carried out microscopic examinations of gastric juice and of chyme formed from various food substances and did some chemical tests which showed that the acid in the gastric juice is muriatic.[76] He took a sample of gastric juice back to Virginia for a more detailed chemical analysis by himself and his colleague John Emmett.[77]

In addition, Dunglison attempted to learn something about the underlying chemical processes involved in digestion. He himself thought that chymification is a process of chemical dissolution, that is, a reduction to a fluid state of the nutritive elements which does not involve their conversion or reorganization into other substances. Some physiologists thought, for example, that various interconversions involving gelatine, fibrin, and albumen take place in the stomach.[78] To test this idea Dunglison subjected separate portions of fibrin, albumen, and gelatine to the action of the gastric juice, both in and out of the stomach.[79] Then each of the solutions was treated with reagents considered specific for precipitating the original substance. In each case it appeared that the original substance could indeed be recovered, and so Dunglison felt justified in holding that the gastric juice simply dissolves food substances without converting them into something else.

Dunglison seems to have realized, however, that 'solution' is not an un-

---

71. The further correspondence between Dunglison and Beaumont has been published by Myer (n. 46), pp. 159–168, and some excerpts are included in Dunglison's *Ana*, pp. 51–53.

72. Dunglison to Lovell, 12 Jan. (Myer, n. 46, p. 156).

73. Beaumont, *Experiments*, pp. 202–206. These experiments, dated 15–17 Jan., were probably performed before Dunglison's arrival.

74. Dunglison to Lovell, 12 Jan. (Myer, n. 46, p. 157); Dunglison to Hays, 5 Feb. (Dunglison, *Elements*, p. 219); Beaumont, *Experiments*, p. 206.

75. Dunglison to Hays, 5 Feb. (*Elements*, p. 219); Beaumont, *Experiments*, pp. 206–207.

76. Dunglison to Hays, 5 Feb. (*Elements*, pp. 219–222); Beaumont, *Experiments*, pp. 233–234.

77. Dunglison to Hays, 5 Feb. (*Elements*, pp. 221–222).

78. Dunglison (n. 63), I, 483; Dunglison to Lovell, 12 Jan. (Myer, n. 46, p. 158).

79. Dunglison outlined these experiments in his letter to Lovell, 12 Jan. (Myer, n. 46, pp. 157–158), and described the results in his letter to Hays, 6 Feb. (*Elements*, pp. 219–220).

ambiguous concept. In subsequent letters he suggested that Beaumont make comparisons between gastric juice and artificially acidified solutions.[80] In particular he asked Beaumont to dissolve gelatine in both gastric juice and acid and to compare the results by treating them with tan, the reagent used to precipitate gelatine. The precipitates obtained in this way differed considerably,[81] and on being informed of this Dunglison replied that it confirmed his suspicion that the action of the gastric juice was not due simply to its acidity:[82]

In the compound gastric fluid the organic constituents, I have no doubt, modifies [sic] the chemical action in a way that cannot be done by any of our artificial menstrums. Still, your experiments appear to me to tend to the result at which we previously seemed to arrive—that the main gastric action is one of solution, not of chemical conversion.

Dunglison's experiments with acids were probably inspired by those of Tiedemann and Gmelin, but significantly the latter did not make direct comparisons between the acids and the gastric juice, and they tended to think that the acidity of the gastric juice may indeed be largely responsible for its solvent properties.[83]

Dunglison did not regard the nature of the action of the gastric juice as completely settled, however, and suggested to Beaumont a further experiment:[84]

On adding the infusion of galls [tan] to the gastric solution of gelatine, and making a similar experiment with gelatine dissolved simply in water . . . , and weighing the precipitate formed in the two cases, you would be able to see whether as much gelatine remained in the gastric solution as was contained in the aqueous solution, or whether a part might not have experienced conversion.

There is no evidence of Beaumont's having carried out this suggestion. Dunglison's chemical experiments were by no means conclusive, as he himself was undoubtedly aware, but they do suggest that he had sensed a line of research which might have produced significant results had it been pursued.

Shortly after Dunglison returned to the University of Virginia from Washington, the February issue of the *American Journal of the Medical Sci-*

---

80. Dunglison to Beaumont, 29 Jan. and 6 Feb. (Myer, n. 46, pp. 160–161).
81. Beaumont to Dunglison, 10 Feb. and 19 Feb. (Myer, n. 46, pp. 163–165); Beaumont, *Experiments*, pp. 225–226, 227–229, 232, describes such experiments for 3 and 14 Feb. and 27 March.
82. Dunglison to Beaumont, 23 March (Myer, n. 46, p. 167).
83. Tiedemann and Gmelin (n. 9), 1, 330–334.
84. Dunglison to Beaumont, 23 March (Myer, n. 46, p. 167).

ences appeared, containing a review of his *Physiology*.[85] The reviewer treated the book quite favorably except for a vigorous objection to Dunglison's endorsement of the gastric juice theory of chymification.[86] He insisted that there is no conclusive evidence that the fluids of the stomach have a unique ability to chymify food or that the products of artificial digestion are chemically identical with those of natural digestion.

On 5 February Dunglison wrote a long private letter to Dr. Isaac Hays, the editor of the *American Journal*, in which he described the observations which he had made with Beaumont and the results of his chemical analysis of the gastric juice.[87] He avoided any direct reference to the recent review of his book, but he undoubtedly had it in mind when he stated:[88]

> I cannot help feeling gratified, that the results of this case should harmonize so well with the deductions, drawn from less evidence in my 'Physiology,' on many points connected with digestion,—a circumstance, which had impressed Dr. Beaumont, before I had the pleasure of being introduced to him.

Dunglison particularly emphasized that the gastric juice obtained from St. Martin had specific and well-defined chemical and physiological properties. He also described the experiments with gelatine, fibrin, and albumen, but he now drew an additional conclusion from them. In each case the original substance had been subjected to both artificial and natural digestion, and the resulting solutions were affected in the same way by chemical reagents regardless of whether they had been formed in or out of the stomach. Thus Dunglison now felt that these experiments, aside from their original purpose of showing that digestion is a process of solution, provided the evidence for the chemical identity of the products of artificial and natural digestion which the opponents of the gastric juice theory had so long demanded.

The following day Dunglison wrote to Beaumont and called his attention to the review of his *Physiology* in the *American Journal*:[89]

> ... the writer accords with Dr. Jackson and others on the subject of stomachal digestion. There is a systematic obstinacy occasionally amongst Physiologists which requires time as well as evidence for its downfall, and one of the first things to be learned is to disinfect the mind of all bias, which is extremely difficult.

85. 'F.' *Amer. J. med. Sci.*, 1833, *11*, 429–449.
86. *Ibid.*, pp. 433–436.
87. Referred to above in note 70.
88. Dunglison to Hays, 5 Feb. (*Elements*, p. 222).
89. Dunglison to Beaumont, 6 Feb. (Myer, n. 46, p. 161).

Samuel Jackson was not actually mentioned in the review. In his reply of 10 February Beaumont commented on the review with characteristic vigor:[90]

> ... though the suggestions advanced by you on that subject [gastric digestion] need nothing but their own correctness to support them, yet I think with your assistance we shall be able to afford the weapons not only to pary their criticisms, but to make them recoil with severity, if you choose, upon the authors themselves, rendering them effectually disinfecting agents of the systematic obstinacy of their selfish minds and Pseudo Physiological Theories on this subject. That ... the Philadelphia Physiologists, as some others, on the subject of Stomach digestion and the gastric juice are radically wrong, I have not the least doubt, but demonstrated and multiplied facts and experiments to prove, ...

The idea that Beaumont's work would confirm Dunglison's views against such attacks was a recurrent theme in the correspondence between the two men, and it appears that Dunglison's book was, indeed, one of the principal sources for the theoretical discussions of digestion in Beaumont's *Experiments and Observations*.[91]

Dunglison clearly hoped to oversee the publication of Beaumont's work, probably in order to ensure that his findings were presented in the best light.[92] Beaumont, however, seems to have realized that as an unknown he only stood to lose by having the name of a prominent authority associated with his investigations. For a time he seems to have considered allowing Dunglison to arrange for publication, but he informed him quite bluntly that he did not want to share the credit for the work.[93] Dunglison readily acceded to his wishes, though he did expect that Beaumont would include their joint experiments in his publication and acknowledge them as such.[94] Whatever agreement they may have arrived at apparently came unstuck, however, for in March 1833 a notice appeared in a Washington newspaper saying that a previous notice, which mentioned Dunglison's involvement in Beaumont's planned publication, carried 'folly on its front.'[95] The ad was signed by S. Beaumont, and we can only surmise that William's cousin Samuel persuaded him to come home to Plattsburgh to publish the *Experiments and Observations* entirely on his own.

90. Beaumont to Dunglison, 10 Feb. (Myer, n. 46, pp. 162–163).
91. See especially Beaumont, *Experiments*, p. 76.
92. The question of publication is discussed in virtually all the letters referred to above.
93. Beaumont to Dunglison, 25 Jan. (Myer, n. 46, p. 159).
94. Dunglison to Beaumont, 29 Jan. and 6 Feb. (Myer, n. 46, pp. 160–161).
95. *Washington Intelligencer*, 11 March 1833; referred to by Radbill (n. 54), p. 52, note 12, where he also includes additional details.

When Beaumont's book appeared, Dunglison felt that he had been slighted, as he related in his *Autobiographical Ana*:[96]

It might have been anticipated, however, from Dr. Beaumont's sensitiveness as to his own rights, that he would have been extremely liberal as regarded those of others, and especially of one, of whose services he speaks so highly in the letters referred to above; and with such anticipations I confess, I was surprised, on the appearance of his *Experiments*, to find no allusion whatever to my having visited Washington, by request, in a Virginia winter from a distance of upwards of 100 miles; or to my having made a single suggestion to him, or been associated, in any manner, with his investigations.

Beaumont did include a general expression of gratitude to Dunglison (along with several other men), and quoted his and Emmett's chemical analysis of the gastric juice,[97] but, as Dunglison went on to note in his *Ana*, the only indication of his direct participation in Beaumont's work was a reference to his 'presence' at the microscopic examination of the gastric juice.[98] Moreover, according to Dunglison, he had not just been present for these observations, but the results reported by Beaumont 'were absolutely dictated by me.' Most of the experiments which he had suggested to Beaumont, including those comparing gastric juice with acids, were described with no indication of their source. But what probably annoyed Dunglison the most was that Beaumont did not include the experiments on gelatine, albumen, and fibrin, the ones which Dunglison himself considered so important for establishing the nature of digestion and the chemical identity of artificial and natural chyme.[99]

Beaumont did, however, oblige Dunglison to the extent of consistently supporting the idea that the gastric juice is essentially a chemical solvent and denouncing Montegre, Nathan R. Smith, and Samuel Jackson for having denied the gastric juice theory of digestion.[100] Not surprisingly, in a review of the *Experiments and Observations* in the *American Journal*, yet another of the 'Philadelphia Physiologists' criticized Beaumont for this attack upon 'several of the most cautious and laborious investigators

---

96. Dunglison, *Ana*, p. 52.
97. Beaumont, *Experiments*, pp. 7, 78–79. In addition, Beaumont paid several compliments of a general nature to Dunglison and his *Human physiology*.
98. Dunglison, *Ana*, p. 52, in reference to Beaumont, *Experiments*, p. 233.
99. Beaumont, *Experiments*, pp. 207–208, does describe one experiment involving gelatine for 20 Jan., but it bears only a vague resemblance to the ones described by Dunglison. There is little doubt that the latter were actually performed, since Dunglison referred to them in his subsequent letters to Beaumont.
100. Beaumont, *Experiments*, pp. 97–101.

among the physiologists of this country and Europe.'[101] The reviewer, D. Francis Condie, allowed that Beaumont's work was very interesting, but said that he had not, as he claimed, established the gastric juice theory beyond question because he had produced no evidence that the solution produced by artificial digestion is identical with true chyme. Dunglison must have read this review with mixed feelings, since he and Beaumont had found such evidence, but Beaumont had chosen not to publish it. He might also have taken some satisfaction from the reviewer's complimenting Beaumont for comparing the gastric juice with acids and wondering why this technique had not occurred to him earlier in his work.[102]

Beaumont may have been lacking somewhat in discretion, but he demonstrated thrift and modesty in abundance in a subsequent encounter, described by Dunglison:[103]

Soon after the appearance of his book I saw Dr. Beaumont in Baltimore. As he did not present to me a copy, I offered him payment, which, I think, was *Three Dollars*. He said he thought, under all the circumstances, I *ought* to have a copy gratuitously; but took the money. I did not conceal from him my expectation of seeing in it a more detailed account of our joint labors, and reminded him, that the only allusion to my being concerned in the matter [was the reference to my presence at the microscopic examination] . . .; when he replied, that he did not think I would care to be associated with so humble an individual as himself!

The bounds of Beaumont's impertinence and Dunglison's patience had not yet been reached, however, for in 1834 Beaumont asked Dunglison to write a testimonial on the value of his work to be used to obtain reimbursement from Congress, and Dunglison generously did so, though he doubted the propriety of the request.[104]

In spite of his pique, Dunglison subsequently praised Beaumont's work in print on several occasions and probably recognized that the most important observations made on St. Martin resulted from the relatively unsophisticated experiments conceived of by Beaumont himself. Another

---

101. D. F. C. [D. Francis Condie] Review of *Experiments*, *Amer. J. med. Sci.*, 1834, *14*, 117–149 (p. 118). Montegre and Jackson are cited repeatedly throughout this review.

102. *Ibid.*, pp. 130–132. For a time this rather unenthusiastic review must have been one of the major sources of information about Beaumont's work in Britain since it was reprinted in two British journals in 1834 and 1836, as is reported by George Rosen, 'Notes on the reception and influence of William Beaumont's discovery,' *Bull. Hist. Med.*, 1943, *13*, 632, 635.

103. Dunglison, *Ana*, p. 52.

104. *Ibid.*, p. 53; Myer (n. 46), p. 216. This was not the end of the matter, however, for as Dunglison relates in his *Ana* (p. 53), George Combe, the English phrenologist, in 1841 published a book in which he erroneously quoted Dunglison as having said that he had suggested all of the experiments which Beaumont performed at Washington, and Dunglison felt compelled to publish a disclaimer.

index of the value of Beaumont's work was the attention which Johannes Müller paid to it in his *Handbuch der Physiologie*, published in 1834.[105] Earlier the same year, C. H. Schultz had published yet another long and detailed attack on the gastric juice theory.[106] Müller took Schultz's objections to the theory quite seriously, but he felt that they had been answered conclusively by Beaumont's observations. No one, said Müller, had hitherto examined the gastric juice in such large quantity, in so pure a state, and so frequently, as had Dr. Beaumont, who had thereby provided indisputably affirmative answers to the two fundamental questions of whether the gastric juice really exists and whether it can dissolve food in and out of the stomach. These were simple and repetitive observations which Beaumont had made, but they were just what was needed to confirm the existence of a fluid that had proven so elusive in the half century since the time of Spallanzani. Had Beaumont's work not been channeled by the American version of the gastric juice controversy, had he not been incensed by the Philadelphia Physiologists and encouraged by Dunglison, he might not have made the observations that proved to be of such interest to European physiologists.

Nevertheless, Dunglison's specific suggestions to Beaumont were not without importance. Müller also posed a third fundamental question about the gastric juice, namely, whether its solvent properties were due to its acidity or to other unknown substances.[107] First he reported the results of Tiedemann and Gmelin's experiments with acids on food substances, which did not involve direct comparisons between acids and gastric juice and which led them to think that the solvent powers of the gastric juice might be due to its acidity. At Dunglison's request, Beaumont had made direct comparisons between gastric juice and acids, and tested the results with chemical reagents. In reporting the results of these experiments Beaumont seems to have echoed Dunglison's letter when he commented that the gastric juice probably contains 'some principles inappreciable to the senses, or to chemical tests,' which might account for the clear differences between the effects of the two fluids on food.[108] Müller reported the results of Beaumont's comparative experiments in great detail, and these,

---

105. Johannes Müller, *Handbuch der Physiologie des Menschen* (Coblenz, 1834), I, 496–497, 510–526. On the publication of Beaumont's work in Germany and the reaction to it there, see George Rosen, *The reception of William Beaumont's discovery in Europe* (New York, 1942), pp. 26–41, especially pp. 33–38 on Müller.
106. C. H. Schultz, *De alimentorum concoctione experimenta nova* (Berlin, 1834).
107. Müller (n. 105), pp. 526–534; discussed by Rosen (n. 105), pp. 37–38.
108. Beaumont, *Experiments*, p. 228.

together with some additional experiments of his own, convinced him that Tiedemann and Gmelin were wrong, and that the solvent powers of the gastric juice must be due to some unknown principle. Theodor Schwann likewise credited Beaumont with having demonstrated that the solvent power of the gastric juice is not due to its acidity alone,[109] and it seems possible that these experiments, which Dunglison had suggested to Beaumont, may have had some influence on Müller and Schwann's subsequent discovery of pepsin.

Department of the History of Science and Medicine
Yale University
New Haven, Connecticut

---

109. Th. Schwann, 'Ueber das Wesen der Verdauungsprozesses,' *Müller's Arch.*, 1836, p. 93; referred to by Rosen (n. 105), pp. 39-40.

American Attitudes Toward the Germ Theory of Disease (1860-1880)

PHYLLIS ALLEN RICHMOND*

IN the development of the germ theory of disease, the decades of greatest activity in Europe—about 1850 to 1880—coincided with a period of minimum activity in the United States. A glance at the etiological sections in American books and journals of these decades shows that the old miasmatic and atmospheric theories were still of paramount importance. The familiar explanations recur with monotonous regularity, involving miasmata, epidemic constitution, ozone, poisonous gases, and similar items.[1]

The miasma concept was now related to the notion of filth as an aid in transmission. The third and fourth National Quarantine and Sanitary Conventions, held in 1859 and 1860, gave physicians an opportunity to discuss matters relating to causation and contagion, and the views presented at these meetings show a complete absence of anything resembling an animalcular hypothesis. Each convention had a committee investigating "the nature and sources of miasmata," which faithfully turned in reports attributing fevers to decaying vegetation, to an invisible but detectable (method unstated) "malaria" or miasma, and to the presence of offensive effluvia from slaughterhouses, swamps, cesspools, and sewers—mostly the old factors previously enumerated by Benjamin Rush and other eighteenth century authors.[2] These views were only slightly modified during the following decades.

The prevailing opinions were well displayed in the vast literature on cholera. A rather typical view in 1866 was that of a writer in the *American Journal of the Medical Sciences*. In a general review of work on cholera, "D.F.C." (possibly D. Francis Condie of Philadelphia) noted two current theories:

> The opinion that cholera is propagatable through the medium of a specific poison contained in the dejections of patients labouring under the disease, is one entertained by a large number of writers on cholera, and many very imposing facts have been adduced in support of its correctness. By a

---

* Rochester, New York.
[1] Cf. Allen, Phyllis. Etiological theory in America prior to the Civil War. *J. Hist. Med.*, 1947, 2, 492-98.
[2] *Proceedings and debates of the third national quarantine and sanitary convention.* . . . New York, 1859, pp. 226-27, *passim; Proceedings and debates of the fourth national quarantine and sanitary convention.* . . . Boston, 1860, pp. 6-8, 21-27.

few, however, it is maintained that the recent discharges from cholera patients are not infectious, but become so only after they have undergone decomposition.[3]

These two views will be recognized as those of the British epidemiologist, John Snow, and the Bavarian, Max von Pettenkofer. The cholera hypothesis of Pettenkofer appears to have made quite an impression in America. His work was cited in many of the cholera tracts, and one of his articles appeared in *Public Health* in 1873. Our reviewer, on the other hand, did not take much stock in either of the theories mentioned. He much preferred the view that cholera was a contagious disease, propagated by infected persons or their goods (fomites). The contagious material given off by the patients acted as a ferment in corrupting the atmosphere, particularly if the latter was in an "impure and stagnant state," and turned it into a carrier of the "morbific poison."[4] Such an idea was merely a repetition of an older atmospheric hypothesis. Also it indicates that the quarrel between the contagionists and the anti-contagionists was still going on. This long-term argument could not be settled until the specific causal factors in disease had been discovered.

There was, then, a general acceptance of the same old theories although these were somewhat modified by the newer ideas of Snow, Pettenkofer, or the King's College microscopist, Lionel S. Beale. The modifications appear in the etiologic section of the official report of the House of Representatives. *The Cholera Epidemic of 1873 in the United States,* published in 1875. In this report, a more or less chemical explanation seems to have been intended. The cause of cholera was listed as a specific organic poison, transmitted by the ejections of a person suffering from the disease (Snow's view). This poison went through a period of incubation outside the body in an alkaline environment "needed for renewing activity of the poison" (altered Pettenkofer). Its period of "morbific activity" was characterized by the presence of bacteria, though these were not specific (Beale's concept).[5] This etiological con-

---

[3] D.F.C. Review: Cholera, its pathology and treatment. *Amer. J. med. Sci.*, 1866, n.s. 52, 186.

[4] Pettenkofer, Max von. What we can do against cholera. *Public health: reports and papers 1873*. New York, 1875, pp. 317-35. For examples of the influence of Pettenkofer, see The etiology of typhoid fever. *Bost. med. surg. J.* 1872, 86, 58-60; Brockett, L. P. *Asiatic cholera*, Hartford, Conn., 1866, p. 61; Collins, G. T. *The cholera, a familiar treatise on its history, causes, symptoms and treatment, with the most effective remedies.* New York and Cincinnati, 1866, pp. 50-63; Ely, W. S. *An essay on Asiatic cholera*, Rochester, N. Y., 1872, p. 10; Pancoast, Seth. *The cholera. Its history, cause, symptoms and treatment.* Philadelphia, 1873, pp. 11-18; D.F.C., *op. cit.*, 187.

[5] *The cholera epidemic of 1873 in the United States.* House of Representatives, 43d Congress, 2d session, Ex. Doc. no. 95. Washington, 1875, p. 8.

glomeration was probably as complete a synthesis as one could make without drawing on the germ or zymotic theories.

The atmospheric, chemical, and miasmatic theories so dominated etiological thought in the 1870's that when alternative views arose, as in the instance of a book review of James Ross's *Graft Theory of Disease,* American reviewers were cautious and noncommittal. A wait-and-see policy seems to have been almost universal. The case of Austin Flint, a New York physician noted for his work on diseases of the chest, is an interesting example. Flint was the author of a text, *Principles and Practice of Medicine,* long standard for medical students. As a young man he had reported on a typhoid epidemic near Buffalo in such a manner as to secure the attention of John Snow. In fact, Snow used Flint's report to illustrate the transmission of the disease through contaminated water. Flint himself accepted neither Snow's zymotic explanation nor the germ theory. He thought that water might contain an exciting agent of the disease, but not the specific cause. Yet in 1874, a friend believed that Flint was "strongly disposed to accept" an animalcular view.[6] In 1876, however, he published a popular article on medical and sanitary progress in *Harper's Magazine,* in which he dealt with the germ theory in the following terms:

> It is, indeed, claimed by some that the causation of certain diseases by specific organisms of microscopical minuteness has been demonstrated; by the majority of medical thinkers, however, the demonstrative evidence is not considered as complete.[7]

The germ theory was not introduced into Flint's textbook until the fifth edition (1881), and then it was suggested merely for relapsing fever and anthrax. Thus, following the conservative American attitude, he included the theory only when the demonstrative evidence was complete.

There was, of course, good reason to be cautious in accepting the germ theory. The original theory left much to be desired. It was difficult to understand and even more difficult to prove. Techniques had to be unbelievably exact. There was much in the theory that had to be developed and refined or discarded. It had different

---

[6] Hartshorne, Henry. *Amer. J. med. Sci.,* 1873, n.s. 65, 514-17; Flint, Austin. *Clinical reports on continued fever.* Buffalo, 1852; Relations of water to the propagation of fever, *Public health: reports and papers 1873,* 166-67, 172; Hurd, E. P. The germ theory of disease. *Bost. med. surg. J.,* 1874, *91,* 103. Footnote in this article refers to "Textbook of Practical Medicine, II, 621." This must have been the 1873 edition of the *Treatise on the principles and practice of medicine,* though specificity in etiology is mentioned rather than an actual animalcular viewpoint (4th ed., 105).

[7] Flint, Austin. Medical and sanitary progress. *Harper's Magazine.* 1876, *53,* no. 313, 70-84. Actually the demonstrative evidence was completed in 1876-77 by Pasteur and Koch.

applications to different kinds of diseases, but in the beginning this was not realized because so many maladies yielded their secrets at the first bacteriological onslaught. On the other hand, the problems of the germ theory should not have been beyond the intellectual capacity of a society that could produce a Josiah Willard Gibbs. The chief complaint against the American medical profession in this period (1860 to 1880) is the lack of any attempt at experimental work to prove or disprove the theory. This seems to have fitted the general cultural pattern of that age in science, apparently due partly to the lack of university educational facilities, partly to the pre-eminence of divinity and law as the favored professions for the intelligensia, and partly to the emphasis on applied science over pure science.[8]

Some Americans had been animalculists as students, but then turned away from the theory. Horatio C. Wood, Professor of Botany at the University of Pennsylvania, had such an experience, and his remarks about it give some clue to the reason for deserting the contagium vivum camp:

> In conclusion, perhaps it is allowable to state that some two or three years since the writer of this paper was very strongly inclined to believe in the doctrine of animate contagion, having imbibed it during his student life, and that this essay has not been the result solely of studies especially undertaken for the purpose; but that during the prosecution of other microscopic investigations, the evidence so gathered itself in his mind as to lead him into this by-path, and to leave him no doubt that general diseases are not caused by organic entities. There is a vast accumulation of negative evidence which repudiates the doctrine of animate contagion, either as taught by Linnaeus or by more recent authorities. There are no known facts establishing the doctrine; there are many such which strongly support the negative proposition.[9]

The use of microscopic investigations is interesting because in this case the very instrument that should have aided in proving the germ theory turned Wood against it. One is forcibly reminded that perfection in technique was urgently needed before any success could be obtained in establishing the germ theory.

---

[8] The author is at present compiling a bibliography of American pure research in nineteenth century science in an attempt to ascertain whether this view is justified. So far, a large amount of material has been found in the fields of geology and astronomy, but in the other sciences the yield has been meagre. Theoretical research contributions in geology and astronomy seem to have been incidental to and dependent upon the emphasis on these disciplines as applied sciences. Further work is expected to clarify this tentative conclusion.

[9] Wood, H. C. Examination into the truth of the asserted production of general disease by organized entities. *Amer. J. med. Sci.*, 1868, n.s. 56, 352. At the University of Pennsylvania Wood was Professor of Botany, 1866-76, Professor of Materia Medica, Pharmacy and Therapeutics 1876-1906, Professor of Nervous Diseases 1875-1902, occupying, as Oliver Wendell Holmes put it, "not a chair but a settee."

Wood's conclusion was reiterated as late as 1880 in a study on fever.[10] He admitted that there was a definite poison in cases of fever, "sometimes having formed in the system, sometimes having entered the organism from without." The latter idea was not pursued further, though possibly he might have been hinting at the zymotic hypothesis.

The fact that Americans of good repute professionally, such as Wood and Flint, dropped or failed to accept the germ theory does not mean that the hypothesis was totally lost in America before 1875. It is true that it was not adopted to any great extent. A few men, however, still fostered the concept and one new contribution was added by James Henry Salisbury of Cleveland, also known for his dietary contribution, the Salisbury steak. Salisbury's studies on fungi, which he believed caused various diseases, were probably the only original American papers utilizing the animalcular hypothesis to appear in the 1860-1875 period.

Salisbury began his experiments early in the 1860's and his first paper, on inoculation of measles by means of a straw fungus, appeared in 1862. Several other articles followed, notably the work on the spore of the *palmella* plant as a supposed cause of malaria. In 1868 he published a little volume on microscopic examinations of the blood, in which he presented his views on the various forms of fungi which he thought he had found in the blood in cases of smallpox, cowpox, typhoid, intermittent fever, and the remittent fevers. The form of his argument was logical enough, and his illustrations were interesting. As late as 1883, he put out a pamphlet on his opinions, but by this time they were a little outdated.[11] Of all this work, perhaps that on the *palmella* plant was the most typical.

In the malarious districts along the Ohio and Mississippi Rivers, Salisbury found algae or cryptogamous plants called *palmellae*

---

[10] Wood, H. C. *Fever: a study in morbid and normal physiology.* Smithsonian contributions to knowledge. Washington, 1881, vol. 23, pp. 254-55.

[11] Salisbury, J. H. Remarks on fungi, with an account of experiments showing the influence of the fungi of wheat straw on the human system: and some observations which point to them as the probable source of 'camp measles' and perhaps of measles generally. *Amer. J. med. Sci.,* 1862, n.s. *44,* 17-28; On the cause of intermittent and remittent fevers, with investigations which tend to prove that these affections are caused by certain species of palmellae. *Amer. J. med. Sci.,* 1866, n.s. *51,* 51-68; Description of two new algoid vegetations, one of which appears to be the specific cause of syphilis, and the other of gonorrhoea. *Amer. J. med. Sci.,* 1868, n.s. *55,* 17-25; On the parasitic forms developed in parent epitheliel cells of the urinary and genital organs and their secretions. *Amer. J. med. Sci.,* 1868, n.s. *55,* 371-80; *Microscopic examinations of the blood, and vegetations found in variola, vaccina and typhoid fever.* New York, 1868; Original investigations in diphtheria and scarlet fever, showing their kinship and cause to be the mucor malignans (a fungus in the exudations, blood, urine, and sputa), cured by quinine topically administered in powder, on the tongue and by inhalation. *Gaillard's med. J.,* 1882, *33,* 401-24. Also published in pamphlet form, New York, 1882, 1883, Detroit, 1883.

whose spores were easily discovered in the nearby air. Since these plants were always found in the ague lands, Salisbury came to the conclusion that if he could prove that malarial fevers always occurred after exposure to the spores of the *palmella,* and conversely, if there were no fevers where there were no *palmellae,* then he might have the solution to the malaria puzzle. He therefore made a series of experiments to attempt a proof of his hypothesis. He suspended material in the night air of malarious places and recovered the cells of the *palmella.* He found similar cells in the urine of patients suffering from malaria. To connect the two sets of observations, he tried a more drastic form of experimentation. This consisted in leaving boxes of *palmellae*-infested soil in the sleeping rooms of volunteers (on the window sills with the windows partially open) and these men subsequently caught malaria.[12] We can see, of course, that mosquitoes came in the open windows and bit them, but to Salisbury, whose experimental technique was not fine enough to control all possibilities, the result was adequate proof of his theory. An accidental example encouraged him. He left a box of soil in the office of another doctor by mistake and the doctor was taken ill with malaria. Salisbury used the microscope to search for his cryptogams, though he found the wrong type of organisms for his disease.

Encouraged by the reception given his research, especially in Europe, Salisbury carried his idea over to the etiology of other diseases, but his work was indecisive and not much came of it. As it was, after initial acceptance, his experimental evidence was refuted by others who found the *palmella* in localities where there was no malaria, showing it to be widely spread in nature. One of the most effective refutations was that of Horatio C. Wood, who opposed the cryptogamous theory in general and Salisbury in particular. He cited the work of Joseph Leidy in connection with J. K. Mitchell's hypothesis. Wood himself swallowed the *palmellae* without ill effects, and he used the microscope but could not find any of the cells in question. He was particularly disgusted with Salisbury's contention that he had found the fungi of syphilis and gonorrhea—pointing out that "of all the known diseases, the one, the natural history of which is most irreconcilable with the idea of a fungus as the cause is syphilis. Why is contact necessary for its passage from one individual to the other if spores or fungi be the cause?" Wood's objections were repeated by others, one of whom noted that Salisbury had failed to find *palmellae* in the blood of ague patients—"a

---

[12] Salisbury, On the cause of intermittent and remittent fevers (note 11).

great lacuna in his theory." By 1872, the theory was termed unreliable."[13]

The case of Salisbury illustrates another difficulty in securing the acceptance of the germ theory. Fungi are now known to cause serious illnesses so that he was correct in associating fungi with disease. No fungi, however, are involved in the disease with which he was concerned. In so many instances, the animalculists had the correct idea but the wrong disease. This, perhaps as much as anything, discredited the germ theory. Pasteur and Koch finally were successful when they applied the theory to a relatively obscure disease, anthrax. In addition, the bacillus of this disease is a relatively large one and comparatively easy to cultivate. Problems involving the more common diseases, intermittent, remittent and continued fevers, typhus, and consumption were much harder to solve. Each of these has turned out to be, bacteriologically speaking, a whole collection of diseases, and the bacteriological differentiation, as in the case of pathological anatomy earlier, forced clinical differentiation. A similar situation apparently exists today in the present struggle to discover the causes of cancer.

Salisbury appears to have been the only American to have attempted serious experimental work in connection with the animalcular hypothesis in the period immediately following the Civil War. Most others did only what was necessary (in their own minds) to disprove his conclusions. No school of experimentalists followed him or was inspired by him. The stagnant situation in America continued.

One would have expected the learned journals to have picked up European developments and to have reported them widely, but this was not done. Little attention was paid to European bacteriology during the 1870's. The American journals of 1872, to take a sample year, were characterized by a primary concern with medical affairs in the United States. Foreign intelligence was reported, especially in the *American Journal of the Medical Sciences,* but this was taken in the form of abstracts of books or articles in foreign journals, or as letters from American students abroad. As a rule, there were no foreign contributors or reproductions from foreign work *in toto.* When Americans mentioned foreign work on the

[13] Hirsch, August. *Handbook of geographical and historical pathology.* Tr. Charles Creighton. London, 1883, pp. 289, 291; Proust, A. *Traité d'hygiène publique et privée.* Paris, 1877, p. 728. See also *Canada Lancet,* 1872, *4,* 433-34. Wood. *loc. cit.* (note 9), 333-52. See also W, H. Harkness' Salisbury's ague theory. *Bost. med. surg. J.,* 1879, n.s. 2, (whole vol. 79) 369-75. Leidy, Joseph. *The flora and fauna within living animals.* Smithsonian contributions to knowledge. Washington, 1853, vol. 5, pp. 14-15; Hurd, *loc. cit.* (note 6), 104.

germ theory, a rare occurrence, they often chose to accept the arguments of those opposed to it—Beale, Pettenkofer, and others. The only mention of John Tyndall, in any of the four chief journals examined in detail, related to his visit to the United States, rather than to the particulars of his research.[14]

A few exceptions to this general situation may be found. The second *Annual Report* of the Massachusetts State Board of Health had come out in 1871, and in it anthrax was discussed. The views expressed are interesting:

... it must be acknowledged that there are very strong grounds for inferring that the virus of charbon, like that of vaccine lymph and cowpox, consists of minute matter of unknown origin, which, under certain conditions, instead of undergoing chemical decomposition, is capable of preserving its activity outside the body and of being transferred as solid particles from place to place; but, having been introduced into the blood, becomes developed and multiplied, and thus causes the characteristic symptoms.

This hypothesis, if accepted, is sufficient to enable us to explain how the disease may be communicated, and how, by the aid of certain chemical compounds, contagious matter may be neutralized or destroyed.[15]

Such an advanced outlook was very rare in American medical literature.

Four others added their contributions in the next few years. Christian W. Rauschenberg wrote an article in the *Atlanta Medical and Surgical Journal* for September 1872, on "Microscopic organisms as instigators of disease," which was cautious but favorable towards the germ theory. The article was written "with a desire to consolidate into a palatable form the most important general facts" known at the time, and it certainly achieved its purpose. In the following year, George M. Sternberg, later Surgeon-General, published an article on yellow fever in the *American Journal of the Medical Sciences,* advocating the germ theory in no uncertain terms, but *without mentioning any European work.* This seems odd in view of the wealth of support he could have drawn from this source. The 1873 *Annual Report* of the Smithsonian Institution also contained a favorable description of the germ theory, written by John Dalton, a New York physiologist, and in 1874 a

---

[14] *Amer. J. med. Sci., n.s. 64,* Quarterly summary of the improvements and discoveries in the medical sciences; *Bost. med. surg. J., 86, 87,* Foreign correspondence, Progress in medicine; *Chicago med. J., 29,* Selections. The *Trans. Amer. med. Ass.* for 1872 had nothing about foreign work in it. Tyndall's visit was reported in the *Bost. med. surg. J., 86,* 208. Reports and articles on germs can be found in the *Canada med. J., 8,* 65, 336, and the *Canada Lancet, 4,* 42-43, 554-55, both issued in 1872.

[15] *Second annual report of the State Board of Health of Massachusetts.* Public Doc. no. 37. Boston, 1871, pp. 96-97. In 1874, fungi and ferments were suggested as possible causes of cerebrospinal meningitis in the *Second annual report of the Secretary of the State Board of Health of the State of Michigan for the fiscal year ending Sept. 30th, 1874.* Lansing, 1874, pp. 140-42.

cautious article on the germ theory by E. P. Hurd appeared in the
Boston Medical and Surgical Journal. All these writers, cautious
or otherwise, were extremely courageous even in attempting to
espouse so unpopular a cause.[16]

Throughout the nineteenth century, the few Americans who
accepted the germ theory in one form or another believed in some
sort of animalcular or fungus hypothesis. The zymotic theory was
rarely mentioned, though infectious diseases were often termed
"zymotic diseases." Francis Peyre Porcher of Charleston was an exception to this rule. His book, *Illustrations of Disease with the
Microscope*, appeared in 1861. In the text, he stated that "scarlet
fever, measles, small-pox, are each *sui generis*, are disseminated by
exposure to special morbid poisons, working in the blood in the
nature of a ferment, and which are peculiar in their nature."[17]
Porcher's view is apparently the only American one, with the possible exception of Salisbury, showing acceptance of the doctrine of
causal specificity, and his ferment idea is similar to Farr's early
description of the zymotic theory of disease.

A contemporary of Porcher, E. P. Christian of Boston, wrote of
a theory which he called "zymotic," but which lacked the doctrine
of specificity. This use of the word "zymotic" again illustrates the
confusion still existing in medical terminology. The idea of one
specific "zyme" for each disease entity was not understood at all by
Christian. His view was that "zymosis" was to typhoid, scarlet fever,
erysipelas, diphtheria, and measles what "paludal malaria" was to
intermittent, remittent, and continued fevers. In other words, a
poison of one species (zymosis, malaria) could give rise to a number
of different diseases. Thus the causes of all infectious diseases could
be reduced to two or three basic poisons. Yet the genuine zymotic
theory (involving the concept of a specific causal factor for each
disease) was available in the British and especially in the French
literature of the mid-seventies, if Americans had cared to read it.[18]

At a time when a real science of bacteriology was being developed in Europe, American etiology was virtually in the same

---

[16] Rauschenberg, C. W. Miscroscopic organisms as instigators of disease. *Atlanta med. surg. J.*, 1872, *10*, no. 6, 358-59; Sternberg, G. M. An inquiry into the nature of the yellow fever poison with an account of the disease as it occurred at Governor's Island, New York harbor. *Amer. J. med. Sci.*, 1873, *65*, 398-406; Dalton, John. Origin and propagation of disease. *Ann. Rep. Smithsonian Inst.* [for 1873] Washington, 1874, pp. 226-45; Hurd, E. P. Germ theory. *Bost. med. surg. J.*, 1874, *41*, 97-110.

[17] Porcher, Francis Peyre. *Illustrations of disease with the microscope*. Charleston, S. C., 1861, p. 79.

[18] Christian, E. P. On the epidemic relationship of zymotic diseases. *Amer. J. med. Sci.*, 1862, *44*, 91-95; *Index-catalogue of the Library of the Surgeon-General's office*. Washington, 1888, 1st ser., vol. IX, pp. 259-60.

position it had been in for most of the century. A few animalculists can be found for the 1860 to 1875 period, but comparison of the research of Salisbury, for example, with that of Ferdinand Cohn strikingly shows how elementary this work was. In general, the germ theory was not accepted, and animalculists were either forgotten or mentioned only for ridicule. The earlier interests of the 1840's, which led to scientific experimentation and eventually to the germ theory of disease in Europe, had come to a dead end in America.

The doldrum decades preceding the 1880's are an American phenomenon. Why were American doctors so far behind Europeans in developing systematic medical research? And why did they fail to keep up with European developments in the field of bacteriology after 1860, when originally both had had much the same background? The answers to these questions seem to lie in the cultural scene.

During the first half of the nineteenth century, there was considerable interest in science in the United States. A movement was afoot to set up a national science foundation. The Wilkes Exploring Expedition and others were sent out. The Coast and Geodetic Survey was begun. The Smithsonian Institution was founded and at once began to turn out worthwhile contributions to science. The Lawrence Scientific School at Harvard and the Sheffield Scientific School at Yale were established. The lyceum movement caught the popular fancy and famous scientists like Agassiz and Lyell lectured all around the country. American medicine in this period was on a par with that of the more prominent European countries and American medical contributions of great significance were well received.

Then something went wrong. The scientific movement apparently petered out in the late 1850's. This may be blamed on the Civil War. It may also have been because fewer Americans went to European universities for their education and the native institutions were not strong enough to replace them. At any rate, in the 1870's there was a strong movement to improve the educational level and again to stir up an interest in science. Even as Simon Newcomb and others bewailed the American preoccupation with invention and practical science, the first real graduate school on the German pattern was being started at Johns Hopkins. The Hopkins provided a model for the other colleges and soon was called upon to supply their faculties. The whole American educational level was raised drastically in the last two decades of the century.

Before this movement took place, however, America lagged behind Europe in support of pure science and research. Little organized research was carried on in the United States during the nineteenth century, although there was considerable work on an individual basis. There were few laboratories, little decent equipment, and no funds for hiring capable assistants. Furthermore, no one saw any great need for such luxuries.[19] Practising physicians had no time for research, and emphasis was on practice to the detriment of experimental science.

Some excuse for this state of affairs may be made on the grounds that the country was new and the frontier took up the energies of men who might otherwise have turned to science. The supremacy of theology in the intellectual field may likewise have drawn the bright young men away from science.[20] Cultural independence in the arts and in literature was beginning to be apparent in the mid-century, and possibly this independent, nationalistic spirit was reflected in other fields, such as medicine, where American attitudes were unfavorable towards new ideas just at the time when the greatest advances were being made abroad.

In addition to these factors, there was little prestige to be gained in scientific research because the commercial spirit of the Anglo-Saxon world placed the emphasis on practice—a reflection of the businessman's sense of values. There was no tradition of government support for science, as in France, and the tradition of private support had to wait for a generation of multimillionaires. The thought of patronage was repugnant to democratic ideals, and respect was accorded to the sturdy, self-made scientist, following in the Franklin tradition, but without Franklin's viewpoint on what should be done with amassed wealth.

In such a milieu, even doctors trained abroad were soon absorbed into the general pattern. They found the odds too great and when, as in the case of the "Alabama Student," they tried to apply their acquired knowledge, it was too difficult to transform the whole environment into one more favorable for experimental efforts. To the dismay of European professors, some of their best

[19] For more detail, see R. H. Shryock's *American medical research: past and present*, New York, 1947, chap. 1, 2, and American indifference to basic science, *Arch. int. d'hist. d. sci.*, 1948, no. 5, 50-65. This was probably a matter of education. Few medical students had attended a liberal arts college and fewer still had much acquaintance with the physical and biological sciences. A good proportion of the medical profession lacked the basic knowledge necessary to set up a valid experiment or had any notion of how to interpret the results and data of an experimental proof. Americans were skeptical about the value of microscopy. Cf. Stillé, Alfred, *Elements of general pathology: a practical treatise on the causes, forms, symptoms and results of disease.* Philadelphia, 1848, p. 105.
[20] Hall, W. W. *Consumption.* New York, 1857, p. 223-24.

American students went home and were soon engulfed by their surroundings, making few if any contributions to medical advance.[21]

The emphasis on the practical in the American outlook demanded utility at a time when the doctors could promise the least. Pure science, represented in medicine by etiology and the identification of diseases, was not popular. "Cures" and treatment, based on empirical method, suited the public better. The necessity of following the public demand held back the development of medicine because treatment could not be successful, except by chance, when the causes of disease, or even the nature and identity of the diseases themselves, were unknown. Philosophically speaking, this meant that physicians were asking the wrong questions, so that any possible solution to the problems of etiology was limited in scope by the narrowness of the field of inquiry. For example, the epidemiological approach and statistical surveys had been the methods of the early part of the century and these were continued in professional literature even though they were known not to provide a satisfactory account of the etiology of any disease. The emphasis on applied science over pure science was a case of putting the cart before the horse, but one could scarcely expect the public to realize this when the medical profession itself did not do so.

The intellectual climate was obscured by the use of an inadequate and confusing terminology. The precise meaning of the terms used in science in preceding centuries is difficult for the modern reader to grasp because concepts were expressed in a language which appears tantalizingly vague and inexact when compared with present-day terminology. This is especially true of work in medical theory. A striking example of this may be found in some textbooks of the mid-nineteenth century. J. V. von Hildenbrand of Vienna wrote the following passage on etiology:

> Every contagious miasm possesses the properties, 1, of producing a similar virus in the disease which it had occasioned; and 2, of spreading and extending itself ad infinitum, by virtue of this secondary development, that is so long as there exists a matter capable of receiving the miasm, and of producing a new one. Both these properties are similar, by their power of reproduction, to the germs of animals and of plants; but the last property is analogous to the matter of fire, since a single atom of the contagious virus, like a spark, is capable of spreading itself ad infinitum, and of transversing, when unobstructed in its progress, all bodies that are capable of receiving it.[22]

---

[21] Men coming to this country to teach found things equally difficult, a fact illustrated by the adventures of Charles Edouard Brown-Séquard at Harvard. See J.M.D. Olmsted's *Charles Edouard Brown-Séquard, a nineteenth century neurologist and endocrinologist*, Baltimore, 1946, pp. 123-38.

[22] Hildenbrand, J. V. de. *A treatise on the nature, cause and treatment of contagious typhus*. Trans. S. D. Gross. New York, 1829, p. 73.

The difficulty of expressing scientific ideas with inadequate terminology is well illustrated in this paragraph. Hildenbrand used "miasm," "atom," and "virus" all to convey the same basic idea.

Poor instruments, as well as legal, organizational, and commercial obstructions also hindered medical progress in America. Optical instruments such as microscopes were rare and of poor quality until the last few decades of the century. Their worth as scientific instruments rather than as toys was just beginning to be appreciated. It was unlawful to perform autopsies in some states. American democratic principles would not allow experiments to be made with charity patients. Commercial hindrances came from two sources: the quacks (including patent medicine sellers) who would have lost a good part of their market if the medical profession had been able to satisfy the intelligent members of the general public, and the trading companies, which suffered under the quarantine and public health regulations. The removal of the "brutal" port quarantines from Boston and New York in 1859 was hailed as a great victory for commerce and "the welfare of mankind, second only to the Declaration of Independence in Philadelphia, nearly a hundred years ago."[23]

The lack of the scientific point of view is evident in the case of one scientist who found that he suffered from a headache every time he worked with fungi. So he desisted, saying he was "unwilling to test Mitchell's [cryptogamous] theory by so strictly personal an experiment."[24] How different this attitude was from that of Europeans who were practising self-inoculation for the purposes of answering similar questions.

At this time the quality of personnel in the medical profession was at a low level. All kinds of sects flourished and their existence discredited the profession as a whole. Medical schools were abundant, but extremely poor in both curriculum and students. Small colleges that were virtually diploma mills turned out graduates to "practise" (and learn) on their unfortunate patients. In the present state of medical excellence it is hard to imagine the degree to which the profession had sunk. In the early part of the century, most of the better doctors were educated abroad, at Paris and Edinburgh. In the middle period, few left America. When, in the latter part of the century, it became apparent that Germany and France led the

[23] Jackson, Samuel. *The principles of medicine*. Philadelphia, 1832. Pref., xvi-xvii; N. Y. J. Med., 1859, *4*, 159; Proc. & deb. 4th nat. Quar. San. Conv., 14.
[24] R. So. Quart. Rev. 1850, n.s. *1*, 155-56.

world, students once more went overseas to prepare themselves for careers in medicine.[25]

Finally, whatever American discussion of European work on the germ theory existed (and this was very scarce) generally centered upon the ideas of men who refused to accept the hypothesis, or the opinions of those who espoused some variant of it, because they maintained the older views. Since experiments to prove or disprove etiological theory were performed only rarely in the United States, and were almost total failures when they were tried,[26] American physicians thought they were being very objective and scientific in *not* jumping to conclusions. This was a normal reaction, considering how inconclusive their evidence was, but one wishes some attempt had been made, instead, to improve the experimental level. The Europeans evolved the germ theory because they were looking for it, or something like it, to explain causation in infectious diseases. Americans looked a few times—unsuccessfully—and gave up.

Perhaps it is not entirely fair to place so much blame on the American scientific attitude for the failure to contribute to the early development of the germ theory. Most of the criticisms of the hypothesis were valid. It did not explain the peculiar characteristics we now know are due to rickettsial organisms or viruses, to the fungi, protozoa, and other living organisms, to the insect and animal or even avian vectors, to the concept of the carrier, and to immunity. It took nearly thirty years to demonstrate the correctness of John Snow's intuition concerning the malarial parasite. While eventually there was agreement on the transmissibility of many diseases before the acceptance of the germ theory, on others there was controversy. One finds, for example, elaborate quarantine and sanitary cordons utilized during the early pandemics of cholera, and for yellow fever, but by the mid-century these were dropped. Precautions against person-to-person contact were replaced by sanitary precautions designed to clean up foul miasmata. Where a disease, such as smallpox, measles, or scarlet fever, was accepted as transmissible, the agency of transmission was believed to be an effluvia—a poisonous gas in the breath or exuded from the pores—rather than a living organism. It is interesting that where attempt was made to obtain organisms from the breath of a patient, it was

[25] For details, see Shryock, *Medical research*, chap. 1, 2; for medical education see W. F. Norwood's *History of medical education in the United States before the Civil War*, Philadelphia, 1944.

[26] Experimentalists included Benjamin Rush Rhees, Joseph Leidy, Francis Peyre Porcher, James H. Salisbury, and others. See also Stillé, *Elements of pathology*, p. 105.

done in a case of cholera, or other disease not likely to be spread in this manner. This again illustrates the complexity of the problem. The development of the germ theory also prospered in Europe because of the constant interchange of scientific ideas. Largely for reasons of distance, Americans did not take any share in this spirited idea market.[27]

The lively controversies over the germ theory of disease in Europe should have focused American attention on the hypothesis. Unfortunately, up to about 1875, the American medical profession was not interested. Articles in the journals reflected concern over practical problems, such as treatment and techniques, rather than over theoretical problems, such as the etiology of specific infectious diseases. The old miasma hypothesis was generally accepted and even earlier work on the differentiation of miasmata was forgotten. Classification of disease entities had retrogressed to a point where the phenomenon of typho-malarial fever was frequently encountered, thus ignoring the careful study of Elisha Bartlett thirty years earlier. To judge from American medical periodicals, the new science of bacteriology scarcely existed.

Around 1875, however, this situation began to change. Some knowledge of the work on bacteriology abroad seeped in, although American thinking on the matter was still quite confused. Fifteen medical journals have been examined for the 1875-1880 period to determine the degree to which the germ theory was being publicized. It appears that there were two or three items about the theory in almost every journal—either articles, editorials, book reviews, or bits of news—during the five-year period, *an average of one item every other year*. These references were not necessarily favorable towards the new idea, but at least it was being mentioned, which was more than had been done heretofore.[28]

---

27 [Snow, John.] *Snow on cholera, being a reprint of two papers by John Snow together with a biographical memoir by B. W. Richardson, M.D. and an introduction by Wade Hampton Frost, M.D.* New York, 1936. "On the mode of communication of cholera," p. 133; Fenner, E. D. *History of the epidemic yellow fever at New Orleans, La. in 1853.* New York, 1854. Addendum, p. 84; *Proc. & deb. 3rd nat. Quar. Conv., 1859,* 44, 201, 15-85; *Proc. & deb. 4th nat. Quar. San. Conv.,* 1860, 72-73, 113-17; Buckler, T. H. *A history of epidemic cholera as it appeared at the Baltimore City and County Alms-House, in the summer of 1849, with some remarks on the medical topography and diseases of this region.* Baltimore, 1851.

28 The journals (1875-1880) consulted were: *American Journal of the Medical Sciences* (4 items), *American Practitioner* (2 items), *Boston Medical and Surgical Journal* (5 items), *Detroit Lancet* (4), *Eclectic Medical Journal* (5), *Medical and Surgical Reporter* (7), *Medical Annals: Albany* (1), *Medical News* (2), *Medical Record* (1), *Therapeutic Gazette* (1), *Transactions of the American Medical Association* (2), *Transactions of the Eclectic Medical Society of New York* (2), *Transactions of the Homeopathic Medical Society of New York* (2), *Buffalo Medical and Surgical Journal* (0), *Gaillard's Medical Journal* (0). There are some articles available in medical journals other than these, of course.

Publications such as *The Boston Medical and Surgical Journal, The American Journal of the Medical Sciences, The Eclectic Medical Journal,* and *The Detroit Lancet* each contained four or five articles and news reports on the germ theory—chiefly in opposition to it. *The Medical and Surgical Reporter,* on the other hand, had seven items on the theory during the 1875-1880 period, and all were favorable. Pasteur, Koch, Klebs, and Lister were mentioned, as well as Bastian and Beale. The other journals of the day usually had one or two papers or informative notes on the theory, especially towards 1880, but as yet, etiological references utilizing non-germ explanations outnumbered germ theory citations by at least ten to one.

The real acceptance of the germ theory began with the appearance of an English translation of Hugo W. von Ziemssen's *Cyclopedia of the Practice of Medicine* in 1874-1878. The first volume of Ziemssen employed the germ theory in relation to both anthrax and relapsing fever and suggested its pertinence to several other diseases. By 1878, the Ziemssen influence was apparent at the meetings and conventions, as illustrated by the paper given by John T. Carpenter at the 29th annual session of the Medical Society of the State of Pennsylvania.[29] Before that time, it was a rare American dictionary or encyclopedia or even textbook which contained any mention of the germ theory.

A study of some of the representative textbooks between 1875 and 1885 shows clearly how long it took for the new concept to be presented. Henry Hartshorne's *Conspectus of the Medical Sciences,* in the second edition (1874), contained some interesting comments on the etiological theories of his day. He accepted the usual human effluvia (contagion), or "crowd poison," and filth explanations for the origin of typhus, and miasma for yellow fever. He followed the views of Pettenkofer and Thiersch on cholera, and (interesting point) of John K. Mitchell on intermittent fever.[30] Hartshorne was a well-informed Philadelphia physician and a frequent contributor to medical journals. He knew of the work of most European writers on the subject of etiology, but he accepted only that opposed to the germ theory.

---

[29] Carpenter, J. T. The local origin of constitutional disease. *Trans. med. Soc. St. of Pa. 29th ann. session* 1878, *12*, pt. 1, 140. For opposite view, see Davis, N. S. Does etiology constitute a proper basis for the classification and diagnosis of diseases? *Amer. Practitioner,* 1876, *13*, 343-50. Davis argued that the Ziemssen classification, based on etiology, was erroneous.

[30] Hartshorne, Henry. *A conspectus of the medical sciences, comprising manuals of anatomy, physiology, chemistry, materia medica, practise of medicine, surgery and obstetrics.* 2d ed. Philadelphia, 1874, pp. 592-93, 603, 607, 612, 616.

Some of the texts in the early 1880's illustrate the gradual replacement of old ideas by new ones. Austin Flint finally included the germ theory for relapsing fever and anthrax in the fifth edition of his *Treatise on the Principles and Practice of Medicine* (1881), and in 1883 added Koch's tuberculosis discoveries as an appendix, while retaining the older miasma hypothesis for other infectious diseases. In a different book, *Clinical Medicine. A Systematic Treatise on the Diagnosis and Treatment of Diseases* (1879), Flint called attention to the fact that "a peculiar vegetable organism" had been observed in the blood during paroxysms of relapsing fever. He wrote that "if the demonstration be accepted as regards this disease, reasoning by analogy, it is a logical conclusion that it is merely a question of time in regard to the demonstration of the germ theory in regard to its application to other fevers."[31] The student who used this book was being prepared for the new etiology, and it would have come as less of a shock than to one having a more conservative text.

Other texts were really conservative. In 1884 there appeared an American edition of Edmund A. Parke's *A Manual of Practical Hygiene* intended for military use. According to the preface, some Americans had expressed disappointment because earlier editions did not have any material on the germ theory. By this date they were anxious to hear of this work. The new edition did not answer this criticism, and in spite of the date of publication, there was not one word about the work of Robert Koch on cholera, although Pettenkofer was cited frequently. Where the "germ theory" was mentioned, the author either included material to prove that it was *not* correct, or else he chose examples, such as the Klebs *bacillus malariae,* which had been shown to be incorrect or premature.[32]

The textbook writers were by no means the only ones who were slow in adopting the germ theory. In the 1870's, most Americans who even considered this hypothesis accepted the views of those Europeans, such as Max von Pettenkofer, Charleton Bastian, or Lionel S. Beale, who opposed Pasteur. The most exotic types of theory seem to have made a greater impression in the United

[31] Flint, Austin. *A treatise on the principles and practice of medicine.* Philadelphia. 2d ed., 1867; 3d ed., 1868, p. 103; 4th ed., 1873, p. 105; 6th ed., 1886, preface, p. 3; Flint, *Clinical medicine. A systematic treatise on the diagnosis and treatment of diseases.* Philadelphia, 1879, p. 699.

[32] Parkes, E. A. *A manual of practical hygiene for the use of the medical service of the Army.* Ed. F. S. B. François de Chaumont. New York, 1884, vol. 2, pp. 129-30, 134; Flint, Austin. *A treatise on the principles and practice of medicine.* 5th ed. Philadelphia, 1881, pp. 94-95.

States than the scientific results of Pasteur, Ferdinand Cohn, Joseph Lister, and John Tyndall. Lister gave a paper on the antiseptic system and the germ theory at the Philadelphia Centennial Exhibition, but it was not well received. Tyndall's lectures influenced amateur scientists and were reported extensively in the *Popular Science Monthly,* but not in the more learned and pretentious scientific and medical journals.[33] While one can easily blame this state of affairs on the weaknesses of the germ theory, it does seem rather odd that the general atmosphere in medical circles was so completely hostile to the new views. There was no partisan bickering over the hypothesis as one might have expected. The uniformity of opinion is an American phenomenon.

It was quite possible in the late seventies to write of infectious disease without mentioning germs at all.[34] Some writers cited the theory only to condemn it. In 1879 the *American Quarterly Journal of Microscopical Science* carried a review of an article in the *New York Medical Journal* by Dr. H. D. Schmidt. This physician observed that:

> The microscopical study of disease-germs *has not been very prolific in practical results,* and the question as to the existence of specific germs of this character is yet an open one. Investigations of the causes which produce disease are probably among the most difficult and *unpromising* of any which the microscopist can undertake. . . .
> On the whole, it appears that the application of the hypothesis of contagium vivum to the explanation of the phenomena of disease, has had its day.[35]

The reviewer of the article, presumably a layman, accepted Schmidt's views without question.

While some authors ignored the germ theory, a few were so confusing in their presentation of it that their explanations were a worse hindrance to understanding than total omission would have

---

[33] Bailey, T. H. Water-poisoning as a cause of disease. *The Sanitarian,* 1875, *3,* no. 27, 97-107; Boulden, J. E. P. Cholera—its cause and prevention. *The Sanitarian,* 1873, *1,* no. 8, 362-67; Anonymous. The etology of typhoid fever. *Bost. med. surg. J.,* 86, 58-60; Richardson, Joseph G. On certain human parasitic fungi and their relation to disease. *Bost. med. surg. J.,* 86, 158-60; 2d ann. rep. St. Bd. Health Mass., 1871, 112-14; Lynch, J. S. The germ theory of disease. *Balt. Phys. Surg.,* 1873, *4,* no. 3, 17-18; Jordan, E. O. The relations of bacteriology to the public health movement since 1872. *Amer. J. Pub. Health,* 1921, *11,* 1042-47; *Pop. Sci. Mo.,* 1876, *8,* 686-99; 1876, *10,* 129-54; 1877, *10,* 641-54; 1877, *11,* 236, 363.

[34] Hudson, E. D. The pathology and etiology of pulmonary phthisis in relation to its prevention and early arrest. *Trans. N. Y. Acad. Med.* 2d ser. 1876, *2,* 147-59; Carpenter, *loc. cit.* (note 29), pp. 138-143; Cushing, Harvey. *The life of Sir William Osler.* New York, 1940, p. 164.

[35] Review: Dr. H. D. Schmidt on the nature of the poison of yellow fever and its prevention. *Amer. Quart. micros. J.,* *1,* no. 4, 315-16. Italics mine.

been. Frank Wells, Cleveland Public Health Officer, wrote that Liebig, Virchow and the majority of English writers claimed that

> certain disorders, notably the zymotic diseases, spring spontaneously from filth; and hence, being *entirely* amenable to sanitary laws, have been designated by them "filth or preventable diseases"; the other [school], following Pasteur and upheld by Liebermeister, Pettenkofer, and the greater portion of the German school, believe that filth does not directly originate these affections, but simply increases a tendency to their causation, by furnishing a nidus or resting place, a favorable soil, in which the living organisms of disease multiply and develop and without which they become as a rule inert and inoperative. In other words, the one class believe that filth *alone*, communicating the elements of decomposition, is sufficient to produce disease, while the other hold that there must be something more, viz. filth plus some particular poison. Pettenkofer, the warm supporter of the "germ" theory of disease, says that filth is like the charcoal in gunpowder. *It is necessary to have it, in order to produce the explosion.*[36]

If the first group included were supposed to be zymoticists, the author did not have a very clear idea of the zymotic hypothesis. His whole discussion of the second school of thought shows little knowledge of the germ theory as presented by Pasteur. There is no sign that he saw any difference between the views of Pasteur and of Pettenkofer. The spontaneous generation question is brought in in an unusual fashion to support the epidemiologists. Basically, it would appear that Wells had a fine misunderstanding of all the questions of his day: the germ theory, the doctrines of Pasteur, the zymotic hypothesis, and the relation of the filth theory to epidemiology. The favorable mention of Pettenkofer lends support to the impression that Americans chose the wrong side in the European controversy over the germ theory.[37]

It was during the seventies that there was so much preoccupation with the problem of sewer gas. The *Canada Lancet* reported that the Prince of Wales contracted enteric fever (typhoid) in 1872, while on a visit to the home of Lord Londesborough. It was thought that there must have been some defect in drainage causing water pollution or the generation of sewer gas. The gas was assumed to be dangerous because it smelled unpleasant and, with the development of sanitation, it was now frequently associated with disease, particularly typhoid. Many of the articles in the *Plumber and Sanitary Engineer* for the 1875-1880 period indicated

---

[36] Wells, Frank. *Filth and its relation to disease. A report made to the Board of Police Commissioners of the City of Cleveland.* Cleveland, 1876, pp. 5-6.

[37] There was an article by Max von Pettenkofer, "What we can do against cholera," in *Public health: reports and papers 1873*, 317-35, in which he gave practical directions on the prevention of cholera, stressing the importance of cleanliness of water, soil, and air, although he thought that drinking water had nothing to do with the spread of the disease.

great concern over sewer gas poisoning and its prevention by means of "stench traps."[38]

In 1880, Benjamin Lee addressed the Medical Society of the State of Pennsylvania on hygiene, and he blamed sewer gas for typhoid, rheumatism, pneumonia, parotitis, malaria, croup, and diphtheria. No mention was made of germs or any other possible contents of this gas. He stated:

> Whatever the agency by which it works, we know that it comes with the power and potency of death. Escaping into the free atmosphere, its deadly poison is quickly destroyed by the oxidation of its organic poisons; but when it mingles with the confined air of our unventilated living and sleeping rooms, it retains its deadly power long enough to do its work effectually.[39]

It will be recognized at once that this is merely the old concept of a noxious miasma transferred to a new kind of vapor. An effective refutation of this kind of thinking was made by George Hamilton, and especially by J. M. Keating, in a paper and discussion published in the *Transactions of the College of Physicians of Philadelphia* for 1883.[40] By that time, the germ theory was beginning to be accepted universally.

Another element in the American picture concerns the adoption of the antiseptic system. This method of Lister was used reluctantly in the late 1870's because it worked. Apparently few Americans had any idea why it was effective. From articles on the antiseptic procedure in medical journals during the years 1876 to 1881, one would never guess that the germ concept even existed.[41] This is one of the most interesting illustrations of the general American ignorance of European work in the period following the Civil War. Here the practical and visible results of the germ theory of disease were accepted without the theory itself.

[38] *Canada Lancet, 4,* 233-34. See also, Wells, *Filth and its relation to disease,* 53; Keating, W. V. An epidemic of typhoid fever from defective drainage. *Trans. Coll. Phys. Phila.,* 1879, 3d. ser., *4,* 85-125; Hartshorne, Henry. Preliminary report on the sanitary conditions of American watering places. *Public health: reports and papers,* 2, 56, 57; Noel, H. R. Sewer-gas as a cause of diphtheria and typho-malarial diseases, *ibid.,* 362-67; *The Plumber and Sanitary Engineer,* 1878, *1,* 32, 34; 2, *3, 4, passim.* Later this magazine was called *The Sanitary Engineer.*

[39] Lee, Benjamin. Address in hygiene. *Trans. med. Soc. St. Penn., 13,* pt. 1, 121.

[40] Hamilton, George. Sewer gas and its alleged causation of typhoid fever. *Trans. Coll. Phys. Phila.,* 1883, 3d ser. *6,* 270ff.; Keating, J. M. Discussion, *ibid.,* 301-2.

[41] Pepper, William. The sanitary relations of hospitals. *Trans. Amer. Pub. Health Ass. 1874-5.* New York, 1876, 2, 1-10; Smith, Stephen. Some practical tests of the claims of the antiseptic system. *Trans. med. Soc. St. N. Y. 1878,* 106-30; Parrish, W. H. Puerperal septicaemia. *Trans. med. Soc. St. Penn.,* 1880, *13,* pt. 1, 222; Snively, Isaac. Hygiene in its relation to the medical profession. *Trans. med. Soc. St. Penn.,* 1881, *13,* pt. 2, 666; Ewing, J. H. Cases treated by the antiseptic method in St. Mary's Hospital, Philadelphia. *Amer. J. med. Sci.,* 1879, 77, 416-29.

Very often it seemed as if laymen had a better grasp of the germ theory than members of the medical profession. This was not strange when one considers the low status of medical education in America during most of the nineteenth century. Amateur scientists were also among the forefront of the writers of books on the microscope, but this was partly because microscopy was an interesting hobby. In 1875, President Barnard of Columbia University was called upon to speak before the first convention of the American Public Health Association. His address, "The germ theory of disease and its relation to public hygiene," was extremely enlightening. He described the germ theory and the controversy over spontaneous generation. The latter he regarded as solved by Charleton Bastian, though he recognized that further work was necessary before it could be fully settled. He was well acquainted with the research of Pasteur, and Lister's antisepsis, and he was sure that the germ theory was "at least partially true." He was one of the few Americans to mention such European leaders as Schwann, Tyndall, and Klebs, and he was entirely open-minded about the whole subject.[42]

Laymen did more than accept the germ theory—some of them attempted to make their own contributions. In England, for example, in 1850 John Grove had introduced his theory of vegetable germs, which was strongly influenced by the cryptogamous theory of John K. Mitchell. In America at least three laymen had something to add to the theory. The minute yellow cholera flies of J. Franklin Reigert of Lancaster, Pennsylvania, were an unconscious attempt to link the disease with water. Another layman, William D. Riley, attributed diseases to the metamorphoses in locusts and grasshoppers. He was startlingly ignorant of the elements of biology, and it is doubtful that his essay had much influence.[43]

The most significant development in American microbiology before the general acceptance of the germ theory was the discovery

---

[42] Barnard, F. A. P. The germ theory of disease and its relation to hygiene. *Public health: reports and papers, 1873*, 70-87. Books on the microscope for amateurs included: King, John. *The microscopist's companion; a popular manual of practical microscopy.* Cincinnati, 1859; Mantell, Gideon. *Thoughts on animalcules, or a glimpse of the invisible world revealed by the microscope.* London, 1846; Hon. Mrs. Ward, *A world of wonders revealed by the microscope. A book for young students.* 2d ed. London, 1859; Wood, Rev. J. G. *Common objects of the microscope.* London, 1861; Wythe, Rev. J. H. *Curiosities of the microscope, or illustrations of the minute parts of creation, adapted to the capacity of the young.* Philadelphia, 1852; Brocklesby, John. *Views of the microscopic world. Designed for general reading and as a hand-book for classes in natural science.* New York, 1851. *The amateur microscopist; or views of the microscopic world. A handbook of microscopic manipulation and microscopic objects.* New York, 1871.

[43] Grove, John. *Epidemics examined and explained: or, living germs proved by analogy to be a source of disease.* London, 1850, pp. 88-90, 128-37, 154; Reigert, J. F. *A treatise on the cause of cholera. An interesting discovery.* Lancaster, Pa., 1855; Riley, W. D. *Locusts and grasshoppers. The beginnings and the end of febrile or eruptive diseases in living things.* Philadelphia, 1872, pp. 4-5.

of the bacterial nature of pear blight, made by Thomas J. Burrill in 1878.[44] Burrill, an Illinois biologist interested in bacteria and fungi, did not publish his work fully, and little notice seems to have been taken of it. In 1882, he brought out a small volume, *The Bacteria*, which was of considerable moment. His experimental method was similar to that of Robert Koch, and it is important to note that it may have been thought out independently because it is unlikely that Burrill had seen the Koch postulates (also published in 1882) before the publication of his own work.

Even before Burrill's research on pear blight, William G. Farlow had discovered the causal factors in American grapevine mildew and potato rot. Later Farlow and Arthur B. Seymour were to compile an encyclopedia of the parasitic fungi of the United States, classified according to their hosts. Followers of Burrill included Merton B. Waite (insect transmission of pear blight bacteria), Joseph C. Arthur (further research on pear blight), Newton B. Pierce (California vine disease, walnut blight), and Erwin Frink Smith (wilt disease in curcurbits, *Bacteria in Relation to Plant Diseases*.) The latter is famous as the man involved in the argument (1898-1901) with Dr. Alfred Fischer of the University of Leipzig as to whether bacterial diseases of plants actually exist. In this case Americans had to persuade Europeans to adopt the germ theory for plants![45]

Perhaps as a reflection of the lay interest in bacteria, nonmedical publications often carried news of medical interest. A later paper of Tyndall on germs, read before the Royal Society, was abstracted in 1876 in the *American Journal of Microscopy*, the *Popular Science Monthly*, and the *American Journal of Science and the Arts*. Many lectures of Tyndall were reported in full in the two latter journals. It is interesting to see the degree to which the amateur and professional scientists opened their magazines to news of the germ theory, in contrast to what amounts to a conspiracy of silence on the part of medical editors. The *Popular Science Monthly* had at least one article in each volume, beginning in 1874. This meant

---

[44] Smith, E. F. In memoriam Thomas J. Burrill. *J. Bact.*, 1916, *1*, 269-71. Burrill, T. J. Pear blight. *Trans. Ill. St. hort. Soc. for 1877*. Chicago, 1878, pp. 114-16; Fire blight of pears. *Trans. Ill. St. hort. Soc. for 1878*. Chicago, 1879, pp. 79-80; Anthrax of pear trees; or the so-called fire blight of pear, and twig blight of apple, trees. [1880] *Proc. Amer. Ass. Adv. Sci.*, 1881, *29*, 583-97; Bacteria as a cause of disease in plants. *Amer. Nat.*, 1881, *15*, 527-31; Blight, [1881] *Bot. Gaz.*, 1880-81, 5 & 6, 271-73; Some vegetable poisons [1882] *Proc. Amer. Ass. Adv. Sci.*, 1883, *31*, 515-18, *Amer. J. Micr.* 1882, *3*, 192-97; The bacteria. Springfield, Ill., 1882. 11th Ann. Rep. Ill. Indust. Univ. 65 pp.

[45] Rodgers, A. D., III. *Erwin Frink Smith. A story of North American plant pathology*. Memoirs of the American Philosophical Society, vol. 31. Philadelphia, 1952, pp. 342-44, 346-52.

a minimum of two items *per year* as compared with two or three items for a five-year interval in medical journals. By 1882 (volume XX) no less than ten items on the subject were included. Three of these were articles presenting the researches of Pasteur, while others were notes on nomenclature of microbes, the nature of diphtheria poison, Laveran's discovery of the malarial parasite, and Pettenkofer's soil doctrine.[46] There was no excuse for a reader of the *Popular Science Monthly* not being well informed about the latest developments regarding the germ theory.

The readers of the *Scientific American* should have been equally well informed. This journal not only carried short articles and news items about the germ theory, and especially about bacteria, but in its *Supplement* there appeared longer articles by Pasteur and others on the very latest developments. The *Supplement*, in fact, had more medical articles than the main periodical, very often, as in the *Popular Science Monthly*, written by leading scientists and physicians of the day. While the main section of the *Scientific American* seemed more amateurish and less erudite than the *Popular Science Monthly*, the *Supplement* left nothing to be desired. It contained scientific papers of a caliber one would expect to find in a learned journal.[47] Both popular periodicals were far more receptive to new ideas than the medical journals.

The germ theory also reached the public through newspaper supplements such as the *Tribune Popular Science*. As early as 1874, an account of a lecture on the germ theory appeared. The concept was often presented in a more favorable light in popular accounts, such as this, than in more serious scientific journals.[48]

The *American Journal of Science and the Arts* (Silliman's Journal) was primarily a periodical for physical scientists and biologists, and few articles of medical interest were printed in it. Nevertheless, articles on parasitic worms, cholera, the microscope, diseases caused by fungi, and Tyndall on germs were included. *The Sanitarian*, a public health journal, had some mention of the germ theory, especially in articles on specific diseases, in editorials or book reviews. In spite of this evidence of interest, notice of Koch's

[46] Professor Tyndall on germs. *Amer. J. Micr.*, 1876, *1*, no. 4, 33-46; *Amer. J. Sci.*, 1876, 3d ser. *11*, 305ff.; 1877, *13*, 477, 480; 1879, *15*, 235; *Pop. Sci. Mo.*, 1876, *8*, 686-99; 1876-77, *10*, 129-54, 641-54; 1882, *20:* Max von Pettenkofer, Sanitary relations of the soil, 332-40, 468-77; Sketch of M. Louis Pasteur, 823-29; Louis Pasteur, The germ theory, 801-6; Nature of diphtheria-poison, 714; Vaccination for anthrax, 142-43; Accommodative cultivation of infectious organisms, 424-5; William B. Carpenter, Disease-germs, 244-60; Malarial organisms, 857-58; Glossary of microbes, 718.

[47] *Sci. Amer.*, 1875-1880, vols. 32-43; *Sci. Amer. Suppl.*, vols. 1-10.

[48] *Tribune Pop. Sci.*, Boston, 1874, pp. 59-60.

work on the germ theory was *quoted* from the *American Naturalist*, another scientific magazine, rather than abstracted from any published material of the German scientist. The editors of *The Sanitarian* were physicians, and this neglect was similar to that of their colleagues editing purely medical journals. References about the germ theory were also infrequent in the reports and papers submitted to the American Public Health Association in the seventies. Though there were many articles on individual epidemics and on insanitary conditions and their remedies, little was said regarding the bacteriological factors involved. In this instance, as in the case of the medical journals, other interests occupied the physicians.[49]

Other nonmedical journals carried news of the bacteriological activities in varying degrees. Literary magazines such as the *Atlantic Monthly, Harper's Magazine,* and the *North American Review* had very few articles on scientific subjects. Those of medical interest related chiefly to cholera and yellow fever. *The Nation* had a whole section devoted to scientific news, though it must be admitted that this was mainly about technical improvements and inventions. Articles on disinfection, cholera, and the health of great cities appeared. *The International Review* for 1880 contained an article on yellow fever by John S. Billings, of Army Medical Library fame, favorably mentioning the germ theory. Journals in fields which might be affected by medicine were somewhat unreceptive to the theory. *The Journal of Social Science, The Plumber and Sanitary Engineer,* and *The American Architect and Building News* had very little or nothing on the hypothesis. It was the reader of the popular science magazines who learned the most about it.[50]

All this was changed suddenly in the early 1880's. After the cautiousness of the medical profession in the post-Civil War period, the final acceptance of the theory came almost immediately after Koch's demonstration of the tuberculosis bacillus and the statement of his postulates in 1882. The abrupt change from the skeptical, wait-and-see attitude was dramatic and can clearly be seen in the medical publications of the years 1882 to 1885. The germ theory was now treated as something new and different, just as if it

[49] *Amer. J. Sci.*, 1875, 3d ser. *9*, 478; 1875, *10*, 402; 1877, *14*, 426; *The Sanitarian*, vols. 4-8, *passim*, 1880, *8*, 246; *Public health: reports and papers* 1873ff. An exception to this rule may be found in the *Rep. Nat. Bd. Health 1880*, Appendix H, 387-96.
[50] *Internat. Rev.*, 1880, *8*, 29-49. The lay magazines consulted included: *American Architect and Building News* (0 items); *American Journal of Science and the Arts* (5 items); *American Journal of Microscopy and Popular Science* (3 items); *American Monthly Microscopical Journal* (0); *American Naturalist* (2); *American Quarterly Microscopical Journal* (1); *Atlantic Monthly* (0); *Harper's Magazine* (1); *International Review* (1); *Journal of Social Science* (0); *Popular Science Monthly* (18); *Plumber and Sanitary Engineer* (1); *Scientific American* (without *Supplement*) (26).

had not been available to Americans for the past fifteen years! Furthermore, its acceptance was made with such little fanfare that one finds, for example, no mention of the germ theory in an 1881 article on a specific disease, whereas it is taken for granted in a similar article in 1885.[51]

After Koch's discovery, the medical profession as well as the medical editors accepted the germ theory with alacrity. The change in outlook is illustrated by a discussion which took place in 1882 at the Philadelphia County Medical Society following the presentation of a paper on the bacillus tuberculosis by Dr. H. F. Formad. Formad did not believe that the bacillus had any relation to the disease, in spite of Koch, but by this time the atmosphere was already hostile to those who *opposed* the germ theory, and Formad met rough treatment at the hands of his colleagues.[52]

Not many years after this, things began to get out of hand. Bacteriology became practically a scientific fad. Discoveries came thick and fast, and scientists soon were announcing bacterial causal factors for non-bacterial diseases, such as yellow fever, malaria, and, in veterinary medicine, hog cholera. The "remote" cause—the germs—became the sole factor in disease, and the "proximate" causes—the factors of predisposition, physical and mental condition, age, sex, etc.—were ignored. Fortunately, this fervor, which led early virus discoverers to doubt their own findings, did not cause the repudiation of the germ theory. By the late 1880's there were enough accurate findings available to enable the hypothesis to survive the mistakes of over-enthusiasm.

The sudden appearance of the germ explanation in articles on diseases in the medical publications of the mid-eighties is one of the more interesting mysteries of the whole American scene. One year there is scarcely a word about the theory in any of the journals, and the next year it is included as an accepted fact as if it had been known all along. The papers given before the medical societies offer the best clue as to how the abrupt acceptance took place. Evidently the etiological problem presented by the germ theory was argued out in these local groups and the results of the discussion were similar all over the country: the men who presented the arguments of Pasteur and Koch carried the day. Undoubtedly, the ranks

[51] See, for example, *Phila. med. Times*, 1875-1885; *Trans. med. Soc. St. of Pa.*, vols. 12-15; *Trans. Coll. Phys. Phila.* 3d ser. vols. 4-6; *Trans. med. Soc. St. of N. Y.*, 1878-1886; *Trans. med. Soc. St. N. J.*, 1888; *Trans. N. H. med. Soc.*, 1883, etc.

[52] Formad, H. F. The bacillus tuberculosis, and some anatomical points which suggest the refutation of its etiological relation with tuberculosis. *Proc. Phila. Co. med. Soc.*, 1882, 5, 29-41; Discussion, 41-42.

of the victors included the men who had studied abroad in recent years, particularly those who had had the opportunity to pursue bacteriological work in France and Germany.

Summary

The lack of interest in the germ theory on the part of the medical profession was a striking example of American neglect of research in basic science. Up to 1875 only one result of the theory was accepted in the United States: Lister's demonstration of the antiseptic system. His method was adopted because it worked, but the reasons behind it were rejected. This pragmatism in American outlook was matched by a strong intellectual conservatism. There was a tendency to be ultra-cautious when new theoretical concepts were introduced. The profession opposed innovation and change— it tended to be satisfied with the methods it had.[53]

In the post-Civil War period, however, laymen and scientists were much more receptive towards the new idea. Scientific magazines, especially the *Scientific American* and the *Popular Science Monthly*, brought up questions which were rarely discussed in the more erudite medical journals. Contributors to the popular science publications, moreover, included the leading scientists of the day, Europeans as well as Americans. It is not surprising to find that one must go to these publications and not to the professional ones for the new ideas, the new achievements, and the new frontiers in medical science.

The popular science magazines, of course, could afford to print more sensational articles because their editors faced a less critical audience. Editors may also have been influenced by the reputation of famous scientists, such as Tyndall, and so gave space to all their ideas, even those outside the writer's main field of research. In addition, the type of paper published in a popular journal could be more imaginative than one in a professional periodical because the authors were not risking their professional reputations in the process. It is also possible that physicians had more to *unlearn* than laymen, and the new doctrine was rejected because it did not conform with the accepted concepts of what disease was and how it spread.

[53] Both, Carl. *Consumption and its treatment in all its forms.* Boston, 1873. Appendix, 151, 154. Both speaks at length about the difficulty of introducing new ideas into the United States. He blamed this on the lack of a national science foundation and on the fact that "in America nothing theoretical was wanted, but only that which was practical."

On the other hand, leading scientists may have used the popular journals as outlets for speculations they did not care to publish in learned journals. Some physicians, who published very cautious articles on the germ theory in professional medical periodicals gave a much more optimistic opinion of the same thing in the popular magazines.[54] It is entirely possible that these men were trying to goad the cautious physicians into seriously considering the new ideas. Whatever the motive, the net result was a series of competent, informative, and interesting papers in the popular science magazines. The way in which the germ theory was presented in these periodicals stands in marked contrast to the few references found to it in the professional medical journals of the same period.

Finally, after the general acceptance of the germ theory, things happened quick and fast. The general improvement in medical education, especially after the establishment of the Johns Hopkins Medical School, and the development of an increasingly scientific outlook in medicine helped America to catch up with Europe. With the great struggle to establish the germ theory over, Americans soon joined the forefront of the movement to increase knowledge in the sciences of bacteriology, virology, and immunology.

Acknowledgment

The writer wishes to thank Dr. Richard H. Shryock for his encouragement and helpful criticism of this work in all its stages.

---

[54] Compare the article of L. A. Stimson: An experimental inquiry into the value of the carbolic acid spray as a preventive of putrefaction, *Amer. J. med. Sci.*, 1880, *79*, 83-89 with his Bacteria and their effects, *Pop. Sci. Mo.*, 1875, *6*, 399-405.

Poliomyelitis and the Rockefeller Institute: Social Effects and Institutional Response

SAUL BENISON

NO one knows when poliomyelitis first appeared in the United States. There are case histories in American medical literature which suggest that polio in a sporadic form was known in the United States as early as 1841.[1] It wasn't until the 1890s, however, that the disease became a public health problem. In 1894, a polio epidemic struck Otter Creek Valley in southern Vermont, leaving 122 victims in its wake. The Vermont outbreak was the first recognized and reported polio epidemic in the United States.[2] Between 1894 and 1907 seventeen polio epidemics of varying degrees and intensity occurred in a number of regions in the United States.[3] The epidemic of 1907 is of particular importance. It was not only the most severe outbreak to that time in the country (leaving well over 2,500 victims in New York alone), it also provided the impetus that spurred Dr. Simon Flexner to undertake experimental research on the disease.[4]

When Flexner began his polio research in 1907, he was forty-four years of age and Director of the Rockefeller Institute for Medical Research. In a period of little more than fifteen years following his training as a pathologist at the Johns Hopkins Medical School, he had become, as a result of his

---

1. G. Colmer, 'Paralysis in Teething Children,' *Amer. J. med. Sci.*, 1843, 5, 248. For an excellent account of Dr. Colmer's medical career see A. E. Casey and E. H. Hinden. 'George Colmer and the Epidemiology of Poliomyelitis,' *Sth. med. J.*, 1944, 37, 471.

2. C. S. Caverly, 'Preliminary Report of an Epidemic of Paralytic Disease, Occurring in Vermont in the Summer of 1894,' *Yale Med. J.*, 1894, 1, 4; 'Notes of an Epidemic of Acute Anterior Poliomyelitis,' *J. Am. med. Ass.*, 1896, 26, 1.

3. L. E. Holt and F. H. Bartlett, 'The Epidemiology of Acute Poliomyelitis, a Study of Thirty-Five Epidemics,' *Am. J. med. Sci.*, 1908, 135, 74. The chronological listing of epidemics at the end of the paper includes European outbreaks as well. An excellent supplement to Dr. Holt's and Dr. Bartlett's listing is to be found in the appended chronology accompanying *A Monograph on the Epidemic of Poliomyelitis in New York City in 1916* (New York, 1917).

4. The best analysis of the New York epidemic of 1907 is the Collective Investigation Committee, *Epidemic Poliomyelitis: Report on the New York Epidemic of 1907*, Nervous and Mental Disease Monograph Series, n. 6 (New York, 1910).

research in diphtheria, bacterial and plant toxalbumins, dysentery, plague and cerebro-spinal meningitis, one of the leading representatives of pathology and bacteriology in the United States. In 1898, in recognition of his many achievements, he was appointed professor of pathological anatomy at Johns Hopkins. Two years later he was called to the University of Pennsylvania Medical School as Professor of Pathology. In 1903, he was appointed Director of the Rockefeller Institute for Medical Research, a post he then held until his retirement in 1935.[5] In one sense, Flexner's professional development represented the continuity of a tradition that Dr. William Welch had helped establish at Johns Hopkins, namely, that bacteriology in relation to experimental medicine, held out the promise of solving age old problems in clinical medicine. In another sense, it mirrored the growing importance of experimental pathology and bacteriology as tools for medical research.[6]

The first breakthrough in polio research did not occur in the United States but rather in Vienna. In the late fall of 1908, Dr. Karl Landsteiner, the brilliant and taciturn prosector of the Wilheminin 'Spital, succeeded in transferring polio from a human victim to an experimental monkey. Although there is no denying Landsteiner's achievement, it was but half a success, for when he tried to pass the disease to other monkeys, he failed.[7] In 1909, Flexner, following Landsteiner's lead, not only succeeded in transmitting polio from humans to monkeys, but from monkey to monkey as well, demonstrating what many physicians had long suspected but had been unable to prove, namely, that polio was an infectious disease. Within months Flexner was also able to demonstrate that no matter how he inoculated his monkeys, whether intracerebrally, or interperitoneally, or into the sciatic nerve, the disease invariably established itself in the spinal cord and medulla of its victim. Further, he discovered that polio was far more

---

5. The best short published account of Dr. Flexner's life is P. Rous, 'Simon Flexner,' *Obit. Not. Fell. R. Soc., Lond.*, 1949, 6, 409. S. Flexner and J. T. Flexner, *William H. Welch and the Heroic Age of American Medicine* (New York, 1941) has some material on Dr. Flexner's years at the Johns Hopkins Medical School, see especially pp. 160–63; 169–73. George Corner, *Two Centuries of Medicine* (Philadelphia, 1965), pp. 205–207, tells of some of Dr. Flexner's achievements at the University of Pennsylvania Medical School. George Corner, *A History of the Rockefeller Institute, 1901–1953* (New York, 1964), carries the story through his directorship of the Rockefeller Institute. Some years before Dr. Flexner died he began to write an autobiography. He finished eight chapters at his death in 1945. These essentially deal with his boyhood, early education and professional career. While they are essentially a first draft, they are nevertheless candid and revealing.

6. S. Flexner, 'William H. Welch: A Biographical Sketch,' *Papers and Addresses by William H. Welch*, 2 vols. (Baltimore, 1920), I, 11–34.

7. P. Rous, 'Karl Landsteiner 1868–1943,' *Obit. Not. Fell. R. Soc., Lond.*, 1947, 5, 295; K. Landsteiner and E. Popper, 'Übertragung der Poliomyelitis Acuta auf Affen,' *Z. fur Immunforsch. Exp. Ther.* (1909–1910), 2, 377.

severe when induced experimentally than when it occurred naturally in man. Finally, Flexner was able to show that polio was not caused by a bacterium or a protozoan, but rather by a filterable virus. Flexner's last discovery, however, was little more than a suggestion, that a new previously unknown agent might be the cause of polio. Little was known about viruses at the time save that they were ultramicroscopic and passed through filters which normally held back the smallest of bacteria. No one knew if they basically differed from bacteria.[8]

By the fall of 1910, Flexner was face to face with the key question—how was the virus transmitted and how did it enter the body? At the time it appeared that he was on the verge of solving this problem.[9] Indeed, it seemed to many that it was only a matter of a year or two before Flexner would conquer polio. Had he not just vanquished cerebro-spinal meningitis in relatively short-order? Increasingly in 1910 and 1911, when physicians, public health officials, and ordinary men and women, were faced by polio, they turned to Flexner for guidance and advice. When polio struck the three-year-old son of Mrs. Elizabeth Kane in Providence, Rhode Island, during the fall of 1910, the grieving mother sent a letter about her son's case to Flexner, addressing him as a discoverer in medicine. 'I hope' she wrote, 'that if you have not already found the cure for this awful disease you will be given the light to find it.'[10] Dr. H. G. O'Neill of St. Joseph's Hospital in Memphis, Tennessee, was even more positive. Speaking of his anticipations for Flexner's polio research he told the investigator, '... There is a great hope for some serum that will prevent or modify the disease such as we now have in anti-typhoid serum and this the world will expect at your hands.... I believe,' he concluded, 'in the work of the

---

8. Dr. Flexner's early polio research can best be followed in S. Flexner and P. A. Lewis, 'The Transmission of Acute Poliomyelitis to Monkeys,' *J. Am. med. Ass.*, 1909, *53*, 1639; 'The Transmission of Acute Poliomyelitis to Monkeys, a Further Note,' *J. Am. med. Ass.*, 1909, *53*, 1913; 'The Nature of the Virus of Epidemic Poliomyelitis,' *J. Am. med. Ass.*, 1909, *53*, 2095; 'Epidemic Poliomyelitis in Monkeys,' *J. Am. med. Ass.*, 1910, *54*, 45; 'Experimental Epidemic Poliomyelitis in Monkeys,' *J. Exp. Med.*, 1910, *12*, 227.

9. Dr. Flexner at the time appeared to have established by experimental means that the portal of entry of poliovirus in man was through the olfactory lobes. He was mistaken. The error persisted until the late 1930s when Dr. Charles Swan in Australia, and Dr. Albert Sabin in the United States, presented evidence that the olfactory pathway was not the usual portal of entry for poliovirus in man. See further, S. Flexner and P. A. Lewis, 'Epidemic Poliomyelitis in Monkeys: A Mode of Spontaneous Infection,' *J. Am. med. Ass.*, 1910, *54*, 535; C. Swan, 'The Anatomical Distribution and Character of the Lesions of Poliomyelitis,' *Aus. J. exper. Biol. med. Sci.*, 1939, *17*, 345; A. B. Sabin, 'The Olfactory Bulbs in Human Poliomyelitis,' *Am. J. Dis. Child.*, 1940, *60*, 1313.

10. All letters hereinafter cited, unless otherwise noted, are to be found in the Simon Flexner Papers now preserved in the Library of the American Philosophical Society in Philadelphia. Mrs. Elizabeth Kane to Simon Flexner, 18 Sept. 1910.

Rockefeller Institute.'[11] If the hopes in these letters expressed faith in Flexner, they were no less an expression of the great expectations that many people had of the future successes of the experimental research that Flexner, as Director of the Rockefeller Institute, had come to epitomize. There was, however, no gainsaying the enormity of the problem polio increasingly represented.

Between 1910 and 1913, polio appeared in every state of the United States and in every province in Canada, affecting well over 25,000 children and adults.[12] Although much useful clinical and pathological information about the disease had been gathered and disseminated by Flexner and others during these years, polio fundamentally remained a vast terra incognita to practising physicians. Many doctors could not even recognize the disease when called upon to treat it.[13] This medical deficiency was but one of the problems that Carl Carstensen, age six, faced when he entered the S. R. Smith Infirmary on Staten Island, the afternoon of 15 August 1911.

The Smith Infirmary was a familiar place to Carl. Two weeks earlier his tonsils and adenoids had been successfully removed at the hospital. Since that time he had been in good health. He had no physical complaints, his appetite was good, and he ate and played as vigorously as any other six-year-old. The night before he reentered the hospital, however, he suddenly began to vomit and had difficulty breathing. The next morning when his mother found he also had a fever, she called the family physician, Dr. Joseph Bryan.

Initially Dr. Bryan found little that disturbed him. Although the little

11. Dr. H. G. O'Neill to Simon Flexner, 3 May 1910.
12. The figures given above for the early incidence of polio in the United States and Canada are at best impressionistic, given the difficulty that doctors at the time had in making a diagnosis and the lack of an accurate and consistent reporting system. Poliomyelitis was first made a reportable disease by the State of Massachusetts in 1909. Although twenty-four states made the disease reportable in 1910, only three states made such reporting mandatory by name. In other states it was reportable under the broad rubric of infectious and contagious disease. In part, the problem of reporting polio was related to the general neglect at the time of collecting morbidity statistics. See further, J. Collins, 'The Epidemiology of Disease,' *J. Am. med. Ass.*, 1910, 54, 1925; J. W. Trask, 'Morbidity Statistics in the United States,' *Trans. a. Conf. St. territ. Hlth. Offrs.*, 1910, 8, 37–50; C. H. Lavinder, A. W. Freeman, and W. H. Frost, 'Epidemiologic Studies of Poliomyelitis in New York City and the Northeastern United States, During the Year 1916,' *Publ. Hlth. Bull. Wash.*, 1918, no. 91, pp. 50–55, puts the reported figures for polio in the United States between 1910–1913 at 16,579. They do not report figures for the incidence of polio in Canada during these years although Canada was racked by severe epidemics.
13. Doctors frequently had difficulty in differentiating cerebro-spinal meningitis and diphtheria from polio. For examples of the problems they ran into in making diagnosis see further, Dr. W. B. Hambidge to Simon Flexner, 15 Oct. 1909; Simon Flexner to Dr. W. B. Hambidge, 19 Oct. 1909; Dr. Henry W. Elsner to Simon Flexner, 26 Oct. 1909; Simon Flexner to Dr. Henry W. Elsner, 27 Oct. 1909; Dr. C. F. Williams to Simon Flexner, 15 Sept. 1910; Simon Flexner to Dr. C. F. Williams, 19 Sept. 1910; Dr. C. I. Redfield to Simon Flexner, 12 Oct. 1910.

boy had a fever, he did not seem to be seriously ill. His throat was clear, the vomiting had stopped and he did not appear to have any difficulty breathing. When Dr. Bryan asked him to walk, the little boy walked around the room in a normal fashion. As the examination continued, however, Dr. Bryan found two things which gave him pause. He discovered that Carl had difficulty speaking, and when he tried to drink a glass of water he could not swallow and instead regurgitated the water through his nose. Dr. Bryan diagnosed Carl's condition as bulbo-paralysis affecting the pharyngeal muscles and advised his mother to take him to the hospital.

It is not known whether Dr. Bryan informed Mrs. Carstensen of his diagnosis, or whether she gave the physician who admitted Carl to the Smith Infirmary any more information than the immediate history of his illness. It is known that the admitting physician reexamined Carl and on the basis of his examination came to the conclusion that the boy was suffering from laryngeal diphtheria. Following the examination the house physician was called to look at the patient. When he concurred in the admitting officer's diagnosis, Carl was transferred to the contagious disease ward where he was put under the care of Dr. Charles E. Donovan. Dr. Donovan, following the hospital diagnosis, took a throat culture and as an added precaution gave Carl 4,000 units of diphtheria antitoxin.

Save for a rise in temperature, the evening hours passed without incident. During the night, however, Carl became increasingly restless. His body twitched incessantly and he seemed unable to find a position in which he could breathe more easily. At one point Carl's body movements became so violent that Dr. Donovan assigned a nurse to watch him through the night lest he squirm out of bed. The next morning when Dr. Donovan examined Carl during his rounds, he found that the little boy had great difficulty in breathing, and while the twitching had subsided a new and disturbing sign had appeared. 'His legs,' he later noted in the case history, 'were flexed on the thighs, and the thighs on the abdomen, and the hands showed athetoid contractions.' A sponge bath and enema were ordered. While the nurse administered the enema, Carl died.

Carl's death was so unexpected and sudden that Dr. Donovan immediately asked for and received permission to do an autopsy. Within an hour of the patient's death he removed and examined a portion of the brain, the larynx, esophagus and other thoracic organs. It is clear from the organs examined that Dr. Donovan, still following hospital diagnosis, looked for evidence of diphtheria. He was disappointed in his search. The autopsy examination gave no indication of a diphtheria infection. Later that afternoon, when Dr. Bryan informed hospital authorities of his diagnosis of a possible high lesion of anterior poliomyelitis, Dr. Donovan performed a second autopsy. This time he removed the spinal cord; however, he did not stop to examine it. Instead, he wrapped the cord in sterile gauze and drove to the Rockefeller Institute, where he gave it to Dr. Flexner. That evening, almost twelve hours after death, Flexner examined the cord and found the typical lesions of polio in both the anterior and posterior horns. Carl had died of polio, not diphtheria.[14]

It is doubtful whether, if the staff at the Smith Infirmary had made an accurate diagnosis of polio, they could have saved Carl Carstensen's life. Even when physicians had the ability to make a correct diagnosis, they frequently could not either predict the course, or alter the outcome of the disease.[15] There was no effective treatment.

Fortunately, during early polio epidemics death was not very frequent, occurring in only ten to fifteen per cent of all reported cases. A larger number of those who contracted polio (between twenty-five and thirty per cent) recovered from the infection without any outward effects. The majority, however (between sixty and sixty-five per cent), were left crippled.[16] Some with faces frozen in a perpetual grimace, or, ironically, in what appeared to be a smile. Others were left with bent spines that recalled the twisted rails of war-destroyed railroads. Still others were left with shortened and contracted hands useless for feeding, playing, or holding a loved one, or with wasted thigh and leg muscles that left legs hanging like flails unable to support body weight and useless for movement.

Death and crippling were not the only legacies of polio. The protean nature of the disease, coupled with the apparent inability of physicians to mitigate or cure the infection, left another legacy in its wake, a legacy as unpredictable, as savage and as crippling as polio itself—namely, fear. One cannot mark the date when the fear of polio first appeared in the United States. At the beginning of the early epidemics there was but a vague public apprehension of the disease. To be sure various individuals expressed

14. The details of the Carl Carstensen case can be followed in Dr. C. E. Donovan to Simon Flexner, 22 Aug. 1911, with attachment of Carl Carstensen Case History, S. R. Smith Infirmary, 15–16 August 1911. Dr. C. E. Donovan to Simon Flexner, 12 Sept. 1911; Simon Flexner to Dr. C. E. Donovan, 2 Oct. 1911.

15. For examples of physicians who correctly diagnosed their patients to have polio and subsequently lost them see, K. C. Mead to Simon Flexner, 24 Sept. 1910; Dr. M. E. Armstrong to Simon Flexner, 7 Nov. 1911; Simon Flexner to Dr. M. E. Armstrong, 29 Nov. 1911.

16. The figures given for the outcome of early polio epidemics are at best approximate. See further, I. Wickman, *Acute Poliomyelitis* (Nervous and Mental Disease Monograph, no. 16), (New York, 1913), pp. 91–98.

concern about polio, but these expressions were not as solemn, awesome, or as frequent as those made about other diseases such as tuberculosis, pneumonia, or diphtheria. However, as polio became more widespread in 1910 and 1911, and as an increasing number of cripples joined the victims of previous outbreaks, the disease became more visible and menacing. The fear expressed privately by individuals became public and pervasive, and all too soon a common component in analysis of the cause of the disease, or suggested action against it.

The expression of the fear varied from individual to individual, and frequently it mirrored concerns with other problems that beset contemporary American society. Following the appearance of an article by Dr. John Huber on Infantile Paralysis in the November 1910 issue of *Review of Reviews*, Mrs. A. O. Longmuir of Chouteau, Montana, decided to write a letter to Dr. Simon Flexner at the Rockefeller Institute. The failure of doctors to explain satisfactorily the appearance of polio encouraged Mrs. Longmuir to believe that her own observations might prove to be of some help to Flexner in his research. Briefly Mrs. Longmuir thought the cause of polio was to be found in the habits and customs of her Norwegian neighbors.

> One year ago, [she wrote], we had an epidemic of this disease. It attacked children from one to sixteen years of age. Out of thirty-six cases there was only one American child that had it. As I know nothing about the scientific side of the disease, I wish to write about their (Norwegian) mode of living.
>
> They seem to know very little about sanitation or ventilation. I have seen the father, mother, and four children sleeping in a room twelve by fourteen with every door and window closed and a big fire burning in the stove. They all sleep about the same way.
>
> Under the kitchen floor they dig a cellar with neither light nor air. In this they keep bread, butter, meat, milk and potatoes. It seems to me this alone would be a source of infection. They care very little for fresh fruit or vegetables. Their diet consists chiefly of bread, pork, potatoes, cake and coffee. Even the children drink quantities of coffee. As a rule they have no power of resistance when attacked by disease. More than one half of them suffer from some form of kidney disease.
>
> If this should help in the least to solve why 'more cases of infantile paralysis develop among the Scandinavians than other people [Mrs. Longmuir continued] I shall be glad that I wrote.'[17]

Dr. Flexner's reply was cordial and noncommittal. 'I want to thank

17. Mrs. A. O. Longmuir to Simon Flexner, 14 Nov. 1910.

you,' he wrote, 'for your very valuable letter describing the conditions you have observed among the Norwegian immigrants in connection with the epidemic of infantile paralysis.'[18] It is not Mrs. Longmuir's fear of the life style of her Norwegian neighbors or Flexner's temperate reply to her letter that disturbs. What is unsettling is the seeming reasonableness of Mrs. Longmuir's analysis. The earliest recognized polio epidemics occurred in Norway and Sweden in the late nineteenth and the early twentieth century. What more reasonable supposition for the appearance of polio in the United States than the alien habits and living conditions of recent Scandinavian immigrants. Sometimes immigrants were blamed for no other reason than the fact that they were strangers, and as strangers were thought to be responsible for a wide variety of crimes.[19] In other places, it was not the immigrant who was blamed for the dissemination of polio, but the dispossessed, and, in particular, blacks.[20]

There can be no doubt that one of the effects of polio epidemics was that it helped reinforce existing social fears. But this should not obscure the fact that, once polio invaded an area, no one was exempt from becoming a victim of the fear generated by the disease. Even in relatively homogeneous and well educated communities neighbor turned on neighbor.[21] In the absence of an understanding of the nature of polio, men and women became their own physicians, weaving out of old medical beliefs and half understood social observations, a dark embroidery of explanations—explanations that created a pathology as surely as that caused by polio virus. Inexorably, these explanations became a part of the disease itself, an added burden to be overcome by the physicians and public health officials called on to treat and care for new crops of polio victims.

18. Simon Flexner to Mrs. A. O. Longmuir, 22 Nov. 1910.
19. During the first two decades of the twentieth century, Italian immigrants were blamed for a wide variety of crimes ranging from murder and arson to the dissemination of pellagra and polio. For a typical example of ethnocentric thinking on the part of a physician in rural New York State see Dr. Milton Gregg's case record of the polio illness of Mary Hill of Eldridge, New York, where the blame for the disease is placed on 'an Italian road construction gang in the neighborhood.' (Case Records - Polio - 1911) Flexner papers.
20. Following an outbreak of polio in St. Mary's County, Maryland, on 1 Sept. 1910, the blame for the dissemination of the disease was placed on a black farmer named Cotton Yates. See further, Dr. W. C. Rucker to The Surgeon General, 8 Oct. 1910; *The Baltimore News*, 8 Oct. 1910; *The Baltimore Sun*, 8 Oct. 1910 (General Classified Records of the United States Public Health Service 1897–1934, Record Group 90, National Archives).
21. During a polio epidemic in Princeton, New Jersey in the summer of 1910, the family of Professor Christian Gauss of Princeton University was ostracized by colleagues and neighbors after Professor Gauss' young son was stricken by polio. The ostracism continued long after the boy recovered. Christian Gauss to Simon Flexner, 30 Sept. 1910; Simon Flexner to Christian Gauss, 3 Oct. 1910.

Much has been written of how children were and are prized in the United States. Some historians have even argued that this celebration of children is one of the distinguishing features of the American character. Although the theory is attractive and provocative, there is little evidence to sustain it, especially for the period of the first two decades of the twentieth century. Indeed, for this period, the weight of evidence suggests not a celebration but rather an extraordinary exploitation of children. In 1910, for example, the United States census reported that approximately two million children under the age of sixteen were employed in the nation's industries.[22] Dr. Walter Trattner in a grim litany, has described the legal relations which guided child labor in various states at the time.

> Twenty-two states (including the four leading southern textile producing ones) still permitted children under fourteen to work in factories; thirty states still allowed boys under sixteen to work in mines; thirty-one states still authorized children under sixteen to work more than eight hours a day; twenty-eight states still let children work at night; twenty-three states still did not require adequate documentary proof of age. The employment of children in the street trades—with the exception of the night messenger service—in the canneries and in tenement sweatshops were still virtually unregulated. Child labor on the nation's farms had eluded legislation altogether.[23]

The reality and meaning of these figures is seen in the photographs by Lewis Hine, Jacob Riis, and Arnold Genthe, showing eight and nine-year-old girls tending rooms of cotton spindles in Georgia; begrimed 'breaker boys' working coal cars in the half dark of Pennsylvania mines; and, abandoned waifs sleeping in the stairwells leading to the cellars of New York tenements.[24] Communities of children without childhood. These were the healthy ones. What of the attitudes towards those children who were left crippled and deformed by polio?

There is no known scale by which one can measure the bewilderment and despair of families whose children were left paralyzed by polio. Very often when polio struck, whole families rallied around the victims and fought the disease with every means at their disposal. When polio crippled the ten-year-old daughter of the Hausen family in Winnipeg, Manitoba,

---

22. Department of Commerce, *Thirteenth Census of the United States, Population: Occupation Statistics*, 1910, 4, 168–181 (Washington, D.C., 1914).

23. W. Trattner, *Crusade for the Children* (Chicago, 1970), pp. 115–16.

24. J. M. Gutman, *Lewis W. Hine and the American Social Conscience* (New York, 1967); J. A. Riis, *How the Other Half Lives* (New York, 1971). This is a special edition published by Dover books and contains 100 photographs from the incomparable Riis photographic collection in the Museum of the City of New York.

Mr. and Mrs. Hausen took their child to more than a score of physicians seeking relief in electricity, massage, and braces. When these remedies failed, the child's grandfather took up the cudgels, writing for advice to physicians both in Canada and the United States and finally to Dr. Flexner at the Rockefeller Institute. After recounting his granddaughter's case history, Mr. Hausen bluntly asked Dr. Flexner:

Now what I would like to know is, do you treat these cases in New York? Do you take the patient in charge, board them, etc. and do they get any teaching? How long would the child have to be there, and what would be [the] cost per month during her stay? No doubt it will take at least a couple of years' treatment, but if you can hold out any hope that she might be cured sufficiently to help herself, even if she should show some defects I should like to assist her parents to send her to New York for treatment.[25]

Mr. Hausen's response to the crippling of his granddaughter was not unique. It was shared by others facing similar problems. A Mrs. Louis Weil in St. Louis, a Mrs. Albert E. Hackney in Washington County, Pennsylvania, a Mr. Barry Clemente in New York.[26] How many others is not known. There are no figures. Man's humanity, his capacity for love, his devotion in the face of adversity has not been quantified. There were, however, other responses to crippling. On 3 September 1910, Dr. F. F. Attix, a graduate of the University of Pennsylvania Medical School telegraphed his former teacher Dr. Flexner from Lewiston, Montana.

'Have a brilliant patient age 7, attacked eight days ago with acute infantile paralysis, both lower limbs involved, parents are willing to submit case to you for experimental work. If I bring the case to you, will you accept case, wire reply my expense.'[27]

'I very much regret to say that there is nothing I can do for your patient,' Dr. Flexner replied. 'The subject of the serum treatment is not yet on a basis that would justify its application to human beings, and there is no other way in which I could be of help to the patient.'[28]

In the first decade of the twentieth century numerous petitions were presented to the federal government and various state legislatures to restrict or prevent animal experimentation.[29] One can only imagine the de-

---

25. H. P. Hausen to Simon Flexner, 26 Sept. 1910.
26. Mrs. Louis Weil to Simon Flexner, 11 Nov. 1910; Mrs. Albert E. Hackney to Simon Flexner, 9 Nov. 1910; B. Clement to Simon Flexner, 17 Oct. 1910.
27. Dr. F. F. Attix to Simon Flexner, 3 Sept. 1910 (Telegram).
28. Simon Flexner to Dr. F. F. Attix, 3 Sept. 1910.
29. W. J. Schultz, *The Humane Movement in the United States, 1910–1922* (New York, 1924), pp. 141–61.

spair that moved these unknown parents to offer their child for experiment. Yet there were others who, losing hope, or perhaps lacking a sense of responsibility, acted as desperately. In 1909 Miss Elland Yandell, the daughter of Dr. Lunceford Yandell Jr. of Louisville, while visiting the local poor house with a friend, found Bennie MacLain, age six, hopelessly crippled 'creeping on the floor like a baby.' He had been abandoned by his mother several years before, following an attack of polio. Touched by the boy's condition, the two women sought out the mother and asked if they could take him to a hospital in New York. Bennie MacLain was fortunate; Miss Yandell and her friend took him to the New York Hospital for the Ruptured and Crippled, where Dr. Virgil Gibney, one of the finest orthopedists of the day, undertook a series of reparative operations. After the operations, the two women sought further help from Dr. Flexner. '. . . . Do you think you can do anything for the child,' they asked, 'he is very clever, very fine, and well worth all the help he can receive.[30]

In a deep sense Bennie MacLain's case epitomizes the problems of those afflicted by polio. By some mischance, an unknown agent had brought them to a strange world. It had not only succeeded in transforming them physically in unpredictable and even grotesque ways, it had changed the people around them as well. In this new world some parents continued to love and cherish them as before, while others inexplicably became strangers and abandoned them. Sometimes when all hope was gone, a stranger upon whom they had no conceivable claim, might stop and give them help.

During the first decade of the twentieth century, there were few people in the United States who had as keen an appreciation as Simon Flexner of the medical and social problems caused by ignorance of the clinical nature of polio. Although Flexner was primarily a pathologist, he deemed clinical knowledge to be so important for the eventual control of polio, that in the spring of 1911, he decided, as Director of the Rockefeller Institute, to commit the resources of the then recently opened Rockefeller Hospital to an investigation of the clinical aspects of polio. To insure a flow of patients to the Hospital, he circularized physicians, hospitals, and public health officials in and around New York City about the projected investigation.[31]

---

30. Miss Elland Yandell to Simon Flexner, 25 Nov. 1910; Simon Flexner to Miss Elland Yandell, 26 Nov. 1910.

31. There are many letters to physicians and public health officials during June and July 1911 of Flexner's projected plans to study polio at the Rockefeller Hospital during the summer months. For a typical letter see the one addressed to Dr. William A. Howe, Deputy Commissioner of Health for N.Y. State, 20 June 1911.

'I am planning to spend the summer in town in order to study acute cases of poliomyelitis,' he wrote one physician friend. 'I may add,' he continued, 'that acute cases of infantile paralysis will be admitted to the Rockefeller Hospital and that we would like to have you refer them there if you can. You probably know that no charge is made for medical service, room or nursing, and the facilities are excellent for the care of the patients.'[32]

Many of the responses to Dr. Flexner's circular were enthusiastic. Linnaeus La Fetra, one of the leading pediatricians in New York, replied, 'You may be sure that I will do everything I can to cooperate with you in the matter of referring cases of poliomyelitis to the Rockefeller Hospital. I will speak to the men at the Vanderbilt Clinic as well as be on the lookout at my own service at Bellevue.'[33] Many public health officials from nearby states and cities replied in the same vein. Still there were a number of physicians who found that they could not fully cooperate with Dr. Flexner's plans. Dr. S. S. Goldwater, the Director of the Mt. Sinai Hospital in New York, promised to send patients to the Rockefeller Hospital only when his own wards were full. His reasons were simple and direct. 'We must recognize the prior rights of our own staff,' he informed Dr. Flexner.[34] Others like Dr. Charles C. Caverly of the Vermont State Board of Health questioned the wisdom of transporting acute polio cases to the Rockefeller Hospital from out of state. '. . . . Let me ask,' he wrote, 'if such cases would be admitted after the four weeks quarantine has been raised? We quarantine strictly for four weeks. It would hardly be safe to move them to New York on a railroad train prior to that.'[35] Flexner was well aware of the problem. '. . . . I realize the difficulties in sending us cases earlier in the course of the disease,' he replied. 'I would appreciate it very much if you would inform me of any considerable number of cases occurring together during the summer, which I might be able to study by going to that section where they prevail.'[36]

If Flexner's plans for a clinical study of polio created dilemmas in the medical community, it also brought to a head a problem that had agitated the Rockefeller Institute from the inception of the Rockefeller Hospital. In 1908 when the Rockefeller Hospital was originally planned, Dr. Flexner and Dr. Christian Herter, the two members of the Board of Scientific Directors who were most intimately concerned with the definition of the

---

32. Simon Flexner to Dr. Louis Fischer, 29 June 1911.
33. Dr. Linnaeus E. La Fetra to Simon Flexner, 1 June 1911.
34. Dr. S. S. Goldwater to Simon Flexner, 7 July 1911.
35. Dr. Charles S. Caverly to Simon Flexner, 7 July 1911.
36. Simon Flexner to Dr. Charles S. Caverly, 11 July 1911.

role of the Hospital within the structure of the Rockefeller Institute, saw the duties of the physicians and the laboratories of the Hospital as being chiefly clinical. In their view, research on diseases treated at the Hospital was to be initiated and conducted by members of the various existing laboratories of the Institute.[37] Dr. Rufus Cole, who became the first director of the Rockefeller Hospital in 1909, saw the matter in a different light. For Cole, both the physicians and the laboratories of the Hospital, in addition to their clinical duties, were also to have the responsibility of initiating and conducting basic scientific research.[38]

The debate on the research functions of the Hospital staff continued for the better part of two years. Ironically, it was Flexner's decision to open the Rockefeller Hospital for a study of the clinical aspects of polio, that finally resolved the debate in Cole's favor. Although it was tacitly recognized at the Institute that Flexner's laboratory had primacy in polio research (and while Flexner himself later participated in the clinical investigation as a pathologist), the actual conduct of the clinical study became the responsibility of three Hospital residents whom Cole appointed to the task —Dr. Francis Peabody, Dr. George Draper, and Dr. Alphonse Dochez.

The men were well suited to their jobs. Peabody, a graduate of the Harvard Medical School, had interned at the Massachusetts General Hospital and the Johns Hopkins Hospital, and in addition had a term of biochemical research in the laboratories of Emil Fischer. Draper was equally well trained. A graduate of the Columbia College of Physicians and Surgeons, Draper had previously served at the Presbyterian Hospital in New York and the Pennsylvania Hospital in Philadelphia, and had worked with the immunologist, Paul Ehrlich, in Frankfurt. Dochez, a graduate of the Johns Hopkins Medical School, had no clinical experience but was nevertheless superbly trained as an investigator. He had previously engaged in bacteriological research with both William MacCallum at Johns Hopkins and Eugene Opie at the Rockefeller Institute.[39]

In 1911 the investigation got underway slowly. Initially, few polio cases were admitted to the Hospital, so few, that throughout June and early July, Dr. Flexner devoted himself almost exclusively to his ongoing polio transmission experiments, while Dr. Draper was allowed to go off on

---

37. G. Corner, *A History of the Rockefeller Institute, 1901–1953* (New York, 1964), pp. 90–92.
38. *Ibid.*, pp. 93–94; S. Benison, *Tom Rivers: Reflections on a Life in Medicine and Science* (Cambridge, Mass., 1967), pp. 67–70.
39. C. Robinson, *Adventures in Medical Education* (Cambridge, 1957), pp. 94–97; Corner, (n. 5), pp. 100–104; Saul Benison, *The Reminiscences of Dr. A. R. Dochez* (New York, Columbia University Oral History Memoir, 1956), pp. 1–39.

vacation. As late as 4 July, there were but five cases in the Hospital.[40] By 21 July, the figure rose to ten. Although the patients were afflicted with all grades of paralysis, few of them appeared to be in imminent danger of their lives.[41] If there was any problem at this time it was the difficulty Dr. Flexner had in securing permission to perform an autopsy on the one polio victim who had died in the Hospital. Towards the end of the month, however, the situation changed drastically. On 27 July Dr. Flexner in a letter to Jerome Greene, the secretary of the Institute, described the new conditions that obtained at the Hospital.

.... The isolation ward is at present quite full of poliomyelitis cases, and we had to decline two acute cases yesterday. The whole country hereabout is stirred up and we are offered everything. The conditions, therefore, are as good as possible. I hardly know whether the disease is increasing with the advance of the summer or whether more persons are aware of the fact that the Hospital is a center, and therefore, we are receiving a larger number of applications. I was able to secure a very important autopsy Tuesday on an acute case of the disease on Staten Island which will help us very much in our studies.[42]

In another letter to his wife he added, 'The ward is as charming as any hospital ward can be and in most instances the children are improving. It is a stimulating place. Peabody is working well, but he needs assistance which we are trying to get for him.'[43]

Several days later, Dr. Flexner's budget of news was grimmer.

.... The poliomyelitis situation at the Hospital is entering on its tragic stage. The isolation pavilion is full and other quarters will probably have to be found. The tragedy is the severe and fatal cases. One child (an infant) died this morning and I have just come from the side of a lovely boy of five who is dying. My heart has been torn into shreds. The little fellow has extensive paralysis that has affected the nerves of the diaphragm. He is a little pale-haired almost red-haired fellow, obviously the idol of his grief-stricken parents, two simple dear American people. The Hospital staff has suddenly wakened up to the importance and seriousness of the disease—it is a tragedy. And yet there is no epidemic, but many cases scattered through this immense population.[44]

Although in August 1911 a number of well defined groups of polio cases appeared in and around New York, Flexner remained adamant in his con-

---

40. Simon Flexner to Helen Flexner, 24 June, 4 July, 9 July 1911.
41. Simon Flexner to Helen Flexner, 21 July 1911.
42. Simon Flexner to Jerome Greene, 27 July 1911.
43. Simon Flexner to Helen Flexner, 27 July 1911.
44. Simon Flexner to Helen Flexner, 31 July 1911.

viction that there was no epidemic. He felt so strongly on this subject that when the *New York Times* in mid-August reported that there were more cases in New York in 1911 than were reported in the City during the polio epidemics of 1910, Flexner exploded and attacked the editors of the *Times*. To his wife he explained,

There is no indication that polio is increasing although there were four requests for admission yesterday. The Times report about a greater number of cases this year than last is utterly unreliable and caused by the fact that all our cases are reported (which are the only ones reported we are told, and of course last year none were reported, as would also have been the case this year, but for our studies.) All which goes to show there are no real data of the number of cases in the country. All is conjecture except that there appears to be no epidemic outbreak.[45]

Epidemic or not, patients continued to enter the Rockefeller Hospital in a steady stream throughout August. Their presence had an electric effect on Flexner. 'I am conscious of an unfolding of my ideas of the disease which I have not had before,' he exulted in one letter.[46] In another letter he detailed the significance of the autopsies he steadily performed.

To begin I should say that the fatal case of poliomyelitis yesterday on wh[ich] an autopsy was secured will give excellent material both for inoculation and for working out better the nature (pathology) of the human disease. The monkeys inoculated previously from the specimens secured at autopsy have, in several instances, come down with polio in the correct manner. We are learning the limits of the activity of the virus as it comes directly from human beings and before it has adapted to the monkey, which facts will cause me to modify the notions I have had for demonstrating its presence as in the nasal secretions, etc. . . .[47]

If the autopsies helped transform Flexner's ideas about polio, the daily exposure to patients provided an added psychological impetus to the investigation. On 24 August, Flexner wrote of another tragedy at the Hospital.

The work has nothing new except another autopsy . . . on a child (one of the twins I wrote about) of 8 months. It died, as the others, of paralysis of all the muscles of the diaphragm. The parents are young Russian Hebrews. Today they came to take the second child who had developed paralysis of the legs away. They pawned a ring to get money to employ a nurse and get 'a professor from

45. Simon Flexner to Helen Flexner, 20 Aug. 1911.
46. Simon Flexner to Helen Flexner, 9 Aug. 1911.
47. Simon Flexner to Helen Flexner, 10 Aug. 1911. For a letter with similar remarks on the value of autopsies, Simon Flexner to Helen Flexner, 22 Aug. 1911.

Mt. Sinai.' I saw the young distracted father and all he could say was that 'he was a father and felt as one, and having lost the one child he must try to save the other.' I thought it best to let him take the child and did not dissuade him.[48]

Flexner was not the only one touched by these experiences. All of the investigators were affected. Working at both the bedside and in the laboratory, Peabody, Draper, and Dochez made extraordinary efforts on behalf of their charges, often laboring to the point of exhaustion. When it appeared, toward the end of the summer, that a new diagnostic procedure might be developed, Peabody postponed a long needed vacation, and continued to work long hours at the Hospital until Cole, fearing for his health, ordered him to leave for vacation. By early fall the investigation was completed.[49] In all, 161 cases of polio were treated at the Hospital, and of these seventy-one were admitted for stays of from three to four weeks, while the rest were cared for on an outpatient basis in the dispensary. Twelve died.[50]

There can be little doubt that both Cole and Flexner were pleased by the summer's work. In October 1911, Cole proposed to the Board of Scientific Directors that the results of Peabody's, Draper's and Dochez' investigations be published in the form of a monograph. 'No good study of the disease in the English language is now available,' he told the Board, 'and it is hoped that such a work may make a valuable clinical contribution.'[51] Cole had yet another reason. He felt that the publication of such a study would make friends for the Rockefeller Hospital in the medical community and that doctors in future would cooperate more readily with the Hospital in other clinical investigations.[52]

On 1 June 1912, Peabody's, Draper's and Dochez's study appeared as a volume in the Rockefeller Institute Monograph Series under the title *A Clinical Study of Acute Poliomyelitis*. Although the book contained no more than 187 pages, it was packed with an extraordinary amount of information. In addition to a brief historical and epidemiological review of polio, it contained among other things, pathological information on acute cases, detailed analysis of both the blood and cerebrospinal fluid at different

---

48. Simon Flexner to Helen Flexner, 24 Aug. 1911.
49. Simon Flexner to Helen Flexner, 29 Aug. 1911. Some of George Draper's clinical investigations toward the end of the summer of 1911 may be followed in George Draper to Simon Flexner, 13 Sept., 18 Sept., 19 Sept. 1911.
50. F. W. Peabody, G. Draper, A. R. Dochez, *A Clinical Study of Acute Poliomyelitis* (New York, 1912), pp. 1–2.
51. Rufus Cole, 'Report to the Board of Scientific Directors of the Rockefeller Institute: Oct. 14, 1911,' in *Repts. Dir. of the Lab. and Dir. of the Hosp.*, II, 285.
52. Rufus Cole, 'Report to the Board of Scientific Directors of the Rockefeller Institute, April 12, 1912,' in *Repts. Dir. of the Lab. and Dir. of the Hosp.*, III, 68.

stages of the infection, suggestions for making prognoses of various types of polio, therapeutic recommendations, as well as full accounts of thirty-four cases. The heart of the volume, however, lay in its effort to draw a more intelligible clinical picture of polio.

In 1912 there were two major systems of polio classification. The first, a system devised by the Swedish polio pioneer, Dr. Iver Wickman, held that there were eight forms of the disease which he described as spinal, acute ascending, bulbar, encephalitic, ataxic, polyneuritic, meningitic, and abortive.[53] The second, a classification developed by the German clinical investigator Dr. Edward Müller, tried to simplify Wickman's system. He argued there were but four forms of polio which he designated as spinal, cerebral, bulbar, and abortive.[54] While both systems contained a number of common elements, they differed in one fundamental respect. The former was based on a mixture of clinical symptoms and pathological anatomy, while the latter developed almost exclusively from an anatomical basis. For their own part, Peabody, Draper and Dochez maintained that a better appreciation of the clinical nature of polio could be obtained if one recognized but three groups of cases which they characterized simply as abortive, cerebral, and bulbospinal.[55]

In one sense the classificatory system offered by Peabody, Draper and Dochez was a makeshift. They knew full well, for example, that many polio cases were not purely of one type either clinically or anatomically. More important, they realized that it was all but impossible to make a classification that would be applicable to all cases. 'The best one could do,' they admitted in their study, 'is to attempt to reconcile the chief clinical symptoms with the predominant anatomical lesion.'[56] Yet for all of this, Peabody, Draper and Dochez did succeed in clarifying the disease for the practising physician. Their success lay not so much in their simpler system of classification, as in their descriptions and analysis of the symptomatology and the different courses various types of polio took. One measure of the nature of these descriptions is to be found in their characterization of the sensorium of children fatally afflicted with respiratory paralysis.

With the onset of respiratory difficulty, it seems almost as if the children were suddenly awakened and made to realize the struggle before them. Little chil-

53. I. Wickman (n. 16), pp. 38–39.
54. P. H. Römer, *Epidemic Infantile Paralysis* (New York, 1913), pp. 13–19: F. W. Peabody, G. Draper, A. R. Dochez (n. 50), pp. 27–28.
55. F. W. Peabody, G. Draper, A. R. Dochez (n. 50), p. 29.
56. *Ibid.*, p. 30.

dren seem to age in a few hours. One sees a heedless, careless sleepy baby become all at once wide awake, high strung, alert to the matter in hand, and this is breathing. The whole mind and body appear to be concentrated on respiration. Respiration becomes an active voluntary process and every breath represents hard work. The child gives the impression of one who has a fight on his hands, and who knows perfectly well how to manage it. All he wants is to be left alone, not to be interfered with, to be allowed to carry out the fight on his own lines. Instinctively, he husbands his strength, refuses food and speaks, when speech is necessary, quietly and with few words. One little child of four, so helplessly paralyzed that she was unable to move, but with a mind that seemed to take in the whole situation, said to the nurse, clearly but rather abruptly, between her hard taken breaths, 'My arm hurts'; 'Turn me over'; 'Scratch my nostril'; and then when the doctor approached, 'Let me alone, doctor!' 'Don't touch my chest.' Pressure on the chest, tight neck bands, anything that obstructs easy respiration is immediately resented. The child demands constant attention, is irritated unless everything is done exactly as he wishes it, and often shows an instinctive appreciation for some especially efficient nurse. He is nervous, fearful, and dreads being left alone. The mouth becomes filled with frothy saliva which the child is unable to swallow, so he collects it between his lips and waits for the nurse to wipe it away. He likes to have his lips wet with cold water, but rarely takes it into his mouth, for he knows he cannot swallow it. During the whole course it is remarkable that cyanosis is absent. There is a little bluish tinging of the lips and tongue, but much more distinctive is the pallor, which is sometimes striking. Sweating is profuse. Then, as respiration gets weaker, the mind becomes dull, and with the occasional return of a lucid interval, he gradually drifts into unconsciousness.[57]

The clarity and compassion of the descriptions gripped physicians everywhere and following publication, the monograph quickly became the bible on polio throughout the United States.

In 1956, Dr. Dochez, asked to evaluate the research he had participated in forty-five years earlier, bluntly replied, 'I do not think it was a significant contribution.'[58] Compared to Dochez's later distinguished contributions to an understanding of pneumonia, scarlet fever, and influenza, the clinical investigation of polio was perhaps of a lesser order. Nevertheless despite Dochez's judgment, there can be no doubt of the value and importance of that work. Its full significance is perhaps best seen if one examines what led to the investigation. In addition to Dr. Flexner, one of the key physicians was Dr. Rufus Cole. Cole never investigated polio himself,

57. Ibid., pp. 71–72.
58. Benison, *Reminiscences of Dr. Dochez* (n. 39), p. 58.

neither at the Johns Hopkins Medical School and Hospital where he was trained, nor at the Rockefeller Hospital where he served as director. Still Cole was an extraordinary force in Peabody, Draper and Dochez's achievement. It was Cole who had the vision of initiating and carrying out clinical research at the Rockefeller Hospital with the Hospital staff. And it was Cole who infused that staff with the enthusiasm and élan necessary to carry such research forward. Clinical research did not begin at the Rockefeller Hospital. The polio investigation conducted by Peabody, Draper and Dochez had the virtue however of setting a standard for such research. It not only established a model for the future clinical investigation of polio but of other diseases as well.[59] In addition it provided a human dimension to other ongoing polio research at the Institute. In so doing, it helped solidify the status of the Rockefeller Institute as a center for polio research in the United States.

Department of History
University of Cincinnati
Cincinnati, Ohio

59. *Ibid.*, pp. 55–56; C. Robinson (n. 39), pp. 87–89.

Malaria

- African Fever
- Ague & Fever
- Bilious Fever
- Chaugres Fever
- Country Fever
- Genesee Fever
- Hungarian Fever
- Intermittent Fever
- Jungle Fever
- Kentish Disorder
- Lake Fever
- Malignant Fever
- Marsh Fever
- Paludal Fever
- Walchern Fever

Glossary of Historical Fever Terminology

A recurring problem for the medical historian is that of correlating old names for diseases with modern disease entities. When confronted with such puzzles as "gastrointestinal remittent hectic fever," "mucous fever," or "pneumo-enteritis contagiosa," one may feel quite justified in giving way to despair. The following list, compiled as a matter of convenience, may prove helpful in sorting out some of the names for one kind of diseases—the fevers. Multiple definitions are a reflection of the confusion in disease differentiation before the establishment of the germ theory. Readers are invited to contribute additions or corrections to this list. It is hoped that eventually a similar compilation may be made for the names of diseases which are not fevers.

A

ABDOMINAL TYPHUS FEVER—typhoid
ADYNAMIC FEVER—typhus
AFRICAN FEVER—malaria
AGUE—malaria
AGUE AND FEVER—malaria
ANGINA SUFFOCATIVA—diphtheria

B

BARBADOS DISTEMPER—yellow fever
BILIOUS FEVER—typhoid; malaria
BILIOUS OR RECURRENT FEVER—relapsing fever
BILIOUS REMITTENT FEVER — malaria; undulant fever
BLACK DEATH—bubonic plague
BLACK FEVER—leishmaniasis
BLACK VOMIT—yellow fever
BLOODY FLUX—dysentery
BRAIN FEVER—epidemic cerebrospinal meningitis
BREAKBONE FEVER—dengue

C

CALENTURE—yellow fever, deficiency diseases
CAMP FEVER — typhus; typhomalarial fever (obsolete)
CEREBROSPINAL FEVER — epidemic cerebrospinal meningitis
CHANGRES FEVER—malignant malaria
CHARBON—anthrax
CHICAHOMINY FEVER—typhomalarial fever (obsolete)
CHILDBED FEVER—puerperal sepsis
CHILL FEVER—malaria
CHIN COUGH—whooping cough
CHOLERA—cholera Asiatica
CHOLERA MORBUS—24-hour flu
COLD PLAGUE—epidemic cerebrospinal meningitis
CONGESTIVE FEVER—typhoid; epidemic cerebrospinal meningitis
CONSUMPTION — tuberculosis of the lungs; cancer of the lungs
CONTINUED FEVER—typhoid
COUNTRY FEVER—malaria

D

DANDY FEVER—dengue
DEVIL'S GRIP—infectious pleurodynia
DOTHINENTERIA—typhoid
DUMDUM FEVER—leishmaniasis

E

EIGHT DAYS' SICKNESS—tetanus
ENTERIC FEVER—typhoid
EPHEMERAL FEVER—febricula
EPIDEMIC DIAPHRAGMATIC SPASM—infectious pleurodynia
EXANTHEMATIC TYPHUS—typhus

F

FAMINE FEVER—relapsing fever
FEVER AND AGUE—malaria
FLOOD FEVER—Tsutsugamushi fever
FLUX—dysentery
FRAMBOESIA—yaws
FRENCH POX—syphilis

G

GAOL FEVER—typhus
GENESEE FEVER—malaria
GLANDULAR FEVER—infectious mononucleosis
GREAT POX—syphilis

H

HECTIC COMMON INFLAMMATORY FEVER—advanced tuberculosis of the lungs
HECTIC FEVER—fevers from pyogenic infections; advanced tuberculosis of the lungs
HIS-WERNER DISEASE—trench fever
HOSPITAL FEVER—typhus
HOSPITAL GANGRENE—fusospirochetal disease
HUNGARIAN FEVER—malaria

I

ILEO-TYPHUS FEVER—typhoid
INFLAMMATORY FEVER—fevers from pyogenic infections
INTERMITTENT FEVER—malaria
IRISH FEVER—typhus; relapsing fever

J

JAIL FEVER—typhus
JAPANESE RIVER FEVER—Tsutsugamushi fever
JUNGLE FEVER—malaria

K

KALA-AZAR—leishmaniasis
KENTISH DISORDER—malaria

L

LAKE FEVER—malaria
LOCKED JAW—tetanus
LUNG FEVER—pneumonia

M

MALIGNANT BILIOUS FEVER—yellow fever
MALIGNANT FEVER—malaria
MALIGNANT PUSTULE—anthrax
MARSH FEVER—malaria
MEDITERRANEAN FEVER — undulant fever
MEMBRANOUS CROUP—diphtheria
MIXED FEVER—typhus

N

NERVOUS FEVER—mild typhus

P

PALUDAL FEVER—malaria
PAPPATACI FEVER—phlebotomus fever
PESTILENTIAL FEVER—typhus
PETECHIAL FEVER—epidemic cerebrospinal meningitis
PHTHISIS—tuberculosis of the lungs
PLAGUE—bubonic plague
PUTRID FEVER—typhus
PYTHOGENIC FEVER—typhoid

Q

QUINTAN FEVER—trench fever

R

RECURRING FEVER—relapsing fever
REMITTENT FEVER—malaria

S

ST. ANTHONY'S FIRE—erysipelas
ST. VITUS'S DANCE—acute chorea
SANDFLY FEVER—phlebotomus fever
SCARLATINE RHEUMATICA—dengue
SCROFULA—tuberculosis of the lymph glands
SEPTIC FEVER—fevers from pyogenic infections
SEVEN DAY FEVER—relapsing fever; disease caused by leptospira hebdomadis
SHIN-BONE FEVER—trench fever
SHIP FEVER—typhus
SLEEPY SICKNESS—epidemic encephalitis
SORE THROAT DISTEMPER — diphtheria
SPIRILLUM FEVER—relapsing fever
SPLENIC FEVER—anthrax
SPOTTED FEVER — typhus; epidemic cerebrospinal meningitis
SPOTTED TYPHOID—typhus
STRANGER'S FEVER—yellow fever
SWEATING SICKNESS—miliary fever
SYDENHAM'S CHOREA—acute chorea
SYNOCHUS FEVER—fever from pyogenic infections; typhoid
SYNOCHUS-HECTICA—typhoid
SYNOCHUS PUTRIS—yellow fever

T

TABARDILLO—typhus
THREE-DAY FEVER—phlebotomus fever
TICK FEVER—Rocky Mountain spotted fever
TYPHOID AFFECTION OF LOUIS—typhoid
TYPHOMALARIAL FEVER — obsolete combination of typhoid and malaria; (rarely) Rocky Mountain spotted fever
TYPHOUS FEVER—typhoid
TYPHUS BILIOSUS—infectious jaundice
TYPHUS GRAVIOR—typhus
TYPHUS ICTEROIDES—yellow fever
TYPHUS MITIOR—typhoid
TYPHUS PETECHIALIS—epidemic cerebrospinal meningitis

U

ULCERATIVE ANGINA—diphtheria

V

VARIOLA—smallpox

W

WALCHERN FEVER—malaria
WHITE SWELLINGS—tuberculosis of the bones
WOLHYNIAN FEVER—trench fever
WOOL-SORTER'S DISEASE—anthrax

Y

YELLOW JACK—yellow fever

PHYLLIS A. RICHMOND

Smallpox Inoculation in Colonial Boston

JOHN B. BLAKE*

WHEN inoculation of smallpox was first tried in Boston in 1721, it caused a violent controversy. Not only was its medical value disputed, but other issues were also involved, including theology, politics, the interference of the clergy in the secular affairs of the community, and the professional status of the physicians.[1] Many of these complications were peculiar to this incident alone, and within a few years the medical profession and most educated laymen generally agreed that inoculated smallpox was a milder disease than natural smallpox. The basic issue, the value of inoculation for the protection of the community as a whole from a deadly contagious disease, persisted almost until the practice was superseded by vaccination. Could inoculation prevent smallpox epidemics, and if not, could it significantly decrease the death rate of the entire community from smallpox? What were the best methods to achieve these ends?

Before these questions can be answered with regard to Boston, it is necessary to know something about the relation of smallpox to local disease conditions, and the people's reaction to its presence. Although there are no smallpox statistics for the seventeenth century, there is ample evidence of its deadly presence. There are figures on the total number of burials in Boston for each year from 1701 through 1774, and there is enough census material to provide fairly good estimates of the size of the population.[2] One obvious general feature is the high death rate, averaging

---

* Read at the meeting of the History of Science Society, April 5, 1952. The author wishes to acknowledge the generous assistance of the Johns Hopkins University Institute of the History of Medicine in the preparation of this paper. He is indebted to Miss Genevieve Miller for several valuable suggestions.

* Department of the History of Medicine, Yale University School of Medicine, New Haven, Connecticut.

[1] For accounts of the controversy, see Joseph M. Toner, "History of inoculation in Massachusetts," *Massachusetts Medical Society, Publications*, 1867-68, *2*, 153-172; Reginald H. Fitz, "Zabdiel Boylston, inoculator, and the epidemic of smallpox in Boston in 1721," *Johns Hopk. Hosp. Bull.*, 1911, *22*, 315-327; George L. Kittredge. Introduction to Increase Mather, *Several reasons proving that inoculating or transplanting the small pox, is a lawful practice*. Cleveland, 1921, pp. 1-67; John T. Barrett, "The inoculation controversy in Puritan New England," *Bull. Hist. Med.*, 1942, *12*, 169-190; John B. Blake, "The inoculation controversy in Boston: 1721-1722," *New Engl. Quart.*, 1952, *25*, 489-506.

[2] "Account of burials and baptisms in Boston, from the year 1701 to 1774," *Massachusetts Historical Society, Collections*, 1795, ser. 1, *4*, 213-215; Lemuel Shattuck, *Report to the Committee of the City Council appointed to obtain the census of Boston for the year 1845*. Boston, 1846, Appendix, 71-72; Lemuel Shattuck, "On the vital statistics of Boston," *Amer. J. med. Sci.*, 1841, n.s. *1*, 369-373.

for the entire period in the neighborhood of 35 per 1,000. Equally outstanding is the wide annual variation. A change of 5 per 1,000 —roughly equal to that caused in Boston in 1918 by the devastating influenza pandemic—was a common occurrence. In spite of the high and variable death rate, however, smallpox stands out in the eighteenth century like the 1918 influenza in the twentieth. In the epidemic years of 1702, 1730, and 1752, the general death rate nearly doubled, and in 1721 it reached the phenomenal height of 105 per 1,000. No other disease which the Bostonians experienced ever caused such concentrated mortality. It struck swiftly and almost universally, sparing neither age, sex, nor social class. It was a loathsome disease, and of those who survived, many bore the marks of their affliction to the grave. It is no wonder that people lived in constant dread of its approach. Since it was also one of the few clearly recognized specific diseases which both doctors and laymen unequivocably agreed were contagious, the colonists were able to develop certain methods to combat it.

The principles and basic statutes of their policy were laid down before 1721. The first line of defense was quarantine. All incoming vessels which had had smallpox on board during their voyage, or which came from a place where smallpox was known to be prevalent, were required to undergo an examination by the Selectmen or a doctor under their direction. They removed the sick, the exposed, and their possessions to the isolation hospital on an island in the outer harbor, together with any cargo deemed infectious. Not until these goods and the ship had been cleaned and aired and all the crew and passengers were well, did the Selectmen allow them to approach the town. This was not always effective, however, and occasionally cases of smallpox occurred in town. The Selectmen then isolated the patients and their families by removing them to a pesthouse or by surrounding their homes with fences, red flags, and guards.[3]

These policies continued in effect throughout the eighteenth century, with ever-increasing rigor and with many refinements in statutory provision and administrative method. The vigor and comparative success with which they were pursued in the New England Colonies were in marked contrast to the more or less

[3] This account is based primarily on an examination of the statutes found most conveniently in Massachusetts General Court, *The acts and resolves, public and private, of the Province of the Massachusetts Bay* (21 vols., Boston, 1869-1922), and *Acts and resolves, 1780-1805* (13 vols., Boston, 1890-98); of the records of the Selectmen and town of Boston in Boston Record Commissioners, *Report* (39 vols., Boston, 1876-1909; vols. 24 to 39 issued as Boston Registry Department, *Records relating to the early history of Boston*); and of contemporary Boston newspapers.

endemic presence of smallpox in English cities, and to the more frequent presence of smallpox in populous sections of the Middle Colonies. From 1700 to 1775 there were only five epidemics in Boston which quarantine and isolation were unable to prevent or control. The people were strongly devoted to these policies, and as Dr. Benjamin Waterhouse pointed out:

> The inhabitants of New England view the small-pox with singular dread; ... the malady has been kept at an awful distance, by restrictive laws, and still stronger popular impressions; so that in New England, the most democratical region on the face of the earth, the priest, the magistrate, and the people, have voluntarily submitted to more restrictions and abridgments of liberty, to secure themselves against that terrific scourge, than any absolute monarch could have enforced.[4]

The introduction of inoculation in 1721 brought a new factor into this situation which greatly complicated public health policies. To the older possibilities of smallpox or no smallpox was added a third, inoculated smallpox, which was always a premeditated act. The individual's desire to protect himself or his family against a deadly disease came into conflict with the desire of the community to achieve the same end, for while inoculation protected the individual from natural smallpox, unless properly managed it spread the disease to others. Some just method of reconciling this conflict was needed, and the experience of 1721 had failed to provide an answer.

Late in 1729 occasional smallpox cases began appearing in Boston, and although the Selectmen took the usual precautions for isolating the sick, the disease continued to smolder through January. During February it spread slowly and inoculation again became a topic of popular discussion. Even William Douglass, the leading opponent in 1721, recommended it, but many still disagreed. On February 24th several citizens petitioned the town to devise proper methods for preventing the spread of smallpox by inoculation. Before the town meeting convened, however, the disease began to spread more widely and the Selectmen removed the guards from infected houses. Taking the situation into their own hands, a number of inhabitants had themselves inoculated. When the voters met on March 10, it was already too late to do anything about it, and they confined themselves to entreating those who planned to be inoculated to warn their neighbors first and to stay in their homes till they were free of infection. Not ready to

---

[4] Benjamin Waterhouse, *A prospect of exterminating the small pox Part II, being a continuation of a narrative of facts concerning the progress of the new inoculation in America.* Cambridge, 1802, p. 6.

encourage inoculation, yet unable to prevent it, the town of necessity accepted it and tried to minimize its tendency to spread the disease. Altogether, nearly four hundred people were inoculated, of whom twelve died. On the other hand there were about thirty-six hundred cases of natural smallpox, with nearly five hundred deaths.[5]

The figures proved again that the death rate for inoculated smallpox was much lower than for natural. The epidemic also prompted the General Court to pass a law which in effect laid down the first of the basic policies governing the future conduct of inoculation. Among other things it required heads of families to notify the Selectmen whenever anyone in their households came down with smallpox, unless more than twenty families in town were known to have the disease at the same time.[6] Undoubtedly the reason for the proviso was a brief that once the situation was that bad, traditional controls could no longer keep it from spreading. By interpretation and administration, the twenty-family rule became the standard, in the absence of other specific authority, for permitting inoculation.

Although smallpox appeared on incoming vessels and even within the town from time to time during the next twenty years, prompt protective measures prevented the development of any epidemics, and inoculation was never allowed. Then, on Christmas Eve, 1751, when the people of Chelsea went to the rescue of a ship from London wrecked in Nahant Bay, they caught the smallpox. On January 6th the first case appeared in Boston. For over two months the Selectmen were able to keep it under control by their usual methods, and the physicians promised not to inoculate anyone without due notice. Finally, however, the town fathers were forced to admit defeat. On March 23d they announced that there were so many cases they feared "no Method can be taken to prevent the spreading of that Distemper."[7]

This was the signal. Immediately inoculation started, and it proved far more popular than in 1730. Inoculation literature, old and new, was already appearing. Not all of it was favorable. Speak-

---

[5] Mass. Gen. Court, House of Representatives, *Journals*. Boston, 1919-, *9*, 120, 122, 133, 136; *Boston News-Letter*, Oct. 30, 1729, Jan. 8-Mar. 19, 1729-30, Mar. 26, 1730; *Boston Gazette*, Dec. 1, 1729, Jan. 12, 21, Feb. 2, Mar. 16, 1729/30, Mar. 30, 1730; Record Commissioners, *Report*, *12*, 14-15; William Douglass, *A summary, historical and political, of the first planting, progressive improvements, and present state of the British settlements in North-America*. London, 1755, II, 397; Shattuck, "Vital statistics of Boston," 373.

[6] 1731-32, ch. 13, Mass. *Acts and resolves*, 2, 621-622.

[7] Douglass, *Summary, historical and political*, II, 397; *News-Letter*, Jan. 9, 16, 23, Feb. 13, 20, 27, 1752; *Boston Evening-Post*, Mar. 9, 1752; *Boston Post-Boy*, Mar. 16, 23, 1752.

ing for many, no doubt, was the author of a letter published in the *Evening-Post* on April 13th. According to his information, there were by April 6th about six dead, fifty recovered, and forty then sick from natural smallpox, and perhaps twelve hundred inoculated cases. The advocates claimed the more, the better, because it would save lives, clear the town of infection sooner, and let people return to their business. The writer thought it very dangerous, for there were far too many for the physicians to care for should any considerable number of them, as was possible, break out with dangerous symptoms. He continued:

> It may also be worthy of their [the physicians'] Reflection, that as by inoculating such Numbers *at once*, in all Parts of the Town, a vast many will speedily be infected in the *natural Way*, whether *they* will not be chargeable with *increasing the general Distress?* For, if the inoculated (who have many Friends) can scarce procure the necessary Assistance *at this Time*, what will become of the many *Poor (who cannot be inoculated)* in that Time of dreadful Calamity?

To some extent this writer's fears seem to have come true. During January, February, and March there were only five deaths from smallpox, but early in April those who had been inoculated late the month before broke out with the disease, and it quickly spread. Many more people caught it the natural way than by inoculation, and nearly all who died were among the former. The toll mounted rapidly. During April there were 119 deaths from the disease; in May there were 205 and in June 203. By the end of this month, the epidemic was waning, and during July there were only 31 deaths. By July 27th there were only seventeen infected families, and the Selectmen prohibited further inoculation. The reason for the decline is obvious: there were hardly any susceptible people left. By mid-August the epidemic was over.[8]

According to the final statistics, out of a population of 15,684, 5,998 had had the disease before, 1,843 moved out of town, and only 174 remained in town without catching it. There were 7,669 cases of smallpox, nearly half the entire population. Among these were 5,545 cases of natural smallpox with 539 deaths, and 2,124 of inoculated with 30 deaths.[9] Clearly these results added further proof, though it was hardly needed, that the death rate from inoculated smallpox was substantially lower than that from natural. If

---

[8] Thomas Prince, "Observations on the state of the small pox at Boston, in 1752," *Gentleman's Magazine, and Historical Chronicle* (London), 1753, 23, 414; John Tudor, *Deacon Tudor's diary*. William Tudor, Ed. Boston, 1896, pp. 7-8; *Post-Boy*, July 6, Aug. 17, 1752; *Evening-Post*, July 27, 1752; Record Commissioners, *Report*, 17, 283.

[9] Prince, "Observations on the small pox," 414. There are minor discrepancies between his statistics and those recorded by the Selectmen, Record Commissioners, *Report*, 17, 283.

there had been no inoculation, the disease unquestionably would not have spread as fast as it did, and the total number of cases might well have been smaller. Yet it seems safe to say that inoculation of about twenty-two per cent of the nonimmune inhabitants did lower the impact of the epidemic on the community's death rate.[10]

For a decade the Selectmen were able to prevent any more epidemics. Late in December 1763, however, another round of cases began which did not have such a fortunate outcome. By January 17th there had been a total of ten cases, and the people were becoming alarmed. Many of those who were able to do so fled. Some people wanted to start inoculation, and others, among them the governmental officials, feared they would. The Governor and Council issued a proclamation forbidding it until the Selectmen should give permission, and as the number of infected houses approached twenty, the Selectmen got the legislature to pass an emergency act raising the critical figure to thirty. Through February they continued their control measures. More and more cases were reported, but as some went to the pesthouse and others died, the total number of infected families at any one time gradually declined, till on February 23d the Selectmen jubilantly reported that there were only five.[11]

By then inoculation had started outside the town. The issue naturally arose as soon as it became apparent that there was any chance of the disease spreading. There was, moreover, stronger sentiment in favor of the practice than ever before. In part this was due to developments which had taken place in other colonies. Inoculation was introduced to Philadelphia in 1730 and tried again in 1736-37. In 1750 it excited renewed attention, and in that year Dr. Adam Thompson published a tract recommending, on the basis of suggestions in Boerhaave, preparatory treatment with mercury and antimony. Most of his fellow practitioners strenuously opposed this idea at first, but certain New Jersey doctors took it up, among them a Dr. William Barnet. When smallpox struck the Quaker city again in 1759, Benjamin Franklin tried to

---

[10] Assuming that Prince's figures were correct, that all who had inoculated smallpox would otherwise have had natural, and that the death rate for this group would have been the same as it was for those who did have natural smallpox, we may conclude that another 177 people would have died and that the death rate from smallpox would have been 48 per 1000 population instead of 36 per 1000, an increase of 33 per cent.

[11] Record Commissioners, *Report*, *19*, 290-292; *20*, 1-43; 1763-64, ch. 17, Mass. *Acts and resolves*, *4*, 668; *News-Letter*, Jan. 19, 26, 1764; *Gazette*, Jan. 23, 1764; James Gordon to William Martin, erroneously dated Mar. 9, 1764, Mass. Hist. Soc., *Proceedings*, 1899-1900, ser. 2, *13*, 389.

popularize a simpler English method, but the mercury-antimony preparation became the accepted one, and Dr. Barnet was invited to set up a private inoculation hospital in Philadelphia. The successes of those who used these drugs—whether because of them or in spite of them—and treated their patients in private hospitals made it seem to many that inoculation was almost infallible.[12] Now that smallpox had appeared in Boston, about the middle of January 1764 several "Gentlemen of Distinction" invited Dr. Barnet to come there.[13]

Since inoculation within the town was forbidden, strong support for special hospitals grew rapidly. Many people, of course, desired them because they wished to have themselves and their families inoculated before they caught the disease in the natural way. Others advocated them in order to accommodate the inoculationists without endangering the town. They hoped the hospitals would ease the pressure for allowing inoculation within Boston and therefore tend to prevent the spread of the epidemic.[14] In 1761, when there had been grave danger that the smallpox then present might get out of hand, Dr. Silvester Gardiner had proposed establishing a hospital in Boston, but the town had turned him down.[15] In January 1764 the House of Representatives still refused to accept this idea,[16] but shortly after proroguing the General Court, the Governor and his Council on their own authority arranged with the Selectmen and several physicians to open an inoculation hospital on Point Shirley in Chelsea. A special committee devised regulations to prevent smallpox from spreading from the hospital, and on February 20th it was in operation. It cost money of course. The charge was one pound, five shillings, four pence per person for medicines and professional attendance,

---

[12] Henry Lee Smith, "Dr. Adam Thomson, the originator of the American method of inoculation for small-pox." *Johns Hopk. Hosp. Bull.*, 1909, *20*, 49-52; George W. Norris, *The early history of medicine in Philadelphia*. Philadelphia, 1886, pp. 104-113; Adam Thompson, article in *Virginia Gazette*, April 17, 1761, reprinted in *Boston Gazette*, Jan. 30, 1764; Arnold C. Klebs, "The historic evolution of variolation," *Johns Hopk. Hosp. Bull.*, 1913, *24*, 73-82; Carl Van Doren, *Benjamin Franklin*, New York, 1938, pp. 296-297; Whitman M. Reynolds, "Inoculation for the smallpox in colonial America," *Bull. Hist. Med.*, 1948, *22*, 273-276. As an example of how important the use of these chemicals seemed to contemporaries, see the bitter newspaper war engendered in Boston when William Greenleaf, Jr., a druggist, was accused of supplying adulterated calomel to the physician in charge of an inoculation hospital. *Gazette*, Apr. 23-July 16, 1764, *passim*.

[13] *Gazette*, Jan. 23, Feb. 13, 1764.

[14] *News-Letter*, Jan. 19, 26, Feb. 9, 16, 23, 1764; *Gazette*, Feb. 13, 1764; *Evening-Post*, Feb. 6, 20, 1764; Mass. *Acts and resolves*, *4*, 697; Record Commissioners, *Report, 16*, 103.

[15] Silvester Gardiner, "To the freeholders and other inhabitants of the town of Boston, in town meeting assembled, March, 1761," broadside reprinted in Mass. Hist. Soc., *Proceedings*, 1858-60, *4*, 325-328; Record Commissioners, *Report, 16*, 51-52.

[16] Mass. Gen. Court, House of Representatives, *Journal. Boston*, 1763-64, pp. 214-215.

plus three dollars a week for food, nursing, and other necessities.[17] So popular was this development that on February 27th the Governor made the barracks at Castle William available to all physicians for inoculation.[18]

The pressure for allowing inoculation did not ease, however, and early in March, when the situation began to deteriorate again, the Selectmen gave up trying to control the epidemic. The physicians of Boston agreed with the Overseers to treat the poor free of charge, and on March 13th the town voted to allow anyone, inhabitant or not, to be inoculated until April 20th.[19] Boston quickly became one great hospital, as thousands of citizens went through the operation and hundreds poured in from other towns and even from other colonies to take advantage of this opportunity. The physicians did a rushing business, and several professional inoculators besides Barnet came in from outside.[20] Before the epidemic was over nearly everyone who did not flee—or who had not had the disease before—caught it, either naturally or by inoculation. By June 30th, according to the official census, there had been 699 cases of natural smallpox with 124 deaths, and 4,977 cases of inoculated with 46 deaths. Of the latter, 1,025 had passed through the disease under the inspection and care of the Overseers of the Poor and about 400 came from other towns.[21]

Several significant results emerged from this epidemic. For the first time inoculation hospitals were tried in Boston. As usual, the death rate among the inoculated was far more favorable. More important was the greatly increased use of the technique. In 1721 about two per cent of the smallpox cases in Boston were by inoculation, in 1730 ten per cent, and in 1752 twenty-eight per cent. In 1764, excluding the four hundred noninhabitants, the percentage rose to eighty-seven. This lowered the death rate for smallpox so markedly that for the first time a smallpox year failed to stand out as one of unusual mortality. Aside from the fact that more people believed in it, one of the major reasons for this change was that for the first time arrangements had been made for inoculating the poor.

[17] *News-Letter*, Feb. 9, 16, Mar. 8, 1764; *Gazette*, Feb. 13, 1764. The rates for children were slightly lower.

[18] *Gazette*, Feb. 27, 1764.

[19] Record Commissioners, *Report, 16*, 105-106, 109, 112; *20*, 49; *News-Letter*, Feb. 23, 1764; *Gazette*, Feb. 27, Mar. 5, 19, 1764.

[20] *News-Letter*, Mar. 15, 22, 29, Apr. 13, 1764; *Gazette*, Mar. 12, 19, 26, May 28, 1764; *Evening-Post*, Mar. 12, 1764; *Post-Boy*, Apr. 9, 23, 1764; James Gordon to William Martin, Mass. Hist. Soc., *Proceedings*, 1899-1900, ser. 2, *13*, 390.

[21] Record Commissioners, *Report, 16*, 116; *20*, 80.

The aftermath of the epidemic nevertheless showed that the practice was still acceptable to the majority only as a last resort. On April 20th the period allowed for inoculation was over, and the Selectmen were faced with the problem of clearing the town of infection. One difficulty was caused by a number of people who had failed to be inoculated when they had the opportunity, and who were now coming down in the natural way and perpetuating the epidemic. Several began to regret their previous decision, so the Selectmen gave the physicians permission to inoculate those who had been in town on or before April 20th, hoping in this way to speed its passage through the town.[22] A more serious problem was that outsiders persisted in coming in for inoculation, and they were able to find doctors willing to oblige. In town meeting the citizens called on the legislature to act, while the Selectmen warned such people of "that resentment which has risen and is still rising in the Breasts of Multitudes of the Inhabitants against those who attempt so grossly to abuse them as to make this Town a Hospital, not withstanding proper Hospitals are provided conveniently situated to receive such as incline to take the Distemper."[23]

Even the hospitals were now looked upon adversely. Inoculation at Castle William ended May 12th, but with the permission of the Selectmen the attending physicians opened a new hospital on Noddle's Island. Many people, however, believed that these places tended to continue the epidemic, and on May 24th the voters decided not to allow any inoculation hospitals within the town's boundaries.[24] Point Shirley was outside Boston's jurisdiction, and when reports came in that people were returning from there "quite Green with the Small Pox and very infectious," the Selectmen, fearing that the resentful inhabitants would take their own "extraordinary steps," warned Dr. Barnet of an "unhappy event" if he did not make sure that no one left until he was completely free from infection.[25]

On June 15th, in answer to Boston's request, the General Court passed a new law rigidly restricting inoculation. It provided severe penalties for a noninhabitant who was inoculated in Boston without the Selectmen's permission, for anyone who, having had small-

[22] Record Commissioners, *Report, 20,* 59; *News-Letter,* Apr. 26, May 3, 1764; *Gazette,* May 7, 1764.
[23] Record Commissioners, *Report, 16,* 117-118; *20,* 59, 61, 64-65; *News-Letter,* May 10, 1764.
[24] Record Commissioners, *Report, 16,* 123; *20,* 60; *News-Letter,* Apr. 26, May 17, 24, 1764; *Gazette,* Apr. 23, May 21, 28, 1764.
[25] Record Commissioners, *Report, 20,* 69-70; see also, *ibid., 20,* 73; *Evening-Post,* June 11, 1764; *News-Letter,* June 14, 1764.

pox by inoculation or otherwise, moved from the house where he was staying while sick into any town where smallpox did not generally prevail, and finally for anyone who "willfully, wantonly or carelessly" communicated smallpox to another person. The law also forbade the use of any house as an inoculation hospital without the town's prior consent, and all physicians and nurses employed in smallpox hospitals were required to reside there constantly, lest by passing from place to place they endanger others.[26]

Popular opposition continued during the next few years, in Boston and elsewhere in Massachusetts. In 1771 Dr. Samuel Gelston, a professional inoculator, undertook to set up a hospital on a tiny island about a mile west of Nantucket. The people in the nearby town of Sherborn feared this would spread the disease among them, and on their petition the General Court immediately ordered Gelston to stop.[27] An inoculation hospital erected on an island near Marblehead in 1773 was soon after burned to the ground by a mob. When two of the ringleaders were arrested, another mob rescued them from the Salem jail. Popular feeling was with them, and the matter ended there.[28] In Boston, although smallpox threatened to become epidemic early in 1775, the voters decided that as long as there was any chance of controlling it, there should be no inoculation.[29]

The Revolution, however, brought a marked change in the popular attitudes. While Boston was under siege from April 1775 to March 1776, smallpox ran rife in the town, but the revolutionary government was able to keep it from getting into the army or the surrounding countryside.[30] After the British had evacuated, however, it soon proved impossible to maintain isolation procedures, and the disease began to spread. Despite the efforts of the civilian and military authorities, many people, some soldiers among them, faced with the alternative of catching the natural disease, secretly had themselves inoculated instead. Despairing of controlling the disease, the government decided to

[26] 1764-65, ch. 12, Mass. *Acts and resolves*, *4*, 728-729.
[27] Mass. *Acts and resolves*, *18*, 567.
[28] Samuel A. Green, *History of medicine in Massachusetts*. Boston, 1881, pp. 77-78; Mary Vial Holyoke, "Diary," G. F. Dow, Ed. *The Holyoke diaries, 1709-1856*. Salem, 1911, pp. 81-82.
[29] Record Commissioners, *Report*, *18*, 223-224.
[30] Mass. *Acts and resolves*, *19*, 9-10, 15, 17, 95-96, 157, 165, 172; John Morgan, *A recommendation of inoculation, according to Baron Dimsdale's method*. Boston, 1776, p. 11; Allen French, *The first year of the American revolution*. Boston, 1934, pp. 493-495; Louis C. Duncan, "Medical men in the American revolution, 1775-1783," *Army med. Bull.*, 1931, no. 25, pp. 16, 66; James E. Gibson, *Dr. Bodo Otto and the medical background of the American revolution*. Springfield, Ill., 1937, pp. 88-90.

get the epidemic over with as soon as possible, and a general inoculation of soldiers and civilians in Boston followed.[31]

The Bostonians were not the only ones who, prompted by fear of natural smallpox, were secretly taking it by inoculation, for it seemed certain the infected troops would spread it over the countryside. Further pressure came from those who wished to be inoculated without exposing themselves to the penalties of the law. The members of the General Court finally came to the conclusion that the best way to prevent people from performing the operation secretly and thereby endangering their fellow citizens was to legalize and regulate it. On July 9, 1776, they passed a law permitting the county courts to allow inoculation hospitals in such places and under such regulations as they judged most convenient and safe for the inhabitants. Anyone who inoculated or was inoculated elsewhere, except in a town where more than twenty families were known to have smallpox, was subject to a severe penalty.[32]

This hastily contrived legislation soon aroused opposition. Some complained because the justices allowed inoculation hospitals in towns whose inhabitants did not want them, some because the justices refused to allow them where they were wanted, and some because they were improperly managed.[33] It was therefore revised in April 1777 to prohibit the hospitals in any town without its consent. The amendment also stipulated certain basic regulations to which all hospitals must conform. There had to be proper facilities for cleansing all patients of infection before they left, and preference had to be given to local inhabitants and to those who might be soldiers in the coming campaign. Each patient had to give a bond of ten pounds, and the physicians one of five hundred pounds, to observe the requirements.[34] Two months later the General Court passed a special order for military reasons prohibiting any inoculation in the towns surrounding Boston harbor, but when smallpox became threatening the following March, the town voted to allow general inoculation anyway. The legislators quickly abandoned any idea of preventing the practice. They not only repealed the prohibitory order, but passed a resolve tem-

[31] 1776-77, ch. 8, Mass *Acts and resolves*, *5*, 555-557; *ibid.*, *5*, 661-662; *19*, 290; James Thacher, *A military journal during the American revolutionary war*. Boston, 1823, pp. 50, 53-54; Ezekiel Price, "Diary, 1775-1776," Mass. Hist. Soc., *Proceedings*, 1863-64, ser. 1, *7*, 259-260; French, *First year of the revolution*, p. 671; Francis R. Packard, *History of medicine in the United States*. New York, 1931, I, 83-85.

[32] 1776-77, ch. 7, Mass. *Acts and resolves*, *5*, 554-555; *ibid.*, *5*, 661, 663; Morgan, *Recommendation of inoculation*, pp. 11-12.

[33] Mass. *Acts and resolves*, *5*, 663, 713; *19*, 585, 874.

[34] 1776-77, ch. 39, Mass. *Acts and resolves*, *5*, 633-635.

porarily permitting any town in the state to erect inoculation hospitals under the regulation of the Selectmen alone, dispensing in the emergency with the need for a license from the county court.[35]

Obviously, while many still feared that inoculation would spread smallpox, it had become on the whole far more popular since the Revolution began. Even the ordinary folk who had earlier led the opposition, and who were still sometimes suspicious of the private hospitals, seemed ready enough to take the disease this way when it was financially possible and the chances of avoiding natural smallpox were slim. Prior to the Revolution the popular attitude was that inoculation was to be used solely as a last resort, after it became apparent that it would be practically impossible to avoid natural smallpox; during and after the Revolution, the popular attitude became that if there was any chance of getting natural smallpox, it was time to inoculate. The people's confidence in inoculation, and their willingness to be inoculated, had greatly increased.

So well established had the practice become during the war years, that when in 1783 four physicians petitioned Boston for permission to carry on inoculation on Apple Island, though there was then no particular threat of an epidemic, the town readily granted their request. In 1788, when there were several cases of smallpox in nearby towns, the authorities permitted inoculation hospitals in Watertown, Newton, Medford, and Brookline, and in 1789 on Rainsford Island in Boston harbor. Inoculation continued on Rainsford Island for several years, and in Brookline, at Dr. William Aspinwall's extensive establishment, until vaccination rendered it obsolete.[36]

Only once more, in 1792, was there a great epidemic in Boston. When it became apparent that smallpox was spreading, the town voted overwhelmingly for inoculation, and called on the Overseers to employ physicians to inoculate and care for the poor. Of all the smallpox cases among the inhabitants, ninety-seven per cent were by inoculation and only 262 people left town to escape the disease. Like other epidemics, this one, which had affected much of the eastern part of the state, prompted new legislation. It was primarily designed to tighten up the administrative control of natural

[35] Mass. *Acts and resolves, 20,* 15-16, 352, 354; Record Commissioners, *Report, 26,* 14-16.
[36] Record Commissioners, *Report, 26,* 323-324; Registry Dept., *Records relating to early Boston, 31,* 188, 223, 282, 284; Mass. *Acts and resolves, 1788-89,* 368; Benjamin Waterhouse to John Haygarth, October 28, 1788, quoted in John Haygarth, *A sketch of a plan to exterminate the casual small-pox from Great Britain.* London, 1793, II, 325-329.

smallpox, but at the same time it further facilitated the establishment of inoculation hospitals.[37] Unquestionably inoculation had become an accepted practice.

From the introduction of this procedure through the epidemic of 1752, it grew slowly, and it failed to realize its potential ability drastically to reduce the community's death rate. The opposition to inoculation in each succeeding epidemic, though declining, continued strong. Many still did not trust it and preferred to take their chances on getting natural smallpox. Then too, as Benjamin Franklin pointed out, "the expense of having the operation performed by a surgeon weighs with others, for that has been pretty high in some parts of America; and when a common tradesman or artificer has a number in his family to have the distemper, it amounts to more money than he can well spare."[38] These people opposed allowing others to inoculate because, as practised, it did help spread the disease to those who for whatever reason were unwilling or unable to be inoculated. By the 1760's and early '70's, however, its value was more clearly accepted, and arrangements were made to inoculate the poor during an epidemic. This helped substantially in making it far more widespread in the epidemic of 1764 and in greatly lowering the death rate. In each succeeding epidemic the vast majority always took the disease by inoculation.

By the '60's inoculation hospitals, first suggested by an anonymous pamphleteer in 1721, were being tried in other colonies. In Boston in 1764 they were accepted temporarily for special reasons. But in nonepidemic periods they continued to be exceedingly unpopular with the majority. Although far safer than natural smallpox, the inoculated variety was more dangerous and unpleasant than no smallpox at all, and many people hoped, with some reason, that if inoculation was prohibited, they could avoid the disease altogether. Moreover, the practice was time-consuming and expensive. In a general epidemic, when it was freely allowed within the town, this made less difference, since one could go through it at home, and trade and business were completely disrupted anyway. But ordinarily the common citizen could not afford to be absent from his work for the month or more necessary to go through the whole process, much less to pay for the expenses of doctor, nurses, food, and lodging at an inoculation hospital. The latter were of no benefit to the great majority, who saw them only

[37] Registry Dept., *Records, 31,* 302-304, 307-308; 1792, chs. 28, 58, Mass. *Acts and resolves, 1792-93,* 50-53, 85-88.
[38] Quoted in Van Doren, *Franklin,* p. 297.

TABLE 1

Year	Population	Natural Cases	Natural Deaths	Natural Deaths per 1,000 cases	Inoculated Cases	Inoculated Deaths	Inoculated Deaths per 1,000 cases	All cases Cases	All cases Deaths	Deaths per 1,000 cases	Cases per 1,000 population	Deaths per 1,000 population	Per cent of cases inoculated	Left town	Escaped disease	Had smallpox before
1721	11,000	5,759	842	146	287[1]	6[2]	21	5,889	844	143	535	77	2	......	......	......
1730	13,000	3,600	500	139	400	12	30	4,000	500	125	308	38	10	......	......	......
1752	15,684	5,545	539	97	2,124	30	14	7,669	569	74	490	36	28	1,843	174	5,998
1764	15,700	699	124	177	4,977[3]	46	9	5,276	170[4]	32	336	11	87	1,537	519[5]	ca. 8,370
1776	......	304	29	95	4,988[6]	28	6	4,063	57[4]	14	......	......	90	......	......	......
1778	......	122	40	328	2,121	19	9	2,243	59	26	......	......	95	......	......	......
1792	19,300	232	69	298	9,152[7]	179	20	8,346	248[4]	30	432	13	97	262	221	ca. 10,300

[1] Including 157 inoculated in neighboring towns.
[2] Including 4 deaths in neighboring towns.
[3] Including about 400 nonresidents inoculated in Boston.
[4] No allowance is made for the possibility that some of the deaths occurred among nonresidents inoculated in Boston.
[5] Most of these were out of town during most of the epidemic.
[6] Including 1329 nonresidents inoculated in Boston.
[7] Including 1038 nonresidents inoculated in Boston.

as possible sources of infection, threatening death to those who were susceptible and economic distress to the whole community.

The Revolution helped greatly to popularize the practice. The disruption of ordinary government together with the movements of troops, recruits, and returning veterans played havoc with the old preventive measures and spread smallpox widely. Massachusetts was forced to devise a policy for permitting inoculation under proper supervision. With the return of peace, this system of inoculation hospitals was allowed to continue. It certainly benefited the individuals fortunate enough to be able to pay. It was perhaps a source of some protection to others by removing in part the temptation to inoculate secretly and by relieving the pressure to allow general inoculation whenever there was the slightest possibility of an epidemic.

From the point of view of the community, however, the hospitals were unable to protect a sufficiently large number to be of much significance. They were obviously unable to prevent epidemics among the general population. When properly regulated by governmental authority, as, in time, they were, they were no danger to the community and could therefore be safely permitted. From the community standpoint, what inoculation could do, and did do from 1764 on, when the government arranged to inoculate the poor, was to lower the death rate markedly when a smallpox epidemic became inevitable. Inoculated smallpox was not a pleasant affair. It caused some loss of life and brought in its train great personal suffering, especially among the poor, and great economic loss to the entire community. It certainly was not the equivalent of universal protection by vaccination. But compared to an epidemic of natural smallpox, it was indeed a blessing.

NOTE ON TABLE 1

At least three similar tables have been printed: by Thomas Pemberton in "A topographical and historical description of Boston, 1794," Massachusetts Historical Society, *Collections*, 1794, reprinted 1810, ser. 1, *3*, 292; by "Investigator," *Columbian Centinel*, July 24, 1802; and three times by Lemuel Shattuck, "On the vital statistics of Boston," *Amer. J. med. Sci.*, 1841, n.s. *1*, 373; *Report to the Committee of the City Council appointed to obtain the census of Boston for the year 1845*. Boston, 1846, p. 144; *Report of a general plan for the promotion of public and personal health* . . . Boston, 1850, p. 70. Only "Investigator" gave the sources of his information.

1721: In February, 1721/22, the Selectmen took a census of the population, including the number of smallpox cases and deaths. They reported that 10,567 people continued in Boston, that there were 5,889 cases and 844 deaths (*Boston News-Letter*, February 26, 1721/22; William Douglass, *A summary, historical and political, of the first planting, progressive improvements, and present state of the British settlements in North-America.* London, 1755, II, 396). Douglass's statement that there were 5,989 cases is an error, perhaps a misprint. Zabdiel Boylston recorded his 247 inoculated cases and 39 performed by other physicians both in Boston and neighboring towns in *An historical account of the small-pox inoculated in New England, upon all sorts of persons, whites, blacks, and of all ages and constitutions* . . . 2d ed., Boston, 1730, p. 34. He later recorded one additional case not in his book, bringing the total in and about Boston to 287 (*News-Letter*, Mar. 5, 1729/30). It is apparent from Boylston's records that between 121 and 138 only of his detailed cases in the *Historical account* were residents of Boston. If the figure is set at 130, this, added to the 5,759 cases of natural smallpox stated by Boylston to have occurred in Boston (*Historical account*, p. 33), gives the total of 5,889 cases recorded by the Selectmen. Boylston gave the number of deaths from natural smallpox as 844. It seems probable, however, that the Selectmen included in this total the two Boston residents among Boylston's six fatal cases, so I have listed deaths from natural smallpox at 842. None of the other three tables takes into account the 39 cases inoculated by other physicians, nor the fact that many of Boylston's patients were not residents of Boston. I have included the six people inoculated by Boylston in May 1722, but have not included the scattering of natural cases in April and May 1722 (John B. Blake, "The inoculation controversy in Boston: 1721-1722," *New Engl. Quart.*, 1952, *25*, 497).

1730: The population is estimated from the censuses of 1722 and 1742 (Shattuck, *Census of Boston 1845*, pp. 3, 5). The other figures are only approximate estimates given by Douglass (*Summary, historical and political*, II, 397).

1752: The statistics used here were given by Thomas Prince, "Observations on the state of the small pox at Boston, in 1752," *Gentleman's Magazine, and Historical Chronicle*, 1753, *23*, 414. There are minor discrepancies between them and those recorded by the Selectmen (Boston Record Commissioners, *Report*, *17*, 283) taken before the epidemic was completely over. Pemberton and "Investigator" gave the Selectmen's figures, Shattuck, Prince's. Although there may have been some nonresidents inoculated in Boston during the epidemic, Prince's statistics apparently applied to the local population only.

1764: The population is estimated from the census of 1765 (Record Commissioners, *Report*, *20*, 170). My figures are those given by the Selectmen (*ibid.*, *20*, 80). Pemberton listed 669 natural cases, probably a misprint. Shattuck, in giving the total number of cases, did not subtract the number of nonresidents.

1776: My figures are those given by Pemberton and "Investigator." Shattuck gave only 18 deaths from inoculated smallpox and included nonresidents in his total number of cases. He did not indicate how he obtained his population estimates for 1776 or 1778 and I have found no reliable figures. The disruption caused by the Revolution makes any estimate highly speculative, so I have given none.

1778: My figures are from the Selectmen's enumeration as reported in *Boston-Gazette*, May 18, 1778. "Investigator" did not list any figures for this epidemic. The other tables list 42 deaths from natural smallpox.

Shattuck gave 29 deaths from inoculated smallpox, perhaps a misprint. No information was given on nonresidents inoculated in Boston. However, the town voted to allow ten days for inoculation of the inhabitants only (Record Commissioners, *Report, 26,* 15-16), and the number of nonresidents, if any, was probably negligible.

1792: The population is estimated from the United States censuses of 1790 and 1800. The other figures are from the Selectmen's enumerations. After the first one, taken October 5-6, 1792, when 181 people were still sick, they reported only 33 deaths from natural smallpox and 165 deaths from inoculated, and these numbers were used by Pemberton, "Investigator," and Shattuck. They must be revised, however, because another count two weeks later raised the mortality figures to 69 natural and 179 inoculated, with 62 people still sick (Boston Registry Department, *Records relating to the early history of Boston, 31,* 307-308). In this connection see the comment on "Investigator's" table that not less than 30 people died after the first enumeration, in *Columbian Centinel,* July 28, 1802. This time Shattuck subtracted the number of nonresidents from his figures for inoculated and total cases.

The Medical and Surgical Practice of the Lewis and Clark Expedition*

DRAKE W. WILL**

I

ON the last day of February in 1802 Thomas Jefferson wrote, in part, to Benjamin Rush in Philadelphia: "I wish to mention to you in confidence that I have obtained authority from Congress to undertake the long desired object of exploring the Missouri and whatever river, heading with that, leads into the western ocean ..." He briefly delineated the plans for the expedition and introduced the member of his own official household, Meriwether Lewis, who was to lead this long-cherished project, from whom he requested that:

It would be very useful to state for him those objects on which it is most desirable he should bring us information. For this purpose I ask the favor of you to prepare some notes of such particulars as may occur in his journey and which you think should draw his attention and inquiry. He will be in Philadelphia about 2 or 3 weeks hence and will wait on you."[1]

The busy, hard-working doctor-statesman, always behind in attending to his correspondence, had already received a cordial and flattering letter from the President the previous summer, telling in detail of his distress from a recurrent diarrhea which had plagued him for some two years.[2] Dr. Rush set about to correct his tardiness toward an illustrious patient and wrote immediately to the capital, killing two birds with one stone. In a few lengthy paragraphs, he advised Mr. Jefferson on the means of treating his gastrointestinal disease[3] and inserted another short paragraph in which he acknowledged the President's later request, writing: "I shall expect to see Mr. Lewis in Philadelphia and shall not fail of furnishing him with

---

* John Farquhar Fulton Medal Essay, 1957, of the Society for the History of Medical Science, Los Angeles.
** Department of Pathology, School of Medicine, University of California, Los Angeles 24.
[1] Ford, Paul L., Ed. *The works of Thomas Jefferson.* New York, Putnam, 1904-05, IX, p. 452.
[2] *Ibid.,* VIII, pp. 219-221.
[3] Jefferson's lack of sympathy with the medical practice of his day, particularly to treatment with drugs, was well known to Rush, and the letter contains very general directions but does venture to recommend some spirits.

a number of questions calculated to increase our knowledge of subjects connected with medicine."[4]

Several days later, Dr. Rush entered in his "Commonplace Book," an extensive, highly personal diary, a list of questions for Mr. Lewis against his arrival for the personal conference that Jefferson wished. Jefferson had also sent similar requests to aid Lewis to several other Philadelphians, including Caspar Wistar, professor of anatomy in the medical school, and Benjamin Barton, professor of natural history, who was to succeed to Rush's chair on his death in 1813.

The young soldier, whose family were Virginia neighbors of Jefferson's, had just spent two years as the President's personal secretary in Washington, watching the events unfold which led to the exploration that he was now appointed to direct. He was as familiar as anyone could be with Jefferson's private and public conceptions of the western exploration and, with his own love of the wilderness, a recent tour of frontier military duty, and intense personal loyalty for the President, was well-fitted for the task. At this early stage, he was not only to be the leader of the expedition but was also the quartermaster, engineer, and general factotum. Jefferson had sent him with ample letters of credit in his own hand to the government arsenals and depots to assemble supplies and instruments before he sought out a group of scientists in Philadelphia who were to tutor him, at the President's request, in the essentials of scientific observation.

But Lewis was delayed by miscalculations and misfortune. He was detained a month at Harper's Ferry, supervising the building of the frame for the iron boat that was to carry the expedition down the broad, wide, supposedly rapid-free Columbia to the western ocean. On 20 April he was only at Lancaster as a letter to the President vouches,[5] and he apologized to Jefferson for the delay. He added that he would spend ten or twelve days with Andrew Ellicott, who was at that time Surveyor General of the United States, studying surveying and the use of mathematical instruments.

When Capt. Lewis finally reached Philadelphia, the immediate necessity was the gathering of equipment and supplies. His letter of credit and orders were submitted to the federal purchasing agent who began to assemble and issue the necessary materials. Lewis then was able to turn his attention to his most recent communica-

[4] Butterfield, L. H., Ed. *The letters of Benjamin Rush*. Published for the American Philosophical Society by Princeton University Press, Princeton, N. J., 1951, II, p. 858.
[5] Thwaites, R. G., Ed. *Original journals of the Lewis and Clark expedition*. New York, Dodd, Mead, 1904, VII, pp. 213-216.

tion from the President. Jefferson sent a rough draft of the official instructions for the expedition and proposed, in addition, "your instructions being known to Mr. Patterson, Docrs. Wister, Rush, & Barton these instructions may be submitted to their perusal. . . . These gentlemen will suggest any additions they will think useful as has been before asked of them."[6] He began working with Robert Patterson, an Irish physician and professor of mathematics at the University, who gave him intensive instruction in navigation and astronomical measurements.

Though it is highly probable that Lewis saw Dr. Rush very shortly after his arrival in Philadelphia in early May, Rush waited before he wrote to the President, apparently shortly after another call by the young explorer, perhaps the last. Enthusiastic about the expedition, Rush also noted that Lewis appeared admirably qualified to lead it. Of greater interest, he wrote:

I have endeavored to fulfill your wishes by furnishing Mr. Lewis with some inquiries relative to the natural history of the Indians. The enclosed letter contains a few short directions for the preservation of his health, as well as the health of the persons under his command.[7]

Rush gave Lewis a personal copy of the "Questions"[8] and of the "Directions" reproduced below, and another copy of the "Directions" was appended to his letter to Jefferson.[9]

Questions to MERRYWEATHER LEWIS
before he went up the Missouri[10, 11]

I. Physical history and medicine
  1. What are the acute diseases of the Indians? Is the billious fever attended with a black vomit?
  2. Is apoplexy, palsy, epilepsy, madness, rheum[atic] disease, goitre known among them?
  3. What is the state of life as to longevity? At what age do the women *begin* and *cease* to menstruate?

---

[6] *Ibid.*
[7] Butterfield, *op. cit.*, II, p. 868.
[8] The list of questions was similar to those Rush had previously prepared for Alexander McGillivray in 1790, and again, in 1791, for Timothy Pickering, who had been adjutant-general on Washington's staff when Rush was physician-general of the Middle Department. See Corner, George W., Ed. *The autobiography of Benjamin Rush. His "Travels Through Life" together with his Commonplace Book for 1789-1813.* Princeton, N. J., American Philosophical Society by the Princeton Univ. Press, 1948, p. 189; Butterfield, *op. cit.*, I, pp. 480-481.
[9] The President kept a personally transcribed copy of the "Directions" when he returned the Rush letters in his possession to the family after the physician's death.
[10] Corner, *op. cit.*, pp. 265-267.
[11] The preparation of the scientific reports of the expedition was never undertaken, due to personal and political difficulties of Lewis, the logical author, and his tragic death in 1807. Only Jefferson's great personal efforts saved the journals for preservation. There is no evidence that the "Questions" were ever answered, except indirectly in the journals.

4. At what age do they marry? How long do they suckle the children? What is the provision of their children after being weaned?
5. The rate of the pulse as to frequency in the morning, at noon, and at night, before and after eating?
6. What is its state in childhood, adult life, and old age? Is it ever subject to intermissions? The number of strokes counted by the quarter of a minute by glass, and multiplied by four will give its frequency in a minute.
7. What are their remedies?
8. Are artificial discharges of blood ever used among them?
9. In what manner do they induce sweating? Do they ever use voluntary fasting? At what time do they use their baths?
10. What is the diet, manner of cooking, and times of eating among the Indians? How do they preserve their food?

II. Morals
1. What are their vices?
2. Is suicide common among them? Ever from love?
3. Do they employ any substitute for ardent spirits to promote intoxication?
4. Is murder common among them, and do they punish it with death?

III. Religion
1. What affinity between their religious ceremonies and those of the Jews?
2. Do they use animal sacrifices in their worship?
3. What are the principal objects of their worship?
4. How do they dispose of their dead, and with what ceremonies do they inter them?

May 17, 1803   B. RUSH

In the manuscripts belonging to the Clark family, a long list of questions in Clark's handwriting entitled "Inquiries relitive to the Indians of Louisiana" embodies the queries of Rush verbatim or with some changes in phraseology, apparently transcribed from instructions of Jefferson to the captains.[12] As would be expected, several of Rush's questions relate to bilious fevers, diseases with which his name and reputation are associated in the history of American medicine. Included among the questions in Clark's "Inquiries" are several which Rush might have been expected to ask but inexplicably did not, e.g., "What is their mode of treating the Small pox particularly?" One strongly suspects that this last query is Jefferson's own addition.

On the same day that he wrote to Jefferson of Lewis' visit, Rush had made a rough copy in the "Commonplace Book" of a simple

[12] Thwaites, *op. cit.*, VII, pp. 283-287.

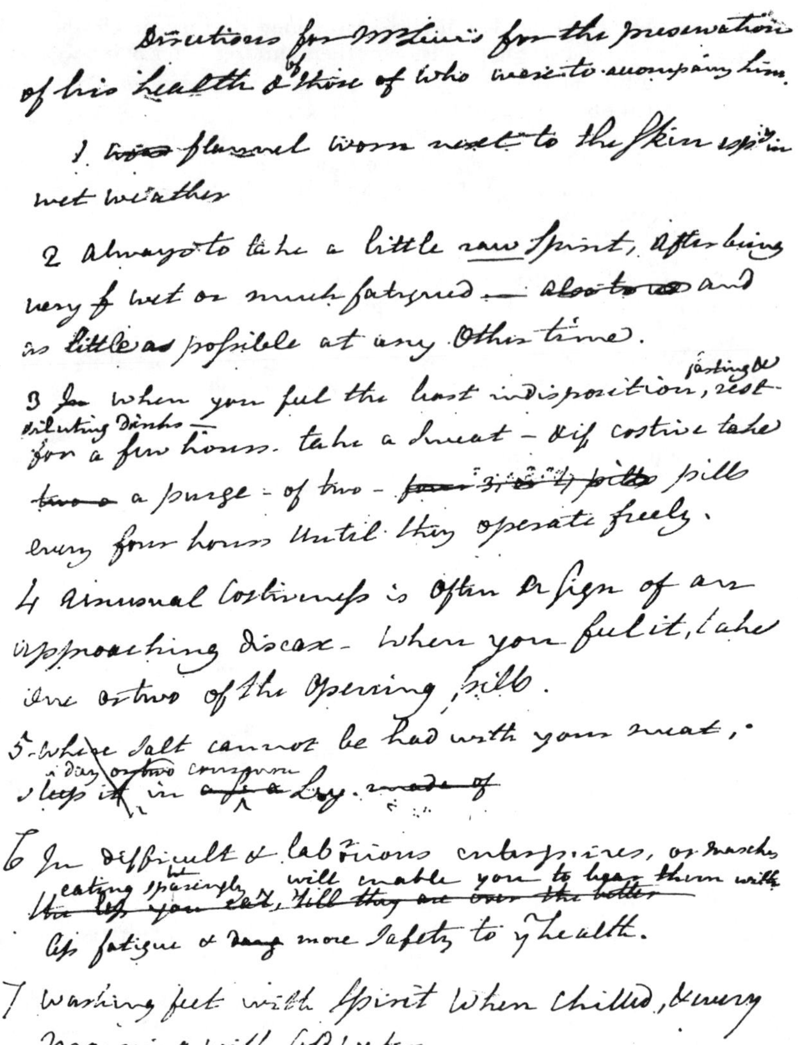

FIG. 1. Rush's first draft of the Directions for Mr. Lewis in his *Commonplace Book*, 11 June 1803. By permission of the American Philosophical Society, Philadelphia.

set of rules which he entitled "Directions for MR. LEWIS for the Preservation of his Health and of those who were to accompany him."[13] In Jefferson's papers, under the same date, 11 June 1803, is a copy in the President's own hand of the same directions rearranged and somewhat expanded, which is assuredly a transcription of the final draft sent to Jefferson by Rush as previously described. The originals of the "Directions" and the "Questions," which were given to Lewis, have never been found. The final draft, from Jefferson's copy, is reproduced here (Figs. 1 and 2):

Dr Rush to Capt. Lewis. for preserving his health. June 11. 1803[14]

1. when you feel the least indisposition, do not attempt to overcome it by labour or marching. rest in a horizontal posture.—also fasting and diluting drinks for a day or two will generally prevent an attack of fever. to these preventatives of disease may be added a gentle sweat obtained by warm drinks, or gently opening the bowels by means of one, two, or more of the purging pills.
2. Unusual costiveness is often a sign of approaching disease. when you feel it take one or more of the purging pills.
3. want of appetite is likewise a sign of approaching indisposition. it should be obviated by the same remedy.
4. in difficult & laborious enterprises & marches, eating sparingly will enable you to bear them with less fatigue & less danger to your health.
5. flannel should be worn constantly next to the skin, especially in wet weather.
6. the less spirit you use the better. after being *wetted* or *much* fatigued, or long exposed to the night air, it should be taken in an undiluted state. 3 tablespoonfuls taken in this way will be more useful in preventing sickness, than half a pint mixed with water.
7. molasses or sugar & water with a few drops of the acid of vitriol will make a pleasant & wholesome drink with your meals.
8. after having had your feet much chilled, it will be useful to wash them with a little spirit.
9. washing the feet every morning in *cold* water, will conduce very much to fortify them against the action of cold.
10. after long marches, or much fatigue from any cause, you will be more refreshed by *lying down* in a horizontal posture for two hours, than by resting a much longer time in any other position of the body.
11. shoes made without heels, by affording equal action to all the muscles of the legs, will enable you to march with less fatigue, than shoes made in the ordinary way.

The medical and surgical materials which Lewis required were assembled without difficulty. An initial list of drugs and supplies drawn up in Washington or enroute to Philadelphia is quite brief;

---

[13] Corner, *op. cit.*, pp. 265-267.
[14] Papers of Thomas Jefferson, Library of Congress, dated 11 June 1803 (see illustration).

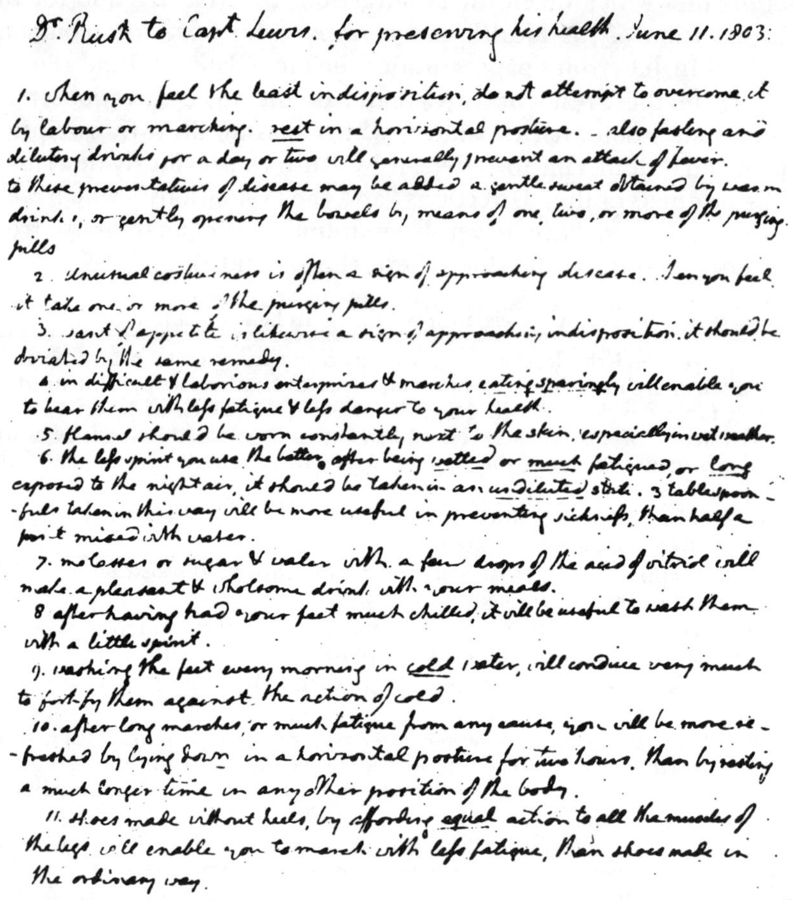

FIG. 2. A final draft of Rush's directions for Lewis in the Jefferson Papers, Library of Congress, transcribed by the President in his own hand.

the final bill is far more detailed.[15] It seems probable that Rush made up or at least edited this final order Lewis gave to the suppliers since an item of fifty dozen bilious pills, made to his prescription, was included. Only $55 was budgeted for medicine, and Lewis must have been somewhat disturbed at the final bill of $90.69 which dipped further into his total appropriation of $2,500 than he

[15] In personal correspondence of R. G. Thwaites in the possession of the Wisconsin State Historical Society a letter from E. C. Stacey in Washington, D. C., dated 26 May 1904, to H. C. Powers, Sioux City, Iowa, describes the original search for the papers. Stacey learned from the War Department that the Tripolitanian piracy expeditions were outfitted at Philadelphia. The Depot Quartermaster in that city "had the matter carefully looked up and furnished me with copies of the records as specified. . . ." Mr. Victor Gondos, Jr., Archivist, Old Army Branch, General Services Administration, after prolonged search, has rediscovered these documents in the National Archives and they are illustrated here.

had planned. The medical supplies were delivered to Lewis, who receipted the bill personally, on 27 May 1803. The invoice is reproduced in its entirety (Figs. 3 and 4).

The bill does not seem great in comparison with other costs.[16] Presents for the Indians, which included such an unknown commodity as "2 doz. Nonesopretty" at $2.94, or 2800 "Fish Hooks assd." at $8.00, cost nearly $700 and even this proved to be entirely insufficient. The single most expensive item was the $250 chronometer. Lewis added an expensive item to the medical bill a little later when he purchased two pounds of tea at nearly two dollars per pound, a luxury which was to be saved for medicine alone, its cost being equal to that of the best powdered Peruvian bark available.[17]

Some items on the list of medicaments require further explanation. Saccharum saturni (lead acetate) was used as an urethral injection in gonorrhea, though for this purpose balsam of copaiba was felt to be more specific. Sugar of lead was also an important part of Rush's armamentarium, used extensively by him for infantile epilepsy, chorea, and hysteria, but this substance was to play the most important part in the preparation of the expedition's collyrium, which the explorers made in large amounts and dispensed freely. Elixir of vitriol, or ethylsulfuric acid flavored with cinnamon and ginger, was given with cinchona as a tonic and was described in a prominent dispensatory of the day as valuable in weakness, relaxations of the stomach, and "decays of the constitution."[18] "Columbo Rad.," an esteemed astringent and bitters, was prepared from the roots of species of *Frasera* from Ceylon (Colombo, "the root") or from the Ohio Valley (columbo of Marietta). Balsam traumatick, originally known as Turlington's balsam, was an American formulation for compound tincture of benzoin which, with basilic ointment (rosin cerate), calamine ointment, and diachylon (lead oleate), comprised the drugs used in wound dressings.

Nothing was used more often, to judge by the expedition's journals, than Rush's potent bilious pills. In his famous battle with yellow fever in the Philadelphia disasters which began in 1793, Rush came to feel that the effluvium of bile in the fevers accompanied by jaundice must be relieved by prompt evacuation and in 1793 described his powerful remedy.[19] Known as "ten and ten," an

[16] Thwaites, *op. cit.*, VII, pp. 238-246.
[17] Thwaites, *op. cit.*, VII, pp. 238-246.
[18] Thacher, J. *The new American dispensatory.* 4th ed. Boston, T. B. Wait, 1821, p. 559.
[19] Butterfield, *op. cit.*, II, pp. 648 cf.

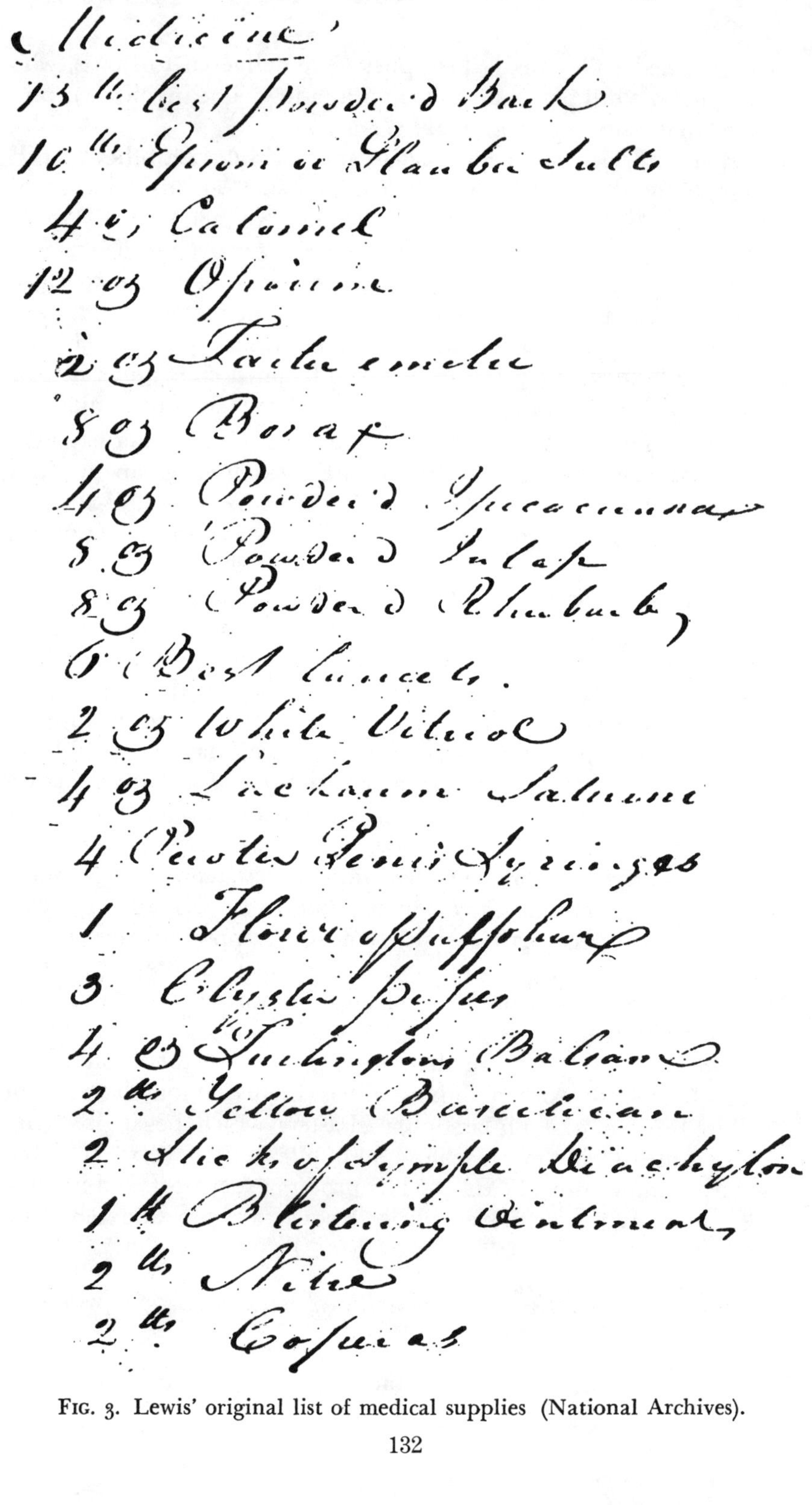

Medicine

15 lb best powder'd Bark
10 lb Epsom or Glauber Salts
4 oz Calomel
12 oz Opium
2 oz Tartar emetic
8 oz Borax
4 oz Powder'd Ipecacuanha
5 oz Powder'd Jalap
8 oz Powder'd Rhubarb
6 Best Lancets
2 oz White Vitriol
4 oz Lacteum Saturni
4 Pewter Penis Syringes
1 Flower of Sulphur
3 Clyster pipes
4 oz Turlington's Balsam
2 lb Yellow Basilicum
2 Sticks of Symple Diachylon
1 lb Blistering Ointment
2 lb Nitre
2 lb Copperas

FIG. 3. Lewis' original list of medical supplies (National Archives).

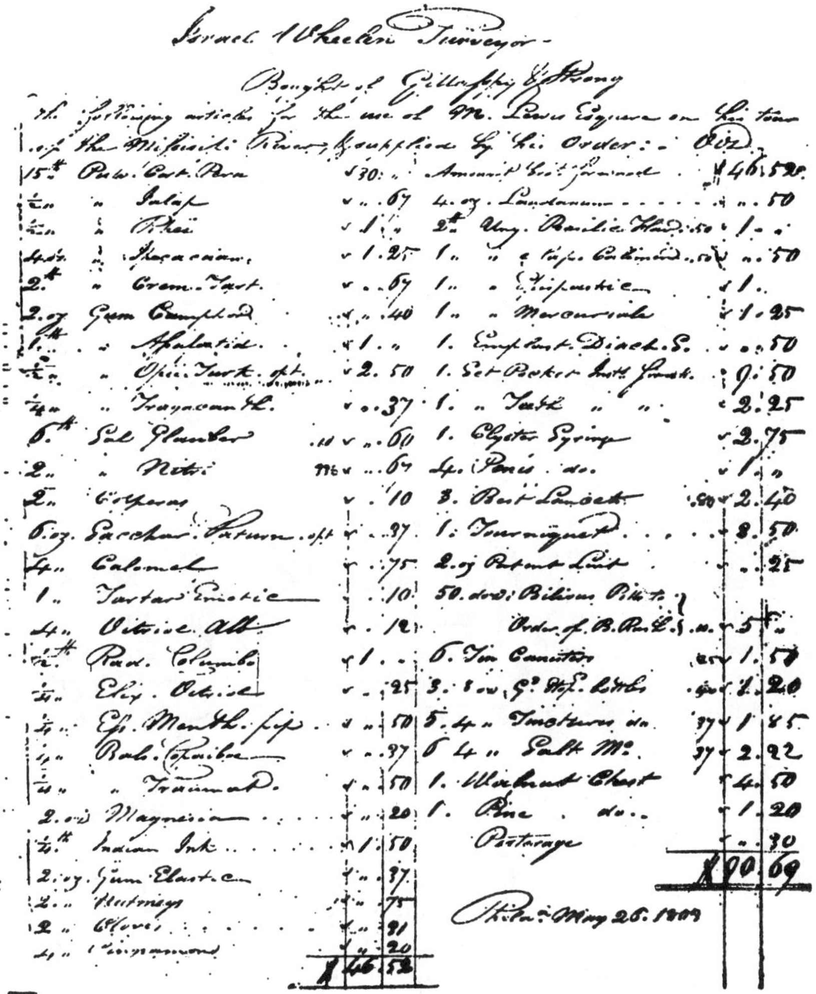

Israel Wheelen Purveyor

Bought of Gillaspy & Strong

the following articles for the use of Mr. Lewis Esquire on his tour up the Missisippi River, & supplied by his Order :- Viz.

15 lb	Pulv. Cort. Peru	$30. —		Amount brot forward	$46.52
1/2 "	" Jalap	" .67	4. oz.	Laudanum	" .50
1/2 "	" Rhei	1. —	2 lb	Ung. Basilic Flav. .50	1. —
4 oz	" Ipecacuan	1.25	1 "	" e lapis Calaminar. .50	" .50
2 lb	" Crem. Tart.	" .67	1 "	" Epispastric	1.
2 oz	Gum Camphor	" .40	1 "	" Mercurial	1.25
1 lb	" Assafoetida	1. "	1.	Emplast. Diach. S.	" .50
1/2 "	" Opii Turk. opt.	2.50	1.	Set Pocket Insts. small	9.50
1/4 "	" Tragacanth	" .37	1.	" Teeth " "	2.25
6 lb	Sal Glauber	" .60	1.	Clyster Syringe	2.75
2 "	" Nitri	" .67	4.	Penis do.	1. "
2 "	Copperas	" .10	3.	Best Lancets .80	2.40
6 oz.	Sacchar. Saturn. opt.	" .37	1.	Tourniquet	3.50
4 "	Calomel	" .75	2 oz	Patent Lint	" .25
1 "	Tartar Emetic	" .10	50. doz.	Bilious Pills to Order of B. Rush	5. "
4 "	Vitriol Alb.	" .12			
1/2 lb	Rad. Columbo	1. —	6.	Tin Canisters .25	1.50
1/4 "	Elix. Vitriol	" .25	3.	8 oz. Gd. Stopd. bottles .40	1.20
1/4 "	Ess. Menth. pip.	" .50	5.	4 " Tincture do. .37	1.85
1/4 "	Bals. Copaiba	" .37	6	4 " Salt Mo. .37	2.22
1/4 "	" Traumat.	" .50	1.	Walnut Chest	4.50
2. oz	Magnesia	" .20	1.	Pine do.	1.20
1/4 lb	Indian Ink	1.50		Porterage	" .30
2. oz.	Gum Elastic	" .37			$90.69
2. "	Nutmegs	" .75			
2 "	Cloves	" .31			
4 "	Cinnamon	" .20			
		$46.52			

Philada. May 26. 1803

FIG. 4. Bill of sale for the medical supplies of the Lewis and Clark expedition (National Archives).

equal mixture of calomel and jalap, it was adapted by Rush in 1793 to calomel, gr x, and jalap, gr xv, "to carry the calomel through the bowels." It is known that he also prescribed calomel and gamboge pills, still officially known as compound mild mercurous chloride pills in the American pharmacopeia, "so as to procure large evacuations from the bowels."[20] The 600 pills the explorers packed into their gear were undoubtedly the calomel and jalap

[20] *Ibid., II,* pp. 699 cf.

"Bilious Pills to Order of B. Rush," a quantity sufficient to have combatted even more than the "unusual costiveness" Rush described in his suggestions to Lewis for his health.

Lastly there were six kegs containing 30 gallons of spirits of wine. With the thoroughly detested dehydrated "portable soup," they were listed as "Provisions &c" in the records still extant.[21] The spirits figure high in the annals of the expedition and were the basis of many remedies and decoctions prepared by the captains and a welcome tonic on many an exhausting, cold, and discouraging afternoon.

His purchases completed, Lewis returned to Washington briefly while the goods and equipment were drayed to Pittsburgh and, on 30 August 1803, after many agonizing delays, the capable and earnest young man, with a platoon of soldiers, cast off in a flatboat into the Ohio River bound for the Mississippi.

William Clark joined Lewis and his party in Louisville. A militiaman like Lewis and brother of George Rogers Clark, William Clark had been Lewis' commander for a short time on the western frontier. A more experienced soldier than the younger Lewis, Clark was Lewis' choice as co-leader, and their great mutual respect and varied gifts led to a joint command of unusual harmony and effectiveness. The explorers continued down the Ohio to Kaskaskia and there Lewis left for St. Louis by land. Clark, the field captain, continued on with the boat to the Wood River, a few miles above St. Louis, where the party was to assemble in winter quarters. From 12 December 1803 until May 14th the following year, the troops trained in the base camp while the captains spent many days in St. Louis, stocking the expedition and learning what they could about the great unknown western river from the numerous travellers in the town who had information to give.

In the crude frontier settlement, their scientific and medical education apparently continued. A family tradition in the Saugrain-von Phul families of St. Louis has led several historians to investigate the contribution that Dr. Antoine Saugrain may have made to the expedition.[22] Perhaps the most prominent scientist in the Mississippi Valley, Saugrain was a European-trained physician who made the first lucifer matches in the United States and was the first to use cowpox vaccine in the Valley, where he inoculated the Kanawha nation. His thermometers and barometers were made for

---

[21] Thwaites, *op. cit.*, VII, p. 241.
[22] Meany, E. S. Doctor Saugrain helped Lewis and Clark. *Wash. hist. Quart.*, 1931, 22, 295-311.

commercial sale and, though the statement is unsupported by any documentary evidence, he is said to have furnished a thermometer, matches, and medicines to Lewis. No thermometer was purchased for the expedition's use by the public stores, yet a thermometer was in use and Pvt. Whitehouse was even sent back to retrieve it one day in 1805 (July 22d) when Lewis left it hanging in the shade,[23] and its later breakage is fully recorded.[24] Portable thermometers were rare instruments in 1803, and Lewis required three in his original lists of scientific instruments and it is entirely possible that one was made for him in Philadelphia. But the family tradition of Dr. Saugrain remains and Lewis' thermometer may well have been made in St. Louis with the mercury scraped from the back of Mrs. Saugrain's best mirror, as the story goes.

In the small camp where the Wood River flows into the Missouri, preparations ended. There was no turning back for supplies, assistance, or further information, spurious or real, about what lay west beyond the Mandans. On May 14th, the small, healthy, well-disciplined party,[25] their admired captains in the lead, shoved off in the small boats and on foot to track the mighty rolling western rivers to the distant sea.

II

As quiet as the gentle rainy spring day on the great flooding Missouri is William Clark's first journal entry for 14 May 1804: "I set out at 4 oClock P.M., in the presence of many of the neighbouring inhabitents, and proceeded on under a jentle brease up the Missouri...."[26]

Meriwether Lewis was in St. Louis on an urgent last-minute business trip and met the party on May 20th at St. Charles. Lewis issued the orders for rations as the party slowly made their way up the broad lower reaches of the muddy river.

The day after tomorrow lyed corn and grece will be issued to the party, the next day Poark and flour, and the day following indian meal and poark; and in conformity to that rotiene provisions will continue to be issued to the party untill further orders. should any of the messes prefer indian meal to flour they may recieve it accordingly—no poark is to be issued when we have fresh meat on hand.[27]

---

[23] Thwaites, *op. cit.*, VII, p. 119 (Pvt. Whitehouse's Journal).

[24] *Ibid.*, III, p. 51; VI, pp. 197, 203.

[25] The permanent party initially numbered 34, including Sacagawea, Indian wife of the interpreter, and Clark's slave, York. Sgt. Floyd's death and the discharge of two soldiers lowered the outbound party to 31, later raised to 32 by the birth of Sacagawea's son, and this remained the expedition's numerical strength. See de Voto, B., Ed. *The Journals of Lewis and Clark*, Boston, Houghton Mifflin Co., 1953, pp. 489-491.

[26] De Voto, B., Ed. *The Journals of Lewis and Clark*. Boston, Houghton Mifflin Co., 1953, p. 3.

[27] Thwaites, R G.., Ed. *Original journals of the Lewis and Clark Expedition*. New York, Dodd, Mead, 1904, I, pp. 33-34.

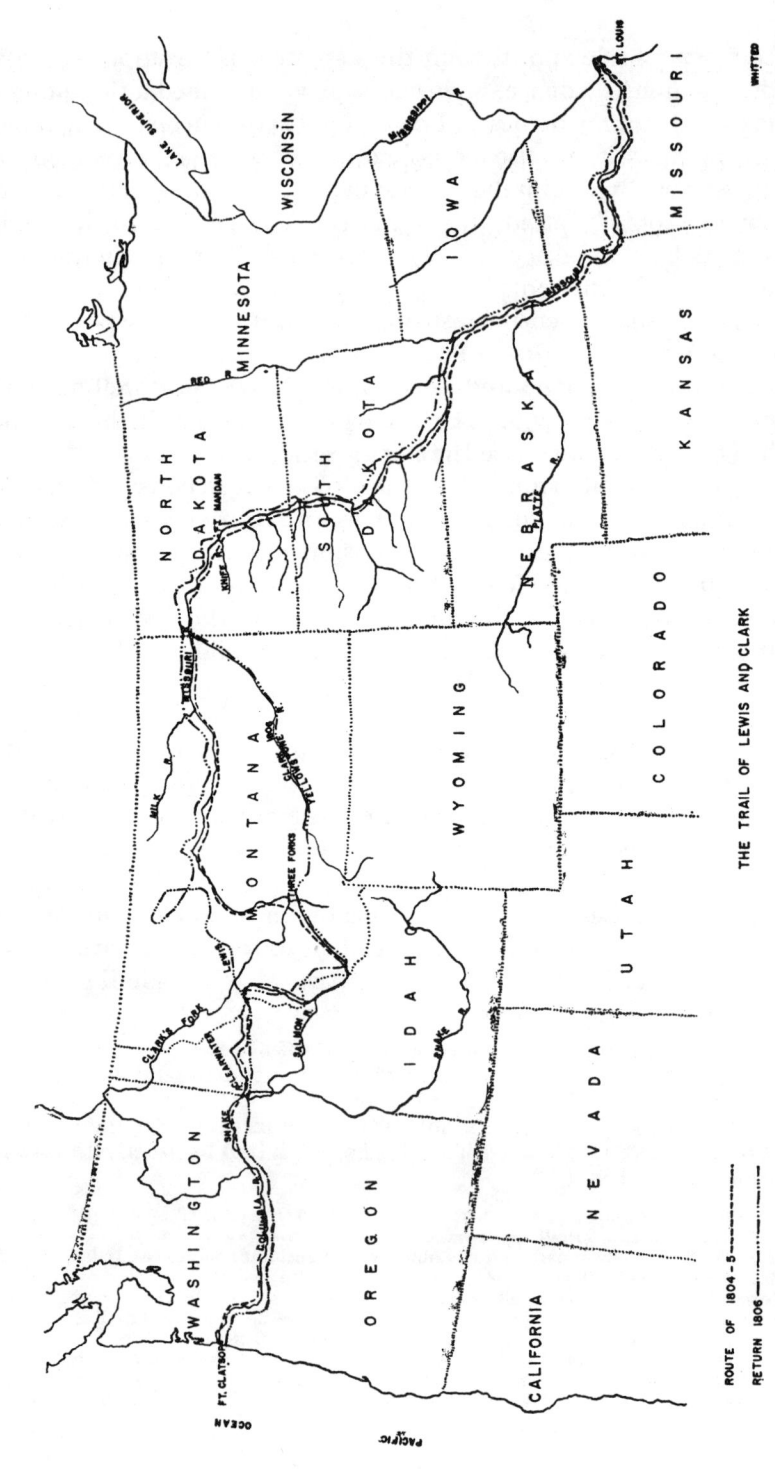

Fig. 5. Sketch map showing the routes of the Lewis and Clark party.

Later, on the upper reaches of the Columbia watershed, when camas roots and poorly dried salmon became the only diet of the Corps of Discovery, this early period would be fondly remembered as one of great luxury. Except for sore eyes from the continual glare of the river and storms of fine dry silt and the grinding physical labor of lifting the laden boats over the continual snags, progress was smooth until Independence Day, 1804, when "Jos Fields got bit by a Snake, which was quickly doctered with Bark by Cap Lewis."[28] Rattlers abounded, and De Voto feels that Joe Fields was bitten by one of these, but one wonders if Lewis' "poultice of bark and gunpowder"[29] would have cured the patient so expeditiously.

A standard treatment of the day is noted several days later by Clark; "one man verry sick, Struck with the Sun, Capt. Lewis bled him & gave Niter which has revived him much."[30] A much graver problem were the "tumers" and "biles" which occurred over the exposed, continually wet skin and produced regional lymphadenitis, often sufficiently painful to keep the men from working. The captains ascribed this disorder to the muddiness of the river water and occasionally were required to resort to more drastic treatment than the usual poultices of elm and cornmeal. Clark notes "I opened the Tumer of a man on the left breast, which discharged half a point."[31] Otherwise Clark was well pleased by the progress of the journey. "It is worthey of observation to mention that our Party has been much healthier on the Voyage than parties of the same number is in any other Situation."[32]

On the 19th of August, however, a major emergency occurred. "Serjeant Floyd is taken very bad all at once with Biliose Chorlick we attempt to relieve him without success as yet, he gets worst and we are much allarmed at his Situation, all attention to him."[33] Floyd, whose brief and pathetic journal is extant, cryptically noted twenty days before, "I am verry Sick and Has ben for Somtime but have Recovered my Helth again."[34] The day following the sudden onset of his illness, which Pvt. Gass recalled as a violent colic,[35] the distressed Clark wrote, "Serjeant Floyd as bad as he can be no pulse

---

[28] Thwaites, *op. cit.*, I, p. 66.
[29] Allen, Paul, Ed. *History of the expedition of Captains Lewis and Clark, 1804-5-6*, (Reprint of edition of 1814, with Introduction by J. K. Hosmer). Chicago, A. C. McClurg, I, p. 22.
[30] Thwaites, *op. cit.*, I, pp. 69-70.
[31] *Ibid.*, I, p. 91.
[32] *Ibid.*, I, pp. 85-86.
[33] Thwaites, *op. cit.*, I, p. 114.
[34] *Ibid.*, VII, p. 22.
[35] Gass, P., *Lewis and Clarke's Journal to the Rocky Mountains in the years 1804-5,-6 as related by Patrick Gass, one of the officers in the expedition.* Dayton, Ells, Chaflin, & Co., 1847 (reprint), p. 29.

& nothing will Stay a moment on his Stomach or bowels. Passed two Islands on the S.S. and at the first Bluff on the S.S. Serj. Floyd Died with a great deal of Composure, before his death he Said to me, 'I am going away I want you to write me a letter.' "[36] Pvt. Whitehouse said, "he was layed out in the most decent manner possable."[37] The probability is greatest that young Floyd died a victim of a perforated gangrenous appendix with generalized peritonitis, and the unfortunate sergeant would have fared little better in Philadelphia with Rush and his colleagues in attendance. Buried with military honors above the Big Muddy he had hoped to ascend and explore with his comrades, Floyd was the first American soldier to be buried in the trans-Mississippi West and his name is commemorated by the commanding bluff on which he lies.

The journey up the Missouri to the Mandan villages[38] and the period spent there in winter quarters, 1804, was marked by no other major medical problems following Sgt. Floyd's death. There were minor difficulties with boils, poisoned water, dysentery, and an acute form of rheumatism of the neck and legs. Clark writes of his co-commander's attempt to treat some violent rheumatic pains in his neck: "Capt. applied a hot Stone raped in flannel, which gave me some tempore ease. . . ."[39] The freezing cold added to the problem of keeping the large party occupied with sufficient work, and frostbite became serious on the hunting and wood-cutting details outside the camps. Clark's journal entries on frostbite are a curious mixture of both reticent delicacy and bald chilling statement. He noted "this day being Cold Several men returned a little frostbit. . . . my Servents feet also frosted and his P—s a little,"[40] or "Snowed last night, wind high from NW. Sawed off the boys toes."[41] The latter referred to the frost-bitten feet of a young Indian lad.

Clark tantalizes the medical reader throughout with entries like the following: "one man taken violently Bad with Plurisie, Bleed & apply those remedies Common to that disorder."[42] Lewis, on the other hand, gives us a brief yet full account of the birth of

[36] Thwaites, *op. cit.*, I, pp. 114-115.
[37] *Ibid.*, VII, p. 51 (Whitehouse's Journal).
[38] Near present Staunton, North Dakota, 45 miles north of Bismarck and 1600 river miles from the Wood River.
[39] Thwaites, *op. cit.*, I, p. 202.
[40] *Ibid.*, I, p. 235.
[41] *Ibid.*, I, p. 252.
[42] *Ibid.*, I, p. 251.

Sacagawea's first child.[43] The Indian girl's labor (she was probably about sixteen) was "tedious and the pain violent"[44] and Jessaume, an engagé of the Hudson's Bay Co. who interpreted for the captains during their stay with the Mandans, gave her powdered snake rattles in water to hasten her labor. Administered at the last moment, "She had not taken it more than ten minutes before she brought forth."[45] Lewis adds "perhaps this remedy may be worthy of future experiments, but I must confess that I want faith as to it's efficacy."[46]

Venereal disease ("Pox," or primary syphilis) was the principal threat to the party's health in winter quarters at Fort Mandan. Sgt. Gass portentously sums up the situation in his own journal, as follows:

It may be observed generally that chastity is not very highly esteemed by these people, and that the severe and loathsome effects *of certain French principles* are not uncommon among them. The fact is, that the women are generally considered an article of traffic, and *indulgence* are sold at a very moderate price. As a proof of this I will just mention, that for an old tobacco box, one of our men was granted the honor of passing a night with the daughter of the head chief of the Mandan nation. An old bawd with her punks, may also be found in some of the villages on the Missouri, as well as in the large cities of polished nations."[47]

Lewis had four or five patients continually. He left no precise statement regarding his anti-luetic regimen other than the simple note that he used mercury. Both mercuric ointment and calomel were included in the medical supplies, and one suspects that he followed the accepted method of the day, e.g. a priming dose of calomel and jalap to "clear the bowels" for the subsequent calomel, in pill form, which was given until sore gums appeared, then discontinued. After the soreness cleared, calomel was readministered until the primary lesion disappeared.

The expedition resumed its journey on 7 April 1805, to venture into country quite unknown to Americans or to the English and French traders north of the river. Beyond the Mandans was mystery and pure conjecture mixed with genuine information provided by the Indians, the interpretation of which was difficult to

---

[43] Charbonneau, French engagé, interpreter to the expedition, and Sacagawea's husband, was probably absent, being of little use during any emergency. He was usually saved from embarrassment by his squaw's quick mind and physical agility.

[44] Thwaites, *op. cit.*, I, p. 257.

[45] *Ibid.*, I, p. 257.

[46] *Ibid.*, I, p. 258.

[47] Gass, *op. cit.*, p. 72. It should be noted that Gass' journal, the first published record of the expedition (Pittsburgh, 1807) was completely rewritten, edited and expanded by David M'Keehan, a West Virginia school teacher. It is subject to both Gass' later thought and to M'Keehan's editorializing.

master in terms of miles and days. During early May, in the turbulent snow-swollen waters, the white perogue capsized and its goods were lost, or, if recovered, were badly damaged, including many of the medical stores. Little is known about the losses but happily the alcohol was not destroyed: ". . . accordingly fixed our camp and gave each man a small dram. . . . such is the effects of abstaining for some time from the uce of speritous liquors they were all very merry."[48]

At Maria's River, where this wide northern stream rolls into the Missouri, an urgent geographical conference took place and the captains separated to determine which of the unnamed, unknown streams was the Missouri. Clark, on the south fork, came to the decision first that he was following the true Missouri, a conclusion with which Lewis shortly concurred, and on 11 June Lewis and several men left the party to ascend the south fork on foot, Clark remaining to follow with the boats. Before he left, the young captain noted in his journal that Sacagawea was ill and that Clark had bled her. Later in the day, Lewis became quite ill himself with abdominal cramps and fever and, having no medicines, he resorted to a bitter thick black mixture made from the twigs of choke cherry boiled in water. By the following morning, he was completely well. Bakeless, in a biography of the expedition's leaders, relates that Meriwether Lewis' mother was known in Albemarle County, Virginia, as a "yarb doctor" and Lewis had been exposed many times to the preparation and use of such simples.[49]

During Lewis' absence, Clark apparently exhausted his store of information in attempting to treat Sacagawea's illness. Lewis returned in time to take over her care. His description of the sickness sheds considerable light on his knowledge and his abilities as physician-in-chief to his party.

. . . about 2 P.M. I reached the camp found the Indian woman extreemly ill and much reduced by her indisposition. . . . I found that two dozes of barks and opium which I had given her since my arrival had, produced an alteration in her pulse for the better/they were now much fuller and more regular. I caused her to drink the mineral water altogether. when I first came down I found that her pulse were scarcely perceptible, very quick frequently irregular and attended with strong nervous symptoms, that of the twitching of the fingers and leaders of the arm/ now the pulse had become regular much fuller and a gentle perspiration had taken place; the nervous symptoms have

---

[48] Thwaites, *op. cit.*, II, 95.
[49] Bakeless, J. *Lewis and Clark, partners in discovery.* New York, Wm. Morrow and Co., 1947, p. 16.

also in a great measure abated, and she feels herself much freer from pain. she complains principally of the lower region of the abdomen, I therefore continued the cataplasms of barks and laudanum which had been previously used by my friend Capt. Clark. I believe her disorder originated principally from an obstruction of the mensis in consequence of taking could.[50]

Sacagawea recovered rapidly, undoubtedly in spite of the somewhat rigorous measures adopted by the captains. Lewis' rather liberal use of opiates helped ease the pain of her acute illness, the total duration of which was six days. Pelvic pain, fever, rapid thready pulse, and menstrual irregularity in a young woman under such circumstances seems most strongly to suggest acute pelvic inflammatory disease, either recently acquired or an exacerbation of a chronic infection. Sacagawea may also, though less likely, have been suffering with an acute exacerbation of latent post-partum infection or from appendicitis. It is regrettable that the account of her illness is so sketchy, but any diagnostic conjectures should be tempered by the fact that this was the only recorded serious ailment Sacagawea suffered during the entire journey.

At Great Falls, Montana, a series of tremendous cataracts ten miles long, made river travel impossible and the party spent an entire month portaging boats and goods on crude wagons to the upper river under Clark's direction, while Lewis, in the upper camp, supervised the setting-up of the iron boat and acted as cook to his own command. His failure to float the iron boat more than momentarily before its covering of larded and tarred skins leaked or completely parted was apparently one of the least of the disappointments. Clark notes "to state the fatigues of this party would take up more the journal than other notes which I find scercely time to set down."[51] Of trouble, distractions and irritations, there were many and Lewis rather floridly wrote: "our trio of pests still invade and obstruct us on all occasions, these are the Musquetoes eye knats and prickley pears, equal to any three curses that every poor Egypt laiboured under, except the Mahometant yoke."[52]
Despite Egypt's burdens, little worse happened during the month of back-breaking labor than the following incident which Pvt. Whitehouse related in his own journal, "I took sick this evening I expect by drinking too much water when I was hot. I get bled &c."[53] Lewis found his pulse full and apologizes for the want of any instru-

---
50 Thwaites, *op. cit.*, II, pp. 162-164.
51 *Ibid.*, II, p. 183.
52 Thwaites, *op. cit.*, II, p. 266.
53 *Ibid.*, VII, p. 108 (Whitehouse's Journal).

ment other than his penknife but notes that, for venesection, "it answered very well."[54]

On 27 July the expedition reached the forks of the Missouri, where Clark, a natural geographer of genius, rightly decided they must ascend the most western of the three converging streams, which they named the Jefferson River, to reach the western mountains. At this point, they were almost exactly 2,500 miles from the mouth of the great river and had now traversed its entire length. Though still exhausted from the arduous portage, the party was very well, but Clark soon fell ill with constipation and aggravated it by continuing his explorations of the other forks of the river. Lewis records: "Cap! C. thought himself somewhat bilious and had not had a passage for several days; I prevailed on him to take a doze of Rushes pills, which I have always found sovereign in such cases and to bath his feet in warm water and rest himself."[55] Lewis' knowledge of Rush's famed remedy was probably better than Clark's notion of the recommended dose, since he enthusiastically took five of the pills at once and recorded no ill effects from this total dosage of, presumably, over 3 grams each of calomel and jalap. It was the last illness of sufficient note to be recorded in the journals until the explorers began their winter encampment at the mouth of the Columbia.

A long land and water trek led the party through the Rockies from the headwaters of the Jefferson by somewhat devious route over the Lemhi, Gibbon's, and Lolo Passes to the Clearwater River. Here, close to the site of modern Missoula, Montana, the log canoes were built which carried the party into the great Columbia and out to the Pacific. Food presented the primary problem, and shortly the situation became extremely serious. Game was very scarce and poor in quality when available, and the expedition's own food stores were badly reduced. The Indian diet became the party's staple and proved both monotonous and debilitating, consisting entirely of edible roots[56] and dried salmon, with occasional wild game or an equally poor dog purchased from the Indians. Diar-

---

[54] *Ibid.*, II, p. 189.
[55] Thwaites, *op. cit.*, II, p. 279.
[56] A variety of these roots and bulbs were used by the Indians, usually made into a gruel or pounded and dried to form a bread. Those mentioned prominently in the journals included camas (*Camassia quamash*), wapato (*Sagittaria latifolia*), and cows or biscuitroot (*Lomatium geyeri*). Probably others were the Indian potato, the cattails, and bitterroot (*Lewisia rediviva*). L. H. Pammell (*A manual of poisonous plants*, Cedar Rapids, Iowa, Torch Press, 1911) has pointed out the long-term severe nutritional disturbances which result from a continual diet of these otherwise nontoxic plants. Utilizable carbohydrate is low and many contain high concentrations of nonmetabolized starches like inulin.

rhea, the low caloric intake, and absence of salt balanced poorly against the hard labor of frequent portaging, and the party found itself poorly prepared for the extreme privations of winter quarters on the low tidelands of the great river. Near-starvation and gloomy weather were unable to stifle the exultant Clark, who, speaking for the entire party, jotted quickly in his notebook on courses and bearings one of the truly unforgettable lines in the literature of exploration: *"Ocian in view- O! the joy."*[57]

Their camp at the mouth of the Columbia, Fort Clatsop, was cold and almost continuously rainy (and its appearance today is no less dismal than 150 years ago). The leather-clad explorers were hardly ever dry or warm, and colds, pleurisy, and severe rheumatism became serious and recurrent complaints. Both Clark and Lewis remained relatively well and bent all their efforts to provide both salt and meat for their weakened command. Four thousand miles of return travel still faced the party, and the store of Indian presents was almost completely gone so that bartering was reduced in order to provide only the most necessary items, and the impoverished thieving Chinooks could produce even few of these. Moreover, trading on their knowledge of white men, the Indians soon started another type of enterprise.

> An old woman & Wife to a Cheif of the *Chunnooks* came and made a camp near ours. She brought with her 6 young Squars (her daughters & nieces) I believe for the purpose of Gratifying the passions of the men of our party and receiving for those indulgiences Such Small as She (the old woman) thought proper to accept of.
> Those people appear to View Sensuality as a Necessary evel, and do not appear to abhor it as a Crime in the unmarried State. The young females are fond of the attention of our men and appear to meet the sincere approbation of the friends and connections for thus obtaining their favours.[58]

Clark's patience was soon stretched to the utmost as we gather from his exasperated "The Chin-nook womin are lude and carry on sport publickly."[59] The captains treated two men with mercury for almost three months. Lewis learned that the Indians had no specifics against the venereal diseases and that lues always lead to decrepitude, death, or premature aging, but he felt that the simples of lobelia and sumac he had seen used by the handsome and intelligent

---

[57] De Voto, *op. cit.*, p. 279.

[58] Thwaites, *op. cit.*, III, p. 241. Robert Gray's discovery of the great river in 1792 in his American ship, the Columbia, had given the Indian Communities ample opportunity to learn how best to capitalize on the needs and weaknesses of white exploring parties. Clark, after describing at length the physical attributes of what he obviously felt were singularly unattractive women, noted a tattoo reading "J. Bowman" on the left arm of one of the maidens in this speedily assembled commercial enterprise.

[59] *Ibid.*, III, p. 294.

Chippewas of the Great Plains were both "effecatious and sovereign" for both lues and gonorrhea.[60]

While a trio of the men set up a salt-making plant and successfully produced nearly a gallon of salt per day, the continual cold rain and fog began to take serious toll. Pvt. Bratton had to be relieved at the salt works because of very severe low back pain. Though many of the men suffered with various rheumatic complaints, Bratton remained seriously incapacitated until late in May, almost four months. Treated symptomatically with barks, laudanum and "some volatile linniment which was prepared with sperits of wine, camphire, castile soap, and a little laudinum," Bratton improved gradually, regaining appetite and strength, but with too much lumbar pain to be a working member of the party.

Speed was absolutely essential in retracing their course[61] because the Indians on the lower Columbia passed on to the captains a rumor that the friendly Choppunish tribes (Nez Percés), who were boarding their horses, were leaving early for the Rockies. The expedition's Indian goods were now dissipated almost completely by trade with canny natives. Most of the gifts the party could use now would be items of their own personal equipment. Lewis knew that the essential boats and horses would take what trinkets were left and the party must find some expedient to increase their purchasing power. The solution was a relatively simple one, an exchange of goods and horses for medical attention. At first, neither Lewis nor Clark recognized that their fame as physicians had filtered down into the Columbia basin from the Nez Percé tribes nor did it occur to them that they might turn this reputation into something tangible. Clark, practical as ever, made the first attempt.

> I saw a man who had his knee contracted who had previously applyed to me for some medisene, that if he would fournish another canoe I would give him some medisene. He readily consented and went himself with his canoe by means of which he passed our horses over the river safely and hubbled them as usial . . . they [Walla-Wallas] brought several disordered persons to us for whome they requested some medical aid. one had his knee contracted by the Rhumitism (whome is just mentioned above) another with a broken arm &c. to all of whome we administered much to the gratification of those pore wretches, we gave them eye water which I believe will render them more essential sirvice than an other article in the medical way which we had it in our power to bestow on them. . . . The man who had his arm broken

---

60 *Ibid.*, IV, p. 16.

61 Jefferson's failure to provide a ship to relieve the party on the Columbia has never been explained, and the party saw no ships during their stay.

had it losely bound in a piece of lether without anything to support it. I dressed the arm which was broken short above the wrist & supported with broad sticks to keep it in place, but [?] in a sling and furnished him with some lint bandages &c. to Dress it in future.[62]

Clark was both more interested and more comfortable with Indians than the introspective and more fastidious Lewis. "My friend Capt. C. is their favorite physician," Lewis wrote, "and has already received many applications. in our present situation I think it pardonable to continue this deseption for they will not give us any provision without compensation in merchandize and our stock is now reduced to a mere handfull. We take care to give them no article which can possibly injure them."[63]

Their practice, assiduously fostered over the entire return route to the Rockies, became large and, on the whole, Clark, with Lewis' advice, provided better care than many of the tribes were to know again until quite recent times. A selection from the captain's notes gives the reader some idea of the problems the frontier physicians faced.

Several applyed to me today for medical aide, one a broken arm another inward fevers and several with pains across the loins, and sore eyes. I administered as well as I could to all. in the evening a man brought his wife and a horse both up to me. the horse he gave me as a present and his wife who was verry unwell the effects of violent coalds was placed before me. I did not think her case a bad one and gave such medesene as would keep her body open and raped her in flannel. left some simple medesin to be taken. we also gave some Eye water 1 G [?] of Ela v V. & 2 grs. of Sacch^m S^{try} to an ounce of water and in that perportion....[64]

At 11 A.M. Thompson returned from the village accompanyed by a train of invalids consisting of 4 men 8 women and a child. The men had soar eyes and the women in addition to soar eyes had a variety of other complaints principally rheumatic; a weakness and pain in the loins is a common complaint with their women. eyewater was administered to all; to two of the women cathartics were given, to a third who appeared much dejected and who from their account of her disease we supposed it to be histerical, we gave 30 drops of Laudanum. the several parts of the others where the rheumatic pains were seated were well rubed with volitile linniment. all of those poor wretches thought themselves much benefited, and all returned to their vilage well satisfyed.[65]

[62] Thwaites, *op. cit.*, IV, pp. 333-334.
[63] *Ibid.*, IV, p. 358.
[64] Thwaites, *op. cit.*, IV, pp. 339-340 (p. 340). Deciphered, the collyrium contained, per ounce of water, 2 grains of lead acetate and 1 grain of zinc sulfate. "Ela" is a corruption of calamine (Zn CO$_3$) and V. probably represents an abbreviation of vitriol. *Calaminae vitriolum* or zinc sulfate was made by dissolving calamine in sulfuric acid or oil of vitriol. The small "v" possibly refers to an impure, "venale," grade of zinc sulfate. This mildly astringent solution was so successful in treating the conjunctivities Lewis and Clark found so commonly that it became their most successful trade item. A vial of eye water was traded for a good horse. Blindness, undoubtedly due to trachoma and venereal disease, was very commonly observed by the explorers, but is distinguished carefully in the journals from the prevalent "soar eyes" which afflicted both Indian and explorer.
[65] Thwaites, *op. cit.*, V, p. 49.

Their satisfaction was all the Americans, impatient to be on their way, could hope for, though neither Clark nor Lewis allowed themselves to be deceived as to the lasting value of their therapy. Charbonneau's infant, the bright-eyed Pompey, who was Clark's favorite, developed a severe sore throat and cervical lymphadenitis which was carefully poulticed with wild onions and the youngster subjected to the usual purgative regimen.[66] He recovered rapidly and only one serious problem remained to be solved before the party could leave the camps on the Clearwater for the mountains. William Bratton, his appetite good and his weight recovered, was still so crippled by the rheumatic stiffness and pain in his back that he could neither ride horseback nor walk with any comfort. The worried Lewis notes "we have tried every remidy which our engenuity could devise, or with which our stock of medicines furnished us, without effect. John Sheilds observed that he had seen men in a similar situation restored by violent sweats. Bratton requested that he might be sweated in the manner proposed by Sheilds to which we consented."[67] Bratton was sweated for an hour in an improvised Indian steam bath, which consisted of a large pit previously heated by a roaring fire before the naked victim was lowered into it. Comfortably seated under a heavy blanket "orning," Bratton sprinkled water over the hot stones for steam and was interrupted twice when his companions took him out and dunked him briefly in the icy Clearwater. Shields gave him a strong tea of horsemint, having no snakeroot which he had seen used before. The treatment was remarkably successful and in the following week, Bratton went on a trading party, his first activity in four months.

Bratton's illness remains mysterious. Initially relieved at the salt plant because he was "verry unwell" (?), he remained extremely weak and may have suffered a severe gastroenteritis. The onset of low back pain occurred early in the course of the disease, probably within the first three days and it remained after the other symptoms had disappeared. There is no description of colic, diarrhea or vomiting and the young man had been healthy previously. Bratton outlived many other members of the expedition, dying at about sixty years of age after a busy and useful life. It is not known if he suffered a recurrence of his complaint. With only the meager descriptions of his long illness and his dramatic recovery in the daily

[66] *Ibid.*, V, p. 56.
[67] *Ibid.*, V, pp. 60-61.

diaries of the expedition, Bratton may well have had an infectious arthritis initially related to bacterial gastroenteritis, whose resolution may have been complicated by constant dampness, cold, and the necessity of wearing wet leather clothing continually.

The party, once through the Bitter Root range, divided, Lewis to go directly to the portage at Great Falls by a direct route and explore Maria's River, Clark to explore the Jefferson as far as the Three Forks and then to go overland to the Yellowstone, where the captains would rendezvous. Clark's journey was extremely easy, but the last serious accident of the expedition plagued Lewis and his party. Cautiously stalking an elk in the company of the one-eyed boatman, Cruzatte, Lewis writes:

> I was in the act of firing on the Elk a second time when a ball struck my left thye about an inch below my hip joint, missing the bone it passed through my left thye and cut the thickness of the bullet across the hinder part of the right thye; the stroke was very severe . . . with the assistance of Serg! Gass I took off my cloaths and dressed my wounds myself as well as I could, introducing tents of patent lint into the ball holes, the wounds blead considerably but I was hapy to find that it had touch neither bone nor artery . . . as it was painfull to me to be removed I slept on board the perogue; the pain I experienced excited a high fever and I had a very uncomfortable night."[68]

The following day, the entire party was reunited below the mouth of the Yellowstone, as related by Clark, who now took over the journal entries entirely.

> "I was alarmed" he wrote, "on the landing of the canoes to be informed that Capt. Lewis was wounded by accident. I found him lying in the Perogue, he informed me that his wound was slight and would be well in 20 or 30 days. this information relieved me very much. I examined the wound and found it a very bad flesh wound The ball had passed through the fleshey part of his left thy below the hip bone and cut the cheek of the right buttock for 3 inches in length and the debth of the ball."[69]

As Lewis had accurately predicted, 25 days later Clark was able to note that "My worthy friend Cap Lewis has entirely recovered his wounds are heeled up and he can walk and even run nearly as well as ever he could, the parts are yet tender &c &c."[70]

Thirteen days later, a jubilant company of hardy young men who had gone by land and water to the western ocean and returned, tied up at St. Louis. They had been gone 27 months and travelled 8,000 miles by boat, horseback, and on foot. They returned to the adulation of their countrymen and the fascination of all Americans

---

[68] Thwaites, *op. cit.*, V, pp. 240-242.
[69] *Ibid.*, V, p. 330.
[70] *Ibid.*, V, p. 380.

and Europeans who would follow their epic journey in the pages of the printed journals.

The Lewis and Clark party survived dysentery, malaria, poisonous waters, long periods of semi-starvation, and bitter weather, countless superficial wounds and injuries. Much credit is due their youthful vigor and strength, to the absence of the settlements of the next half-century which would seed the plains and rivers with cholera and the other epidemic diseases of great land migrations, and to the friendliness or confusion of the Indians who claimed none of them. But most credit is due to the unusual vigilance and care exercised by commanders who, in addition to the skills of leadership and practical scientific observation, were often more medically knowledgeable than might have been expected. Indeed, the active practice of medicine, somewhat embarrassing to Lewis, the instinctive physician, but enthusiastically handled by Clark, the more practical field surgeon, undoubtedly eased the party's return journey. The medicine which made allies of the Western tribes was truly medicine rather than the possession of deadly weapons, and the Indians would wait for another thirty years or more for the missionaries to return with medical supplies for such use.

Undoubtedly Lewis and Clark possessed not only extraordinary common sense but also the medical knowledge common to most educated men of the time, particularly to those who had served as military officers and had seen military physicians at work. The therapeutic armamentarium was pitifully small, but its very smallness was an advantage in that its essentials were moderately easy to learn. And to supplement their commonly shared information, the captains could rely on a well-assembled stock of medical supplies, a page of specific, written instructions for the care of their health and undoubtedly other advice given Lewis privately by the ex-officio medical counselor to the expedition, Benj: Rush.

Neo-Thomsonianism in the United States*

ALEX BERMAN†

> ". . . Though somewhat partial to the name Thomsonian, as we look on the discoveries which Samuel Thomson made in medicine to be superior to any and all of the theories of past ages; yet, by assuming his name we make ourselves liable to be accused of advocating his errors (for no one is perfect); and his opposition to education &c., makes this epithet really objectionable . . . It restricts those who assume it, to his notions and views, and rather forbids improvement in our noble science."
>
> *The New England Botanic Medical and Surgical Journal, Worcester, Mass.,* 1848, 2, 13.

I.

STATED in broad terms, Neo-Thomsonianism represented the transformation of a movement which had for its base a mass of uneducated, fanatical patent right-holders[1] into a Botanic cult seeking survival in scientific respectability. This change was very marked by mid-century, and did not escape the attention of the discerning Worthington Hooker, who acutely appreciated the irony of the situation. Here was a group of Botanic practitioners, sheepishly dropping the name "Thomsonian," forming medical schools, state medical societies, boards of censors, and issuing diplomas in imitation of the regulars. Indeed, "they had thus the effrontery," wrote Hooker indignantly, "to ask that they might possess, in common with us, that which they have always branded an unjust and odious monopoly. This is a *morceau* in the history of Thomsonism, too precious to be lost."[2] Besides appropriating some of the organizational and educational trappings of the regulars, Hooker also noted that the Neo-Thomsonians were expanding their materia medica, were using steam and emetics less frequently and with more caution, and were beginning to vaccinate for small-

---

* The activities of American Botanic practitioners were investigated by this writer in a doctoral dissertation entitled *The impact of the nineteenth century botanico-medical movement on American pharmacy and medicine*, University of Wisconsin, 1954. Portions of the sixth chapter of this dissertation form the basis of the present article. This study was supported in part by the Research Committee of the Graduate School from funds supplied by the Wisconsin Alumni Research Foundation. The writer is indebted to Dr. George Urdang, Professor Emeritus of History of Pharmacy, for his comments and suggestions.

† University of Wisconsin, Madison, Wisconsin.

[1] For a discussion of the old Thomsonian movement, see Berman, Alex. The Thomsonian movement and its relation to American pharmacy and medicine. *Bull. Hist. Med.*, 1951, 25, 405-428; 519-538.

[2] Hooker, Worthington. *Dissertation on the respect due to the medical profession, and the reasons why it is not awarded by the community*. Norwich, J. G. Cooley, 1844, p. 15.

pox and employ cathartics, in contrast to the practice of the old Thomsonians.[3]

Not only did the old Thomsonian materia medica and therapeutics begin to undergo transformations during the founder's lifetime, but serious organizational changes had also occurred. Towards the end of his life, the vision that Thomson had so hopefully nurtured over the years, of a gigantic "Friendly Botanic Society" composed of citizens happily treating each other with Thomson's patented system and avidly reading his *New Guide*, was fast fading away. The first serious blow to this dream had been Howard's abortive defection in 1832 and the formation of the dissident "Improved Botanics."[4] Thomson had, however, surmounted this obstacle, only to be confronted six years later with a disastrous split engineered by Alva Curtis, Thomson's most able lieutenant.[5] (See Appendix 1.)

One of Curtis' first acts in 1838 as leader of the formidable rival group, the "Independent Thomsonian Society," was to issue a statement of policy:

> This result is to be regretted, as it has the appearance of a split in the Thomsonian ranks, and affords the regulars a plausible pretext for saying that the opposition to their abominable quackery is already divided, and will soon be conquered . . . They [the regulars] need expect no sympathy from the "Independents" in their battles with Thomsonism, nor any conniving with their quackery and murder. Thomsonians are divided, to be sure, into right and left wings, but the regulars will find the columns in both divisions sufficiently deep, active, and persevering, for all their purposes. The steam and lobelia practice, in its most essential features (which for Dr. Thomson's abuse of many of its purest friends and warmest advocates might forever have been called Thomsonian) under whatever name it may hereafter pass, is destined to outlive all others; and will yet be the fashionable practice of this nation and the world.[6]

Curtis' confident prediction that the two factions would present a solid front to the regulars never materialized; the gap between the "left-wing" Neo-Thomsonians and the "right-wing" orthodox followers of Thomson widened rapidly. For a few years the "old patriarch" was able to retain a modicum of organization among his dwindling followers through his "United States Thomsonian Society." With the death of the founder in 1843, however, disorgani-

---

[3] Hooker, Worthington. *Physician and patient; or, a practical view of the mutual duties, relations, and interests of the medical profession and the community.* New York, Baker & Scribner, 1849, p. 119.
[4] The death of Horton Howard in 1833, leader of the insurgent "Improved Botanics," removed this threat to Thomson.
[5] Berman, Alex. *Op. cit.*, p. 420.
[6] *Botanico-Medical Recorder, or impartial advocate of botanic medicine, and the principles which govern the botanico-medical practice,* 1838-9, Columbus, Ohio, 7 (preface), p. vii.

zation set in quickly among his remaining loyal supporters.

In a little more than a decade after the 1838 schism, a remarkable transformation was discernible. The old Thomsonian crusading zeal, with all its color and fanaticism, was gone. With the abrogation of virtually all restrictive medical regulatory acts, a sense of security permeated the ranks of the Neo-Thomsonian practitioners. To be sure, there were still the "poisons of Allopathy" to inveigh against, but the old cry against the monopolizing schemes of the "Mineral Faculty" was no longer tenable. The mass base of patent right-holders which had formed the strength of the old Thomsonian movement and had given it its impressive grass-roots flavor, had by this time almost melted away. In short, what had been a remarkable socio-medical movement was to become, as the century progressed, merely a small, ineffectual, and pseudo-scientific cult.

A series of important events occurred in 1852. That year, a national meeting of Neo-Thomsonians took place in Baltimore. After debating the adoption of various names, the convention organized itself into the "Reformed Medical Association of the United States," and Alva Curtis was elected as its first president.[7] In addition, Neo-Thomsonian practitioners from the five Eastern states of Pennsylvania, Delaware, New Jersey, Maryland, and Virginia held their first annual meeting of the newly-founded "Middle States Reformed Medical Society."[8] Shortly thereafter, the Neo-Thomsonians in the South formed the "Southern Reform Medical Association."[9]

Probably the most important result of the 1852 meeting of the Reformed Medical Association of the United States was the formulation of the "Baltimore Platform." (See Appendix II.) In the words of one of the speakers at this meeting, its object was to present to the world "a code of medical principles that the community may know what we propose . . . as substitutes for the various systems of medicine popular in our day, and to guard them against the injustice and injury to themselves and us, of attributing to us doctrines which we do not sanction."[10] This document

---

[7] Such names as the following had been suggested: "Thomsonian, Physiological Medical, Physio-Medical, Physiopathic, Anti-Pathic, Physio-American." See *Physio-Medical Recorder, or impartial advocate of sanative medicine and the principles which govern the physio-medical practice*, 1852, Cincinnati, *18*, 97-99.

[8] *The Middle States Medical Reformer and Advocate of Innocuous Medication*, 1854, Milford, Delaware, *1*, 17.

[9] Wilder, Alexander. *History of medicine*. Augusta, Maine, Maine Farmer Publishing Co., 1904, pp. 589-90. This Southern group was composed of members residing in Virginia, Alabama, Mississippi, Arkansas, Tennessee, and Kentucky.

[10] *Physio-Medical Recorder*, 1842, *18*, 101.

provided a significant test as to who was or was not a genuine Neo-Thomsonian and spelled out the basic tenets of Neo-Thomsonian pathology and therapeutics.

A number of important resolutions were adopted by the Reformed Medical Association of the United States:[11] 1. The members present pledged support of the three principal Neo-Thomsonian schools then in existence;[12] 2. It was decided that three specified medical journals should be supported as reflecting the views of the assembled delegates;[13] 3. A resolution was adopted urging "the importance of encouraging the preparation of genuine sanative agents, and that our new school druggists, *in all cases*, should be patronized in preference to those of other schools";[14] 4. A resolution was passed to fix a uniform scale of fees; 5. On motion of one of the attending members, it was resolved that "those members of the Reformed Medical Profession who choose to assume the cognomen of *Thomsonian* or *Physio-Medical,* be considered as advocates of true sentiments, and be eligible to membership with us by signing our platform of principles";[15] and, 6. It was decided to publish a "United States Reformed Medical Dispensatory," with the responsibility for the task assigned to the faculty of the Metropolitan Medical College in New York City.[16] It is interesting to note that the Reformed Medical Association of the United States ceased to exist after its first meeting in 1852, and it was not until 1883 that a small group of Neo-Thomsonian physicians were to organize another national body called "The American Association of Physio-Medical Physicians and Surgeons."[17]

---

[11] Synopsis of minutes of the proceedings of the Reformed Medical Association of the United States. . ., *Physio-Medical Recorder*, 1852, *18*, 97.

[12] The Southern Botanico-Medical College at Macon, Georgia; the Physio-Medical College in Cincinnati; and the Metropolitan Medical College in New York City.

[13] *The Southern Medical Reformer*, organ of the Southern Botanico-Medical College; *The Physio-Medical Recorder*, organ of the Physio-Medical College; and a "journal to be established in New York." The New York journal appeared in 1854 under the name of *The Journal of Medical Reform*, and represented the views of the Metropolitan Medical College.

[14] *Physio-Medical Recorder*, 1852, *18*, 100.

[15] *Ibid.*, p. 99.

[16] This Dispensatory was finally written and published in Cincinnati on the individual initiative of William H. Cook in 1869 under the title of the *Physio-Medical Dispensatory*.

[17] This writer is in substantial agreement with Wilder who points out that the Botanic practitioners of this period, feeling secure in the absence of restrictive medical legislation, became indifferent to the need for organization. (See Wilder, *op. cit.*, pp. 670-671.) Another factor to be considered in this connection was the constant bickering and feuding among the Neo-Thomsonians and Eclectics.

In 1859, the editor of the *Physio-Medical Recorder* vainly chided the faithful for their indifference to national organization: "It seems high time now . . . for the staunch advocates of sanative medication to meet again and compare notes. Many have fallen off from the ranks since 1852; many have supposed that the Baltimore Platform was a thing of moonshine, to be altered and set aside at pleasure . . ." (*Physio-Medical Recorder*, 1859, *24*, 160.)

For several years, the Middle States Reformed Medical Society held annual meetings, but despite its pretentious claims, its membership remained very small. In 1854, the Society's journal, *The Middle States Medical Reformer*, stated that the organization had only fifty members,[18] but hastened to assure its readers that "These however, constitute, by no means, the whole number of New-School Practitioners in the five states composing our organization. The precise numbers we do not know, but so far as our information extends, there are over 500."[19] Requirements for membership in the Society were graduation from "any respectable and regularly organized medical college"; or an apprenticeship of two years with satisfactory evidence of competence as judged by the Society's Board of Censors. Of course, adherence to the principles of Neo-Thomsonianism was a *sine qua non*.

Of particular interest are the relations between the Middle States Medical Society and the Eclectics. In 1854, the Society made an alliance with the Eclectic Medical College of Pennsylvania, in which a "Union Platform of Principles" was signed by representatives of both organizations. (See Appendix III.) This move was greeted by Alva Curtis in the Mid-West with a suspicious outburst: "We are glad to learn that the Eclectic College has adopted this resolution," he wrote, "but we must watch them . . . we have been told that one of the doctrines of Eclecticism is, that every man is responsible only for himself—that they reject all authority, and make no pledges."[20]

At first it appeared as if the Neo-Thomsonians had swallowed up the Eclectics. The editors of the *Middle States Medical Reformer* could not contain their excitement and enthusiasm:

. . . The deep and gaping wound with which our professional body has so long suffered, has been entirely healed, and the body restored to pristine health. The true friends of our cause everywhere will hail this as an auspicious event. Hitherto the two New School factions of the Middle States have operated separately, but where was the necessity of so doing? . . . A new era in medicine has commenced. The great brilliant luminary of a legitimate science of medicine is now rising majestically above the horizon.[21]

The following year, the Middle States Reformed Medical Society appointed five delegates to represent it in negotiations with the National Eclectic Medical Association.[22] As it turned out,

[18] *The Middle States Medical Reformer and Advocate of Innocuous Medication*, 1854, *1*, 28.
[19] *Ibid.*, p. 28.
[20] *Physio-Medical Recorder*, 1854, *19*, 118.
[21] *Middle States Medical Reformer*, 1854, *1*, 54.
[22] *Ibid.*, 1855, *2*, 52.

Curtis' warning should have been heeded, for in the course of a few years, the eastern Eclectics gobbled up the Society and its followers. A similar fate overtook the Southern Reform Medical Association.[23]

All staunch and incorruptible Neo-Thomsonians rallied about Curtis and Cook in the Mid-West, where henceforth the sect demonstrated its greatest strength. Wounded by the encroachments of the Eclectics in the East and South, Cook could only rage ineffectually: "It [Eclecticism] is today a more dangerous enemy to medical reform than the bitterest Allopathy is . . ."[24]

For years after the "great schism" of 1838, the Neo-Thomsonians faced a dilemma in naming their organization. Immediately after the split of 1838, the followers of Curtis called themselves "Independent Thomsonians," but this designation was quickly changed to "Botanico-Medicals." In 1851 Curtis, disgruntled, announced, "We never liked the name 'Botanico-Medical' because botany includes all vegetables, bad as well as good. Still it answered our purpose well for thirteen years, and we resume it for the sake of uniformity."[25] The following year, just before the Baltimore convention, Curtis issued an *ex cathedra* statement:

> Let the *name,* then, be not Eclectic which signifies merely choosing and refusing (as all doctors do) ; nor Botanic, which signifies vegetable *poisoning* as well as *curing;* nor Thomsonian, which directs the mind as much to Thomson as his principles; nor Physopathic which signifies windy disease—But Physio-Medical, which signifies natural-medical, or curing according to nature . . . This is the most appropriate name yet proposed.[26]

Despite Curtis' attempt to pressure all Neo-Thomsonians to adopt the name "Physio-Medical" at the Baltimore Convention, the majority vote at that meeting was in favor of the name "Medical Reform."[27] In the course of a few years, the appellations "Physiopathic," "Physo-Medical," and "Medical Reformers" assumed by certain Neo-Thomsonians, passed out of existence, and the designation "Physio-Medical" became synonymous with Neo-Thomsonianism.

No further organizational activity on a national level occurred among the Neo-Thomsonians until 1883, when a call was sent out "to every *true and genuine* Physio-Medicalist on the American Continent, to meet in a grand convention in the City of Indianapolis, Indiana, on the first Wednesday in May 1883, for the pur-

---

23 Wilder, *op. cit.,* p. 592.
24 *Physio-Medical Recorder,* 1867, *31,* 228.
25 *Botanico-Medical Recorder,* 1851, *18,* 26.
26 *Physio-Medical Recorder,* 1852, *18,* 1.
27 *The Middle States Medical Reformer,* 1854, *1,* 44.

pose of organizing a National Association."[28] The circular letter announcing this call was initiated by three State Physio-Medical Societies (Indiana, Ohio, and Illinois),[29] and was signed by ninety-three names from "twenty-three States and Provinces."[30] Meeting at the designated time and place, the convention created the "American Association of Physio-Medical Physicians and Surgeons." Forty-eight persons were designated charter members, and a Platform of Principles, Constitution and By-laws," was drawn up. (See Appendix IV.)

There is a record of the American Association of Physio-Medical Physicians and Surgeons meeting for a three-day annual convention in Dallas, Texas, as late as May 1907.[31] After this date, the fate of the organization, if it still existed, is completely obscured through lack of data.

II.

The establishment of the first chartered Neo-Thomsonian medical school by Alva Curtis in 1839 at Columbus, Ohio, was greeted with derision by the regulars and the "Beachites," and became the target of savage and sarcastic criticism by the orthodox Thomsonians. "It appears that the Curtico-Botanico-Medical College has been chartered by the Ohio Legislature," sneered the editor of the *Boston Thomsonian Manual*. "We had heard a great deal about Dr. Curtis and his school, and the wicked Legislature of Ohio, who would not grant him a charter, but we never dreamed that it was his intention to make the healing art an odious monopoly and imitate the regular medical profession by conferring a sheepskin diploma. But so it is; and the Thomsonians must endeavor to rub along as well as they can without the aid of diplomas and colleges."[32]

To make matters worse, all staunch followers of Samuel Thomson were thrown into deep consternation when Dr. Lanier Bankston, the "Curtis of the South," secured a charter from the Georgia Legislature for the Southern Botanico-Medical College at Forsyth,

---

[28] *Cincinnati Medical Recorder*, 1883, *61*, 63. The circular letter defined "true and genuine" Physio-Medicals as "those whose practice conforms to the great Physio-Medical doctrine of rejecting all poisons. And those who are not *true and genuine* in this sense, as also those who have diplomas procured by money or otherwise fraudulently, and those who sell or issue such fraudulent diplomas, and all who procure abortion, or otherwise are guilty of criminal practices, shall be debarred from the deliberations of this meeting." (*Ibid.*, p. 63).

[29] *Ibid.*, pp. 61-62.
[30] *Ibid.*, p. 72.
[31] *Physio-Medical Record*, Indianapolis, 1907, *10*, 72.
[32] *The Boston Thomsonian Manual and Lady's Companion*, 1839, *5*, 171.

Georgia, that same year.[33] Thus, with two Neo-Thomsonian schools opening in 1839, the new trend in education among the "left-wing" Thomsonian faction was off to a good start. In all, eight Neo-Thomsonian schools were chartered before 1861:[34]

1. *Literary and Botanico-Medical Institute of Ohio* (1839), Columbus, Ohio. This institution moved to Cincinnati in 1841. After many vicissitudes and changes of name, it finally became the Physio-Medical College of Ohio, closing in 1880.

2. *Southern Botanico-Medical College,* chartered in 1839 at Forsyth, Georgia. Two grants of $5,000 each were voted to this school by the State Legislature. The name of the college was changed to Reformed Medical College of Georgia in 1854. Suspended in 1861 and revived in 1867, it underwent another change in name, becoming the American College of Medicine in 1874. It finally merged with the Georgia Eclectic College in 1881.

3. *Alabama Medical Institute,* Wetumka, Alabama. Received a charter in 1844, but closed in 1845 after only one session. The faculty had been composed of seceding professors from the Southern Botanico-Medical College.

4. *Botanico-Medical College of Memphis,* Memphis, Tennessee. Chartered in 1846, the faculty had come largely from the defunct Alabama Medical Institute. In 1859 the institution became Eclectic, changing its name to Eclectic Medical Institute of Memphis. The college closed in 1861.

5. *Scientific and Eclectic Medical Institute of Virginia,* Petersburg, Virginia. Chartered in 1847, this school was "Eclectic" in name only.[35] Torn asunder by faculty squabbles, the college lasted only a few years.

---

[33] Wilder, *op. cit.,* p. 500 and p. 525.

[34] Information on these schools was derived in part from the findings of F. C. Waite, American sectarian medical colleges before the Civil War. *Bull. Hist. Med.,* 1946, *19,* 148-166; also from Wilder's *History of medicine;* and from a number of Neo-Thomsonian journals.

[35] For example, it was announced by one of the professors of the school in 1848 that "We are pleased to find all our students to be fully established in the fundamental doctrines of Thomsonism. There are no mongrels amongst us; none that advocate the peculiar notions of the Beachites . . . We are all very far from confounding the *name* of an Institution with the doctrines taught therein. Although our college is called the Eclectic Institute of Virginia, yet our students will all bear witness, that the doctrines herein taught, are in perfect accordance with the fundamentals of Samuel Thomson. They wish it fully understood that our Institute is not the advocate of the peculiar notions of those termed Eclectics in the West, but that we are Eclectics in the broad sense of the word, which leads us to

'Seize upon truth wherever found
On Christian or on heathen ground,'—

to select, from the accumulated wisdom of the past . . ." (*New England Botanic Medical and Surgical Journal,* 1848, 2, 14.)

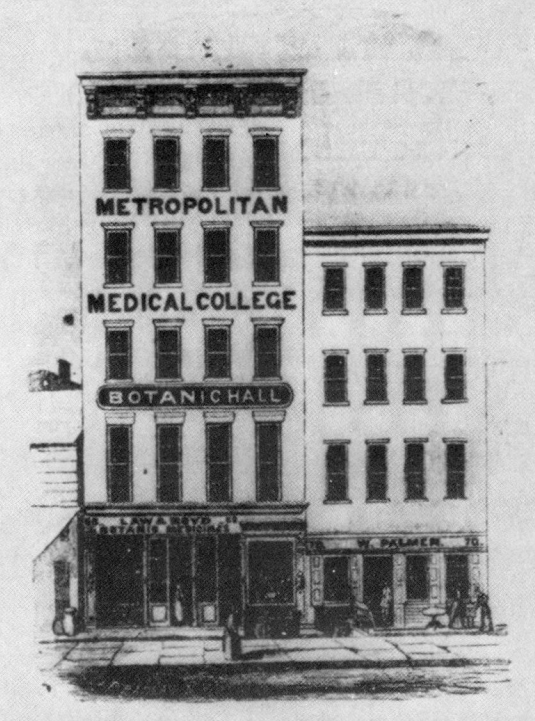

An advertisement of the Metropolitan Medical College which appeared in the College's publication, the *Journal of Medical Reform,* Vol. I, 1854. Note the Botanic establishment of Law and Boyd on the street level of the school building.

6. *Worcester Medical School,* Worcester, Massachusetts. This school was established in 1846, but was unsuccessful in obtaining a charter from the Massachusetts Legislature. In order to circumvent this situation, the Worcester school made an ingenious arrangement to become a branch of the Southern Botanico-Medical College, located approximately 700 miles away. In this capacity, and using the name Worcester Botanico-Medical College it was able to grant degrees in 1846 and 1847 under the charter of the Georgia institution. Terminating its connection with the Georgia school in 1848, it entered into a similar arrangement that same year with the Scientific and Eclectic Medical Institute of Virginia. Under the terms of this agreement, the Worcester school again changed its name to New England Botanico-Medical College. Finally, in 1851, it obtained a Massachusetts charter and operated independently until its demise in 1859.[36] It is interesting to note that probably the most erudite Neo-Thomsonian, Dr. Calvin Newton, was the founder of this school and, until his death in 1853, its chief attraction.[37] In 1852, Newton joined the Eclectics and became that year the President of the National Eclectic Medical Association.

7. *Metropolitan Medical College* in New York City.[38] A charter for this school was secured in 1850. During its last few years of existence it was captured by the Eclectics. Dissension among the faculty as well as a scarcity of students caused the school to close in 1862.

8. *Physio-Medical Institute,* Cincinnati, Ohio. Established in 1859 as a rival of the Physio-Medical College, this school closed in 1885. Waite points out that this institution had only fifteen graduates prior to 1861. After the Civil War, the number of graduates continued to be very small.

[36] For an exhaustive study of the history of this school, see Waite, F. C. The first sectarian medical school in New England, at Worcester (1846-1859), and its relation to Thomsonianism. *New Eng. J. Med.,* 1932, *207,* 984-988.

[37] Calvin Newton (1800-1853), graduated from Union College in 1826 and from Newton Theological Institute in 1829; served as Baptist minister (1828-1831); Professor of Rhetoric and Hebrew at Waterville (now Colby) College, Maine (1831-1838); Professor and President of the Theological Institute at Thomaston, Maine; entered Berkshire Medical Institution in 1842 and received M.D. degree in 1844; became a Fellow of the Massachusetts Medical Society (1845); embraced Neo-Thomsonianism and founded Worcester Medical School (1846); President of the National Eclectic Medical Association (1852); editor of *New England Eclectic and Guide to Health,* Worcester, 1846 (title later changed to *New England Botanic Medical and Surgical Journal*).

[38] *The Journal of Medical Reform,* organ of the Metropolitan Medical College, ran an announcement describing the aims of the College as follows: "The teachings of the Metropolitan will be strictly based upon the doctrines contained in the Platform of Principles of Medical Reform, adopted by the National Reform Convention in the city of Baltimore in 1852 . . . for this Reform we claim Dr. Samuel Thomson of New Hampshire, the father and founder . . . we think to Samuel Thomson belongs the honor of being considered the father of this Reform, and to whom the world is indebted." (*J. med. Reform,* N. Y., 1854, *1,* 251.)

No attempt has been made in this study to evaluate the foregoing schools, but Waite has indicated that they were considerably inferior in caliber to those of the regulars, and that the number of graduates was comparatively small. The subjects taught and the duration of study at these Neo-Thomsonian institutions were similar to those of many regular proprietary schools of the period, with the exception of the distinctive therapeutics and pathology.

Three schools listed above continued to operate after the Civil War, with the last one, the Physio-Medical Institute, closing in 1885. As for the few Neo-Thomsonian colleges which came into existence in the post-Civil War period, three were still functioning in the first decade of the twentieth century:[39]

1. The Physio-Medical College of Indiana, Indianapolis, organized in 1873.
2. College of Medicine and Surgery, Chicago, organized in 1885 as the Chicago Physio-Medical Institute.
3. Physio-Medical College of Texas, Dallas, organized in 1902.

By 1910, only the Illinois school was still in existence; after this date, it, too, became defunct.[40]

The ridiculously small number of students graduating from the three combined Neo-Thomsonian medical colleges from 1901-1908 can be seen from the following statistics published in the *Journal of the American Medical Association*:[41]

1901—18 students	1905—22 students
1902—16 students	1906—22 students
1903—24 students	1907—11 students
1904—20 students	1908—12 students

III.

The Neo-Thomsonian trend was accompanied not only by striking innovations in therapeutics, organizational structure, and education, but also by a different kind of pharmaceutical activity. The large-scale manufacture, distribution, and sale of Thomsonian remedies involving numerous agents and many unauthorized persons, which had been such a remarkable feature of the old movement, had disappeared. By mid-nineteenth century, there were no longer thousands of patent right-holding followers of Thomson to support such activity.

---

[39] *J. Amer. med. Ass.*, 1903, *41*, 438-439; 448.
[40] *J. Amer. med. Ass.*, 1910, *55*, 668-669.
[41] *J. Amer. med. Ass.*, 1908, *51*, 607.

Indeed, scrutinizing this trend closely, it becomes increasingly difficult to speak of Neo-Thomsonian pharmacy per se. The old Thomsonians had been able to build up an extensive pharmaceutical apparatus to serve the needs of their adherents, but the Neo-Thomsonian practitioners were too weak and few in numbers to muster pharmaceutical resources comparable to those of their crusading forebears. Moreover, the rapid rise of an impressive Eclectic pharmaceutical industry in the 1850's completely submerged and overshadowed the few ineffectual attempts of Physio-Medical physicians to create a distinctive pharmacy of their own. For a good part of the century, Neo-Thomsonian pharmacy may properly be regarded as an appendage of Eclectic pharmacy, as subsequent discussion will show.

Intense excitement prevailed among the Eclectics in the late 1840's when W. S. Merrell of Cincinnati began marketing "concentrated" Eclectic remedies.[42] Numerous competing manufacturers immediately followed suit, and before long a lucrative industry had evolved. The Neo-Thomsonians were quick to endorse the new "concentrated" remedies. An editorial appearing in the *Physo-Medical Recorder,* organ of the Physo-Medical College of Cincinnati,[43] praised the advent of these medications as "a glorious work of Medical Reform,"[44] without bothering to give the Eclectics credit for this development. "No one is a greater lover of the different baths [vapor] than ourself, or has a higher appreciation of emetics and enemas," the editor reassured his readers.[45] But, if the new "concentrated" preparations worked as well and were easier for the patient to take and for the physician to administer, he argued, then why not adopt them? Attacking the regular physicians for their employment of poisonous alkaloids, the writer conceded that these plant derivatives had done much to make the allopathic practice "acceptable and popular." Then, contrasting the regular alkaloidal pharmacy with the "New School" pharmacy, the editor wrote:

> ... but how different their articles are from ours. They extract proximate principles, many of which are most deadly in their character ... from the

---

[42] Lloyd, John Uri. *The eclectic alkaloids ... etc.,* Bulletin of the Lloyd Library no. 12. (Pharmacy Series no. 2) Cincinnati, 1910; and the condensed version of this work, *A treatise on the American alkaloids, resins, resinoids, oleo-resins and concentrated principles (so-called Eclectic concentrations),* Drug Treatise no. XXIV, Cincinnati, 1909. These two works are authoritative and indispensable histories of Eclectic concentrated remedies.

[43] For a brief period, the name "Physo-Medical" was used, but was subsequently dropped for "Physio-Medical."

[44] *Physo-Medical Recorder and Surgical Journal,* Cincinnati, 1850, *18,* 167.

[45] *Ibid.,* p. 165.

poppy they extract their morphine; from the strychnos (nux vomica), they extract their strychnine, two grains of which will kill; from cinchona, they extract their quinine, etc., etc.

Now our agents are reduced to a concentrated form without breaking up the relations existing between the proximate principles. For example, we reduce lobelia to so concentrated a form, that from three to five or ten drops upon loaf sugar, or dropped into water, are sufficient to produce emesis; still this article is not lobelina, one of the proximate principles of lobelia . . .[46]

Finally the writer, in a burst of enthusiasm, concluded that because of this "great improvement . . . we feel more than ever inclined to the belief that the Physo-Medical Practice will soon, very soon, become the most popular and successful practice of medicine."[47]

As mentioned earlier, a resolution had been passed at the Baltimore Convention urging patronage of "New School Druggists . . . in preference to those of other schools." Who these "New School Druggists" were can be seen by examining the advertisements in the Neo-Thomsonian journals of the period. The Physio-Medical practitioners in the Cincinnati area apparently favored the concentrated remedies of F. D. Hill and Company of Cincinnati, who advertised "the Most Improved Method of preparing the Concentrated Medicines . . . all articles belonging to the list of Drugs and Medicines used by Thomsonian and Botanic Physicians."[48] From the available data, it would seem that the Eclectic establishments were well patronized. For example, the concentrated preparations of the American Chemical Institute, an Eclectic firm controlled by B. Keith and Company, for whom the wholesale botanic house of Coolidge, Adams and Bond acted as agents, were advertised in the *Journal of Medical Reform*. Similarly, the wholesale botanic druggists, Law and Boyd, offered for sale their concentrated preparations in the same journal without, however, divulging the manufacturer.

The *Middle States Medical Reformer* was an ardent champion of concentrated preparations. It taunted the regulars for their reliance on calomel in liver complaints:

We are often gratuitously informed by persons who wish to say something in favor of the crumbling fabric of Allopathy, that nothing will act on the liver but calomel . . . If such persons wish to know better, they can be very easily taught—call upon any New-School Druggist and procure a dose of Podophylline or Leptandrine; the former which will act with much greater

[46] *Ibid.*, p. 167.
[47] *Ibid.*, p. 168.
[48] *Botanico-Medical Recorder*, 1852, *18*, 191.

power upon the liver, exciting copious flow of bile, without poisoning the blood, *as mercury* . . . Will our Allopathic friends try them?[49]

In 1856, the Middle States Reformed Medical Society unreservedly endorsed the use of concentrated medicines at its fifth annual meeting in Philadelphia.[50] By this time, the Physio-Medical practitioners were patronizing Eclectic establishments, wholesale botanic druggists who stocked Eclectic remedies, and even regular drug stores. The new concentrated Eclectic remedies were being sold through regular retail drug channels soon after their appearance on the market. Advertisements for these products are to be found in the very first volume of the *American Druggist's Circular and Chemical Gazette* (1857).[51]

This does not mean that the Physio-Medical practitioners used only Eclectic concentrated remedies. In a report delivered at the convention of the Middle States Reformed Medical Society referred to above, it was authoritatively recommended that infusions, decoctions, and syrups should be retained as "adjunctive aids," and that extracts and tinctures should not be completely abandoned in favor of concentrates.[52]

In the succeeding years, the Physio-Medical physicians occasionally expressed their dissatisfaction at their inability to establish Physio-Medical pharmacies, as well as with the shortcomings of the botanic wholesale houses and regular drug stores. For example, in 1858, a disgruntled Neo-Thomsonian practitioner wrote to the editor of the *Physio-Medical Recorder* to complain about drug adulteration:

> I am satisfied that our Reform physicians are not careful enough in selecting their medicinal agents. The manufacture of botanic medicines has become a lucrative business; and unprincipled men, disregarding the direful consequences, are adulterating our most sanative preparations. It is not uncommon to find, in our wholesale drug stores lobelia seed adulterated with tobacco, pulverized capsicum with logwood, ginger with corn meal, cream of tartar with alum, jalap with sawdust, etc. . . . Brothers in medical reform, if we can not get pure articles prepared for our immediate use, let us go into the laboratory prepared by the God of nature, and find for ourselves, in this crude state, the healing remedies of a beneficent Creator.[53]

It was, of course, commonplace for many of the old "steam and puke doctors" to go out into the country and gather medicinal

---

[49] *The Middle States Medical Reformer*, 1854, *1*, 13.
[50] *Ibid.*, 1856, *3*, 49.
[51] For example: W. S. Merrell and Co. of Cincinnati, on p. 119; B. Keith and Co. of New York on p. 85; Coolidge and Adams, Wholesale Botanic Druggists of New York on p. 85; and Jacob S. Merrell of St. Louis, on p. 57.
[52] *The Middle States Medical Reformer*, 1856, *3*, 60.
[53] *Physio-Medical Recorder*, 1859, *24*, 83.

plants. But these new practitioners were a different breed of men. Many of them were now the proud possessors of diplomas and M.D. degrees, and the threat to "go into the laboratory prepared by the God of nature" was purely rhetorical.

At an annual meeting of the Indiana Physio-Medical Association in 1895, a prominent spokesman of the cult complained rather bitterly that "We are depending too much on the pharmacists of the old school . . . we should have a Physio-Medical Pharmacy."[54] Another speaker joined in to approve the sentiments of his colleague: "We need efficient, conscientious Physio-Medical pharmacists to manufacture and prepare Physio-Medical remedies for Physio-Medical physicians . . ."[55] The Neo-Thomsonians were unable, however, to attain this goal. Unlike their belligerent predecessors, and their Eclectic rivals whose pharmaceutical activities are of considerable interest and importance, these new Thomsonian practitioners caused hardly a stir on the pharmaceutical scene.

IV.

Despite all exhortations and opposition by Thomson, a considerable expansion in the Thomsonian materia medica had already taken place during the founder's lifetime. By 1869, with the appearance of William Cook's *Physio-Medical Dispensatory*, the original core of 70 plant drugs employed by the old Thomsonians had been increased five-fold.

Nor was this all. Samuel Thomson's crude pronouncements about the nature of disease had been elaborately restated by the Neo-Thomsonian practitioners in quasi-scientific and metaphysical terms. A vitalistic pathology was formulated in which disease was regarded as a unit, and fever proclaimed as a beneficent manifestation of the "life principle." The most authoritative expression of these views was presented in the "Baltimore Platform" of 1852 (see Appendix II) and continued to be promulgated with certain refinements by this sect up to the time of its virtual extinction, about 1910.[56]

Great emphasis was laid by Neo-Thomsonians on the use of "sanative" or "non-poisonous" medication. The regular practitioners, as well as physicians of other schools, were accused by Wil-

[54] *Physio-Medical Journal*, Indianapolis, 1895, *21*, 174.
[55] *Ibid.*, p. 174.
[56] There were undoubtedly still some Physio-Medical physicians practicing after this date, but this writer has been unable to find any publications or data which would indicate any organizational activity after 1910.

liam H. Cook of using poisonous and disease-producing remedies. Of the "allopathic" practitioners, Cook wrote as follows:

> The Allopathic rule in treatment seeks the removal of one disease by making another disease in its place . . . and this doctrine permeates everything that comes from Allopathy. Out of this springs its other proposition, *Ubi virus, ibi virtus*—where there is poison, there is virtue. If disease is to be made, poisons must be used for the purpose; and it is only on this ground that calomel, antimony, arsenic, blisters, iodine, opium, veratrum, gelsemium, strychnine and other destructive agents were introduced as remedies . . . Hence while that school has made such progress in Anatomy, Physiology, Symptomology, Diagnosis and kindred topics, it has steadily conformed its Materia Medica to the rule of using poisons; and its entire numbers and influence have ever been used to oppose every suggestion in practice that did not accord with its primeval pathology . . .[57]

In a savage attack against the Eclectics, Cook denounced them for using "deleterious agents," and compiled a list of "poisons" which he claimed the Eclectics were administering.[58]

A pertinent question that might be asked at this point is how the Neo-Thomsonians defined or determined what was "poisonous." All their definitions were obscure and subjective, apparently influenced by either grossly speculative or empirical factors. Definitions such as the following are given for a "poison": "Any article to which human experience attaches the term *poison* is dangerous to the human frame and at war with vitality";[59] or "every means and process, which, in its nature and tendency, in authorized medicinal quantities, degrees or modes of application, has been known to have directly destroyed human life, or permanently injured the tissue or deranged the physiological action." (*Baltimore Platform*); or "Every article, means or process of cure which . . . is directly antagonistic to the laws of vitality" (*Union Platform of Principles,* see Appendix III). For example, during the meeting of the Illinois Physio-Medical Association in 1865, gelsemium and veratrum were considered deleterious within the meaning of these

[57] Cook, W. H. *The physio-medical dispensatory*. Cincinnati, 1869, pp. 5-6.
[58] *Physio-Medical Recorder*, 1865, 29, 189. Cook wrote: "These lists I have prepared with the utmost care from the latest editions of the several Eclectic textbooks." The following is Cook's list of "poisons" used by the Eclectics:

Fowler's Solution	Hyoscyamus
Antimony Chloride	Stramonium
Litharge and lead acetate	Digitalis
Copper Sulphate	Veratrum
Iodine	Aconite
Zinc Salts	Conium
Silver Nitrate	Cannabis Sativa
Bismuth Salts	Bitter Almond
Gold Chloride	Strychnine
Opium and derivatives	Prussic Acid
Belladonna	Ergot

[59] *Cincinnati Medical Recorder*, 1883, *61*, 133.

definitions and officially proscribed.[60] Taunted by his enemies for not having effective drugs in the Physio-Medical materia medica to alleviate pain, Cook retorted:

> It is often charged against Physio-Medicalism, that it cannot relieve pain as effectively as can be done by the narcotics of Allopathy and Eclectism. This is a mistake. Our agents can secure more effective relief . . . the list [Physio-Medical] already known is far greater than is generally supposed. Among them may be mentioned blue cohosh, mullen, bugle weed, cockle burr, greek valerian, twin leaf, yellow poplar, and at least a dozen others. They are positive and reliable in giving relief to pain . . .[61]

Necessity sometimes forced the Neo-Thomsonians to accept medicinal agents or adopt curative measures which had been authoritatively pronounced deleterious by their leaders. An early example occurred in 1837, when the respectable editor of *The Southern Botanic Journal,* Dr. D. K. Nardin, scandalized his Thomsonian colleagues by advocating the use of quinine sulfate in "chills."[62] Nardin was severely scolded by William H. Fonerden, a prominent Thomsonian, who argued that "if Dr. Nardin may add one article to the materia medica [Thomson's materia medica] I may add another, and so may others ad infinitum, until we have a volume as ponderous as Wood and Bache's American Dispensatory."[63] Furthermore, maintained Fonerden, Nardin was violating a basic principle of Thomsonian therapeutics which always called for the use of general remedies. "A local specific is a general poison," Fonerden reminded Nardin. "This is a favorite axiom with Thomsonian physicians. To those I may add, 'a limited remedy is a general bane.' Is the sulphate of quinine, doctor, a limited or general remedy? Would you prescribe it in every case of disease? I know you would not."[64] Other arguments advanced by Fonerden against the use of quinine were: (a) Dr. Thomson forbade the use of minerals, and since quinine sulfate was a combination of "a tonic extract of Peruvian bark and sulphuric acid," it could not be safely administered; and, (b) It was "equivocal" in action, causing many side-effects.

To these arguments Nardin retorted that he could not see why quinine was more "equivocal" than many remedies in Dr. Thom-

---

[60] Illinois P-M Association. Report of Proceedings of Its Eighth Annual Convention. *Physio-Medical Recorder,* 1865, *29,* 197.
[61] *Physio-Medical Recorder,* 1868, *32,* 126.
[62] *The Southern Botanic Journal, Devoted to the Dissemination and Support of the Thomsonian System of Medical Practice,* Charleston, S. C., 1837-8, *1,* 197. This is the earliest example of the use of quinine by a Thomsonian that this writer has been able to discover.
[63] *Ibid.,* p. 402.
[64] *Ibid.,* p. 403.

son's materia medica; that although common table salt was composed of two deadly mineral poisons, and eggs contained sulfur, they were nevertheless consumed by everyone; and finally, that Fonerden's remarks about general remedies were "overstrained." These heretical opinions were concluded with a burst of defiance:

> With regard to our prescribing quinine to stop chills we shall make no further apology, nor assign any other reasons than that of *absolute necessity,* although we had previously subjected our patients to a vigorous course of Thomsonian medicines daily, for many weeks; and we failed several times where quinine given by others performed cures.[65]

As late as 1865, no agreement could be reached at a meeting of Physio-Medical practitioners on whether to sanction the use of quinine,[66] and it was not until 1869 that all taint was removed from the drug, through its inclusion in Cook's *Physio-Medical Dispensatory* as a "sanative" remedy.[67]

There is reason to believe that the influence of independent Botanic leaders such as Elisha Smith and Thomas Cooke served to accelerate the Neo-Thomsonian trend. Smith's *Botanic Physician* (1830) was the first significant attempt at a scientific synthesis of the Botanic practice. This work strongly emphasized the need for an expanded plant materia medica and a judicious inclusion of some mineral remedies. It was noteworthy for its stress on the need to study all branches of medicine, including surgery. This approach was also taken by Thomas Cooke in the pages of his journal, the *Botanic Medical Reformer and Home Physician*. In a significant editorial, Cooke pointed to the contrast between the therapeutic practice of the independent Botanic and the old-fashioned Thomsonian physician:

> The Thomsonian practitioners, it is pretty generally known, adhere strictly to the manner of practice recommended by Dr. Samuel Thomson, (which consists principally of giving *courses* of medicine, such as stimulating, puking, steaming, and the shower bath, with such other directions as Dr. Thomson gives in his "New Guide," discarding in toto Cathertics, Laxatives, and other means recommended by other well experienced Botanic authors. And we will here state that Botanic Physicians make use of all the articles recommended by Dr. Samuel Thomson, when they deem them necessary: hence, a Botanic practitioner has all the Thomsonian remedies, while the Thomsonian has no other except those which are laid down in the "New Guide." And we believe there is not a person living but would rather take any of our more mild remedies, than resort to the *coursing* practice . . .[68]

[65] *Ibid.*, p. 404.
[66] *Physio-Medical Recorder*, 1865, 29, 200.
[67] *Physio-medical dispensatory*, p. 346.
[68] *The Botanic Medical Reformer and Home Physician*, 1841, *1*, 121.

By the 1840's, many Thomsonians had begun to practice what the independent Botanic physicians had been preaching for considerably more than a decade. In 1865, William H. Cook announced heatedly that "very many people still think our system can do little else than give emetics and baths; and only a limited number of persons understand that we have an extended system of scientific principles."[69]

But try as they might, the Neo-Thomsonians could never achieve more than a pseudo-scientific therapeutics. As the century wore on, it became apparent that the dogma-ridden leaders of this ever-shrinking sect were unable to grasp the implications in the dramatic emergence of bacteriology, immunology, and synthetic organic medicinals. As late as 1907, a professor at the Physio-Medical College of Indiana warned his students that "if you ever hope to become expert in diagnosis and treatment of the sick, you must throw aside the pernicious doctrine of *disease-entity*, a *bacterial* pathology or a microbe disease maker, and *chemical therapeutics* or the doctrine that the living body is simply a chemical laboratory to be ruled only by the chemist. I do declare to you that the so-called 'disease germ' is a monumental medical bugbear, it is the greatest romanticism of the age."[70]

In 1906, a woman graduate of the Physio-Medical College of Indiana received permission to matriculate for a course in obstetrics and gynecology in the medical school of the University of Strassburg, on the strength of her diploma and her Indiana State license. In a letter to the editor of the *Physio-Medical Record,* she praised the remarkable technical facilities of the University, but contemptuously dismissed the prevailing therapeutics. "Of course," she wrote, "I would not for all the world give up my knowledge of Physio-Medical treatment for their superior technic."[71] She then proceeded to tell of her successful treatment of patients with "leptandra virg. and zingiber," and "as I had nothing else on hand I made a strong solution of No. 6 and bathed a burned hand ... The patient said 'it was a little hot,' but she thought it healed very fast ..."[72] For a fleeting instant, the ghost of Samuel Thomson, vindicated, hovered over the Medical Faculty of the University of Strassburg!

[69] *Physio-Medical Recorder*, 1865, *29*, 73.
[70] *Physio-Medical Record*, 1907, *10*, 127.
[71] Letter to Dr. Haggard, editor. From Dr. Th. Rimmelin, Schiltigheim. Strassburg, Elsass, Germany. Dec. 12, 1906. *Physio-Medical Record*, 1907, *10*, 42-45.
[72] *Ibid.*, p. 45.

APPENDIX I

(An attack made by Morris Mattson, spokesman for Samuel Thomson, against the Alva Curtis faction which seceded during the seventh national Thomsonian Convention in 1838. From *The Boston Thomsonian Manual and Lady's Companion*, 1838, 5, 8-11.)

The enemies of Dr. Thomson have stated that he urged a dissolution of the old convention, from a desire to monopolize the sale of medicines. It was his principal aim to propose such measures as were calculated to keep his system in the hands of the *people,* and to prevent them from being imposed upon by a junto of designing knaves, who have used every effort to trample Dr. Thomson in the dust.

The individuals composing this *scare-crow* faction were headed by that ineffable nuisance, that notorious drunken sot, Dr. Draper, who had probably procured a short respite from Moyamensing for that important service. After the old convention had dissolved, and the mongrels discovered the impossibility of hanging on any longer by the skirts of the Thomsonians, Dr. Draper interrupted the assembly with one of his billingsgate speeches, in which he proposed that his followers should adjourn to a tavern in Chestnut Street (Philadelphia), and there organize an 'Independent' convention. The suggestion was carried into effect, and after a two days' session, they had matured a constitution, passed sundry resolutions, and adjourned to meet within a year, in New York City.

Now this was all well enough, with the exception that they should not have christened themselves the *'Thomsonian'* society ... If they can do without Dr. Thomson's system, they can certainly do without his *name*. They should have styled themselves the *'butternut society'* or the 'purifying syrup society.' Either of these would have been far more appropriate than the one selected.

This tavern convention, we perceive, consisted of about thirty members. Ephraim Larabee of Baltimore, a notorious vender of secret nostrums, was the president. We find the names, also, of John A. Brown of Providence, R. I., one of the most noted of the mongrels; B. W. Sperry of New Haven, Conn., a man who, unless very much belied, uses opium and laudanum in his practice in disguise, and engaged in printing a *counterfeit* edition of the New Guide; A. C. Draper, of almshouse and Moyamensing notoriety; William Armstrong, a vender of Jewett's liniments; William Burton and Samuel Ross of Philadelphia, well known in that city for their abominable quackery, and sale of secret compounds; James Thorn (called, par excellence, doctor), the Pennsylvania agent for the sale of Howard's *improved* system of medicine; and last, though not least, Dr. Curtis of Columbus, Ohio....

APPENDIX II

(From *The Physio-Medical Recorder or Impartial Advocate of Sanative Medicine*, 1852-53, *18*, 155-6.)

PLATFORM OF PRINCIPLES
ADOPTED BY THE NATIONAL CONVENTION AT
BALTIMORE, OCTOBER 1852

Whereas, There have arisen in different ages and countries, and of every sect in medicine, men of noble minds and benevolent hearts, who exerted all their energies to reform the errors and abuses of what was called the science and practice of medicine;

And whereas, The men of this description of the Allopathic school are still compelled to pronounce their principles as "incoherent assemblage of incoherent ideas;" and their most efficient medication "horrid, unwarrantable, murderous, quackery;"

And whereas, Many modern New School reformers of the same honest intentions, have few fixed principles of practice in which they can agree, and no firm bond of union in effort for the promotion of Reform;

Therefore, It appeared to be the first and most important duty of this convention to point out the generative errors of all the popular systems of the day, and to lay down in clear and unmistakable terms the fundamental principles of true Medical Science and practice, as guides to all who may desire to attain to perfection in the knowledge of the Healing Art, and as a common creed, which all can advocate and defend, and as a bond of union in effort for the promotion of this most glorious cause of science and humanity; Therefore

Resolved, By the Reformed Medical Association of the United States, that medical science pertaining altogether to natural subjects, must be in itself as fixed and definite as any other natural science.

Resolved, That the reason why medical men have not learned it, is they have attempted to base it upon the violation of physical laws, which are ever variable, instead of those laws themselves, which are immutable; they have built their system on what they call pathology—or rather they have pronounced that pathology which is only deranged physiology, and built upon this error.

Resolved, That the Reformers of past times have failed to perfect their practice, because of the impossibility of doing it while they retain the false notion that the science is based on pathology, or the doctrine that physiological derangements are disease.

Resolved, That the fundamental principles of true medical science are not pathological but physiological.

Resolved, That disease is not vital action deranged, or obstructed, increased, or diminished, but any condition of the organs in which they are unable to perform their natural functions: a condition that permanently deranges, obstructs or diminishes vital action, and in this sense is a unit.

Resolved, That irritation, fever, inflammation—terms used to signify increased, deranged, obstructed, or accumulated vital action in the nervous or vascular systems, are not disease, but physiological symptoms of disease; and are not to be directly subdued, but always to be aided in their ultimate design and intention in removing obstructions and restoring the nervous and circulatory equilibrium.

Resolved, That suppuration is to be encouraged and promoted whenever there is accumulated morbific matter to be removed; that gangrene, being no part of inflammation, but a purely chemical process in opposition to all vital action, and occurring only when vital action has wholly ceased, the associating of it with inflammation, and treating the latter as tending to terminate in the former, has been a source of immense mischief in medication.

Resolved, That it is the duty of the practitioner to reject in toto every means and process, which, in its nature and tendency, in authorized medicinal quantities, degrees or modes of application, has been known to have directly destroyed human life, or permanently injured the tissue or deranged the physiological action, and use those only, which have a direct tendency to aid the vital organs in the removal of causes of disease and the restoration of health and vigor.

Resolved, That the agents of this character are not confined to the vegetable kingdom, but are found in every department of nature, and to be "seized upon wherever found."

Resolved, That though we shall exercise charity toward the ignorance and prejudices of all men, we can count no one a true medical reformer who rejects the doctrines of the foregoing resolutions.

APPENDIX III

(From *The Middle States Medical Reformer, and Advocate of Innocuous Medication*, Milford, Delaware, 1854-5, *1*, 52.)

Union Platform of Principles

(Subscribed to by the Middle States Reformed Medical Society and the Faculty of the Eclectic Medical College of Pennsylvania)

Whereas divisions have occurred among medical reformers, and various parties have arisen entertaining different views only upon some of the minor points of true medical science and practice; and whereas these divisions have greatly retarded the progress of scientific medicine: we the members of the Middle States Society of Medical Reform, do agree to unite with our Eclectic friends upon the following platform of principles.

1st. The fundamental principles of true medical science are not Pathological but physiological.

2nd. Disease is not vital action deranged or obstructed, increased or diminished, but disease we understand to be that condition of a part which disqualifies it for the performance of its function in a normal manner.

3rd. Fever is a manifestation of an effort of the system to remove disease, a physiological action under the circumstances—a general or constitutional indication of disease.

4th. Inflammation is an evidence of local disease—an action produced for the restoration of a diseased part—an effort of the vital force to remove disease.

5th. Physiology is the science of life in its modes of being, but is now usually restricted to life in a state of health.

6th. Pathology is the science of life in a state of disease. It is physiology under abnormal circumstances.

7th. Holding these views, which are legitimate teachings of physiological science, we reject from our materia medica every article, means or process of cure which . . . is directly antagonistic to the laws of vitality, and use those and those only which have a direct tendency to aid the vital organs in the removal of the causes of disease, and the restoration of health and vigor.

8th. We cordially invite all medical reformers in the United States to unite with us upon the platform . . .

9th. Upon these principles, as the basis of the science of medicine, as taught in the Eclectic Medical College of Pennsylvania, the society herein agrees to use all its influence to sustain said institution.

10th. We recognize all who stand upon this platform as true medical reformers.

In Witness Whereof, we, the committee representing the Middle States Reformed Medical Society, and the Eclectic Medical College of Pennsylvania respectively, this 18th day of May, 1854.

    For the Middle State Reformed
        Medical Society

                        John Palemon, M.D.
                        John S. Prettyman, M.D.
                        Wm. J. Williams, M.D.
                        Wm. Fields, M.D.
                        Wm. Armstrong, M.D.

    For the Trustees and Faculty
       of the Eclectic Medical
       College of Pennsylvania

                        John Foney, M.D.
                        John Sites, M.D.
                        Henry Hollemback, M.D.

APPENDIX IV

(From *The Cincinnati Medical Recorder*, Cincinnati, 1883, *51*, No. 6, 97-8)

PLATFORM, CONSTITUTION AND BY-LAWS OF THE AMERICAN PHYSIO-MEDICAL ASSOCIATION

Platform of Principles

1. The Science of Medicine, like all other sciences, is based upon the laws of Nature; and Medical Art can be true and reliable only when it is in harmony with those laws.

2. Disease is that condition of bodily structures in which they are unable to perform their functions in a natural manner, which condition disturbs the harmony or equilibrium of the system; and the object of medical science is the restoration of diseased structures to their normal state, as far as possible, that they may be enabled again to perform their offices.

3. Physiological actions are always resistive to the causes of disease, and tend to the restoration of health when it is disturbed; and remedial treatment should harmonize with these physiological efforts, conserving and assisting the inherent curative powers of the system.

4. Observing this physiological standard as the only true guide in the Curative Art, no article should be used in the cure of disease that by its nature tends to damage the integrity of structures, or impair the vitality of tissues; hence all measures that are injurious, and all agents that are poisonous, are to be rejected from medical practice, as being in themselves causes of disease and not promoters of health.

Constitution

1. The name of this organization shall be THE AMERICAN ASSOCIATION OF PHYSIO-MEDICAL PHYSICIANS AND SURGEONS.

2. Among the objects of this Association shall be: (1) The promotion of the principles of Physio-Medical Science, as enunciated in the Platform of Principles adopted by this organization; (2) The enlightenment of public

sentiment upon these principles; (3) The encouragement of all measures that will advance professional education; (4) The mutual benefit of the members of this Association, and resistance to all unjust laws against Physio-Medical Science.

3. Members of this Association shall conform their sentiments and their practice to its Platform of Principles, and their professional life and conduct shall comport with the honor and dignity of this humane calling.

4. The officers of this Association shall consist of a President, two Vice-Presidents, a Secretary, and a Treasurer; to be elected annually, and to remain in office till their successors are chosen.

. . .

7. The membership fee shall be two dollars a year, and thereafter such an amount as may be annually determined upon by the Executive Committee.

8. This Constitution may be altered or amended by a vote of two-thirds of the members present, at any regular meeting of the Association, one year's notice of the proposition to alter or amend having been publicly given to the Association.

By-Laws

1. A Board of Censors shall be appointed by the President, and confirmed by the Executive Committee, who shall examine all applicants for membership of this organization.

2. Gentlemen and ladies who are graduates of a medical college in good standing, or licentiates of a regularly organized Physio-Medical Society, or shall pass an examination before the Board of Censors, may become members of this Association by subscribing to its Constitution, agreeing therein to submit to its principles and by-laws.

3. Applicants for membership in this Association shall make application to the Board of Censors, accompanying the application with a fee of two dollars, and be recommended by two members of the Association.

4. The Board of Censors shall be guided in the examination of applicants for membership by the Platform of Principles, and shall take such measures as said Board may deem best calculated to elucidate facts bearing on the application, and shall present the conclusions arrived at to the Association; and pending the action of the Association any decision of the Censors shall stand as the decision of the Association.

. . .

6. This Association shall be divided into sections, as follows: Theory and Practice, Materia Medica, Surgery, Physiology, Obstetrics, Gynecology, Chemistry, Hygiene, Microscopy, Pathology, and Histology. The President of the Association shall appoint the Chairmen of the above committees on sciences, and these shall report at the next annual meeting.

7. All papers read before this Association shall belong to the Association.

The Medical History of the Fredericksburg Campaign: Course and Significance

GORDON W. JONES*

THE Battle of Fredericksburg was fought on 13 December 1862. It is generally rated one of the worst managed, from the Union point of view, of America's many bungled battles. General Ambrose Burnside has never been forgiven his great losses despite the fact that General Grant's were of much the same unnecessary magnitude at Cold Harbor later in the Civil War. Interesting militarily as the battle may or may not have been, it is of importance in the history of medicine as a turning point in the care of the wounded. Beginning with Fredericksburg, there was less confusion than before in the handling of the injured, and, perhaps, more mercy.

When the Civil War broke out, the military was served by a body of physicians whose horizons had been restricted by many years of dull routine in a tiny professional army. Few of the higher ranking doctors were equal to the demands of the vast Civil War mobilization. Their imaginations could not grasp the military medical implications. It took the North many months to find able physicians. Those in charge early in the war fumbled. Hygiene in the camps was terrible. The suffering of wounded men, left neglected on the fields, was a national disgrace. The fault lay largely in the fact that the medical service was, in accordance with tradition, organized by regiments instead of by larger units.

This poor organization had prevailed in 1861 and in the earlier fighting of 1862. It will be recalled that 1862 had already seen the fierce Seven Days' Battles east of Richmond in June, the Second Battle of Manassas in August, and the Battle of Antietam in September. It was after the Richmond battles that there was public demand for reform in the North because of the treatment of the wounded in the Union army. The handling of the Confederate wounded had been no better despite the fact that Richmond and its hospitals were close at hand. Dr. Lafayette Guild, Medical Director of Lee's Army of Northern Virginia, had reported his grave concern.[1]

* Fredericksburg, Virginia.
[1] *War of the Rebellion, official records.* Washington, D. C., various dates (hereafter cited as *O.R.*) Ser. I, vol. 11, pt. 3, p. 633.

This scandal of 1862 strengthened the hand of the U.S. Sanitary Commission (forerunner of the Red Cross) which had been created in 1861 over the opposition of the old-line medical bureaucracy. This organization independently inspected troop facilities, criticized sanitary arrangements, collected and distributed supplementary supplies, and succored the troops. Without this great citizens' group the medical débacle would have been appalling indeed. In addition to increasing the popular support of the Sanitary Commission, the experiences east of Richmond forced an internal reform in the medical department of McClellan's Army of the Potomac.

In June of 1862 General McClellan performed what was perhaps his greatest single service to his country. On advice from that favorite of the Sanitary Commission, the new Surgeon General William A. Hammond, he appointed Jonathan Letterman Medical Director of the Army of the Potomac. Letterman was a Pennsylvanian and a graduate of Jefferson Medical College. He was one of those who for twelve years had been in the medical department of the regular army, their talents hidden in various obscure posts. But army routine had not blunted his abilities. In his new position Letterman reorganized the chaotic medical service effectively.

Before he came to power, each regiment had had its own medical service with its own regimental hospital. Its wounded were cared for by its surgeons, whose competence had varied greatly from regiment to regiment. Line officers had used the regimental medical transport to carry their personal effects. Also, in emergencies, the medical transport had been freely used for purposes other than medical. In time of battle the regimental musicians, largely untrained, had acted as litter bearers; often unharmed soldiers had carried their slightly or severely wounded comrades to the rear, using this opportunity as an excuse to get to safety. Perhaps all this had been well enough in battles involving a few regiments, as in past wars. But when several hundred regiments were thrown into battle, the whole system had broken down into an incredible shambles.

Such was the situation that Letterman reformed. In general, he reorganized the medical department by division rather than by regiment. However, his first step was to set up an ambulance service by an even larger army unit, the corps. This service was directed by a captain who was responsible to the medical director of the corps, not to a line officer. This was an innovation. Previously, medical officers had not had line officers under their command. Under the captain there were first lieutenants in charge of ambulances serving divisions and second lieutenants in charge of those serving brigades. All these officers were mounted for the sake of mobility. Enlisted men trained as litter bearers rode the ambulances and went into battle with the troops. Two medical officers were assigned to the corps ambulance train on the march. The ambulances of each division were kept together. Measures were employed to prevent the use of ambulances by line officers not attached to the medical department. In practice the quartermaster corps retained more control over these ambulances than Letterman liked.

Next Letterman planned a reform in supply so that there might be one wagon per regiment for hospital purposes and one wagon per brigade for bulk supplies. These wagons were placed under medical, not quartermaster, command.

Finally he reorganized the field hospital system. He ordered that, before an engagement, there be a field hospital for each division, conveniently situated in a sheltered spot, with a surgeon in charge, an assistant surgeon to provide food and shelter and one other to keep records. He arranged that there be three medical officers to do the operating and three officers to assist each of these operators. Most of these doctors were regimental surgeons who were ordered to leave their regiments at time of battle and report to the division hospital. Letterman insisted on appointing as operators only the most capable, no matter what their rank or seniority. This policy created irritation among men who felt they deserved the glory, not the drudgery, of field hospital work. One assistant surgeon in each regiment was ordered to go forward with trained litter bearers (no longer necessarily the musicians) and establish a first-aid station near the front and send wounded back to the field hospital of the division to which his regiment belonged.[2]

The above is a brief résumé of extensive and detailed orders. On paper it all looks simple enough. But at the time it meant a big change, and such Washington bureaucrats as General Halleck were contemptuous. Secretary of War Stanton joined the opposition, largely because of his dislike of Letterman's superior, the Surgeon General. It took months to put the reforms into effect.

[2] Letterman, Jonathan. *Medical recollections of the army of the Potomac.* New York, 1866, pp. 24-63.

They were delayed by the fact that Letterman was not in charge of affairs during Pope's disastrous Campaign of Second Manassas in August 1862. Confusion, and the fact that most of the ambulances had been left behind at Fortress Monroe when much of McClellan's army was sent to General Pope, made care of the wounded in that fighting as disgraceful as ever. When Pope was dismissed and McClellan reinstated, Letterman too came back as medical director of the army. He found an almost total loss of medical supplies. The ambulances were still missing, and only a few arrived before the Battle of Antietam. All arrangements had to be made in haste during the September advance on the enemy. Field hospitals were set up in barns and manned by surgeons assigned to them without any particular system. After the battle, wounded were scattered, by wagon and railroad, literally all across Maryland. With this confusion as a stimulant, Letterman quickly completed his plans for a field hospital system and let them be known in a circular dated 30 October 1862.[3] His system came into its first full operation at Fredericksburg, six weeks later, making this battle of great significance to medicine.

The military aspects of the Fredericksburg Campaign may be summarized briefly. It was begun late in November 1862, shortly after General Burnside had been made commander of the Federal Army of the Potomac to succeed the slow-moving General McClellan. The first move was a quick change of base from north-central Virginia to the area about Falmouth, a village lying on the north side of the Rappahannock River opposite Fredericksburg. Burnside's plan was then to move quickly across the river, seize the heights west of Fredericksburg, and then move south on Richmond. But these plans were put into operation too slowly and he thereby gave his opponent, General Lee, time to occupy the heights.

On 11 December 1862 Burnside managed to throw three sets of pontoon bridges across the river. The upriver bridge, located between the two present highway bridges leading into Fredericksburg, was laid in the face of great Confederate resistance. In laying the second one, below the railroad bridge, and the third, a mile farther downstream, his men met only token resistance. The town was finally seized and the defenders pushed back to their main lines on the heights. December 12th was spent in a ponderous

[3] O.R., ser. I, vol. 19, pt. 1, pp. 106-117.

movement of the Union army over the pontoons and in their leisurely deployment.

On 13 December the battle began (Fig. 1). If it had been managed correctly, the left wing, deployed in the region of Smithfield Plantation (the present Fredericksburg Country Club), might have been able to crush Lee's right wing and fold it back. But it was poorly directed and was repulsed. The Federal right wing, attacking from Fredericksburg proper, was sent against the impregnable line on the hills where stood thousands of well-protected and well-managed Confederates. The result was a bloody defeat.

December 14th saw no military activity of note. Lee made no counterattack. Burnside's officers persuaded their commander that the whole thing was hopeless. By late on December 15th the army had been drawn back across the river to Falmouth (Fig. 2). No advantage had been derived from the loss of 1,284 killed and 9,600 wounded. The Confederates had lost 458 killed and 3,743 wounded.[4]

It would appear that ineptness as well as lack of speed in executing his plans lost the battle for Burnside. However, the weeks wasted gave Letterman opportunity to reorganize and make plans for a medical campaign almost unique in the Civil War for their effectiveness.

He had many problems. Not the least of these was the quality and discipline of his medical officers. There were slightly more than 550 of them in his service. Some were worthy, some not. In our day when medical training is remarkably uniform it is hard to realize the variation in competence which existed a century ago. Though there were many able commissioned physicians, the official records and memoirs are full of the complaints of the competent against the dullards and know-nothings who somehow got commissions. In the National Archives are the service records of all. It is not unusual to find a curt note on the final card of a doctor's record, "Dismissed from service." Such men were not usually the graduates of the city medical schools of the day nor of the better "country" ones (Dartmouth, Yale, University of Virginia, etc.). Many physicians were mere ex-apprentices. In addition, there were the botanics, the eclectics, and the home-

[4] A very readable recent book on the battle is E. J. Stackpole's *The Fredericksburg campaign*. (Harrisburg, Pennsylvania, Military Service Publishing Company, 1957, 297 pp.). Obviously, only the barest essentials are noted in this article. Other secondary sources used in the preparation of this paper are W. Q. Maxwell's *Lincoln's fifth wheel*. (New York, Longmans, Green and Co., 1956, xii, 372 pp.) and G. W. Adams's *Doctors in blue* (New York, Henry Schuman, 1952, xii, 253 pp.).

opaths, all anathema to the regulars. However, relatively few actual "quacks" got into the Union armies and none received the highly desirable U.S. commissions as Surgeons of Volunteers, the physicians assigned to the Surgeon General's office for duty anywhere he saw fit. Nevertheless, at times the governors did appoint sectarians and incompetents to state regiments before they were mustered into the Federal service. In contrast, the Confederate armies did use more of the botanics at least.[5]

A few of Letterman's subordinates at Fredericksburg may be mentioned as examples of the more competent officer. J. H. Brinton, Surgeon of Volunteers, Jefferson graduate, was there as an observer, surgical preceptor, and collector of material for the Army Medical Museum of which he was then in charge. His prominence and reputation during the war were great. We find him frequently quoted as an authority. He has left an interesting account of conditions in Fredericksburg. P. A. McConnell, Harvard graduate, medical director of the Ninth Army Corps (of the Federal right wing) held a state commission. Because of his effective service at Fredericksburg, Letterman strongly endorsed his later application for a Federal commission. Assistant Surgeon R. O. Craig, Albany graduate, also holder of a state commission, was an example of Letterman's interest in ability rather than rank. He was appointed medical director of the Fifth Corps although many outranked him. Charles O'Leary, medical director of the Sixth Corps and formerly a professor at Ohio Medical College, was, however, a Surgeon of Volunteers.[6] There were three other corps medical directors, each in charge of a large number of doctors. For example, O'Leary commanded 100, McConnell, 74, and Craig, 71. There seemed to be no real relationship between the number of medical officers and the size of the corps concerned.[7]

Military physicians had, of course, many other duties besides treating the wounded. They were busier, by far, treating men sick with the illnesses of armies. The best of them interested themselves in preventive medicine. In this they had to have the co-operation of their colonels. Though the health of the army was his problem, Letterman had little effective control over regimental

---

[5] Much interesting material on the sects is to be found in Alexander Wilder's *History of medicine* (Augusta, Maine, 1901), especially pp. 427 ff., and about the utilization of botanics and eclectics in the Civil War armies, p. 666.

[6] In this paper practically all the information about individual doctors that is not relatively common knowledge was obtained from their service records in the National Archives.

[7] Letterman, *op. cit.*, pp. 76-78.

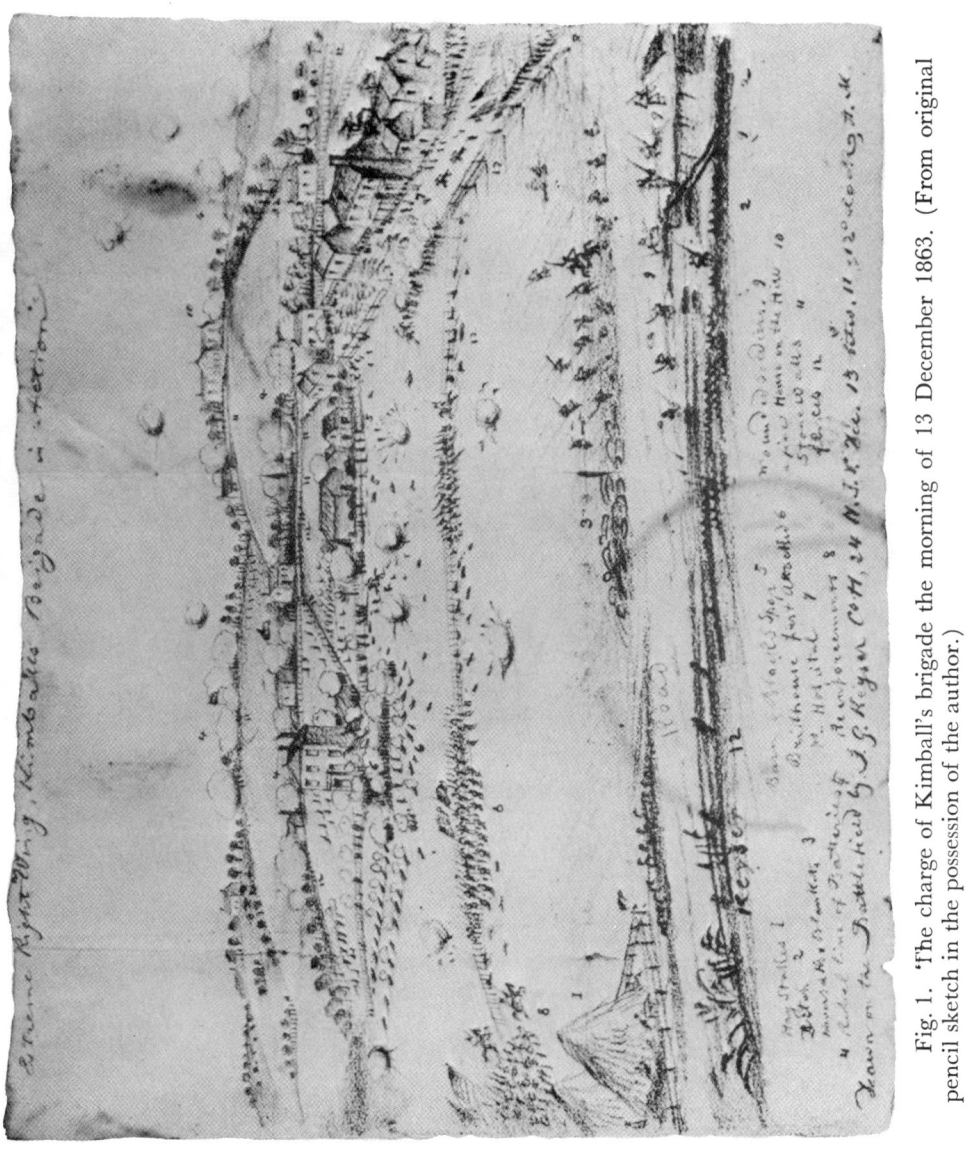

Fig. 1. 'The charge of Kimball's brigade the morning of 13 December 1863. (From original pencil sketch in the possession of the author.)

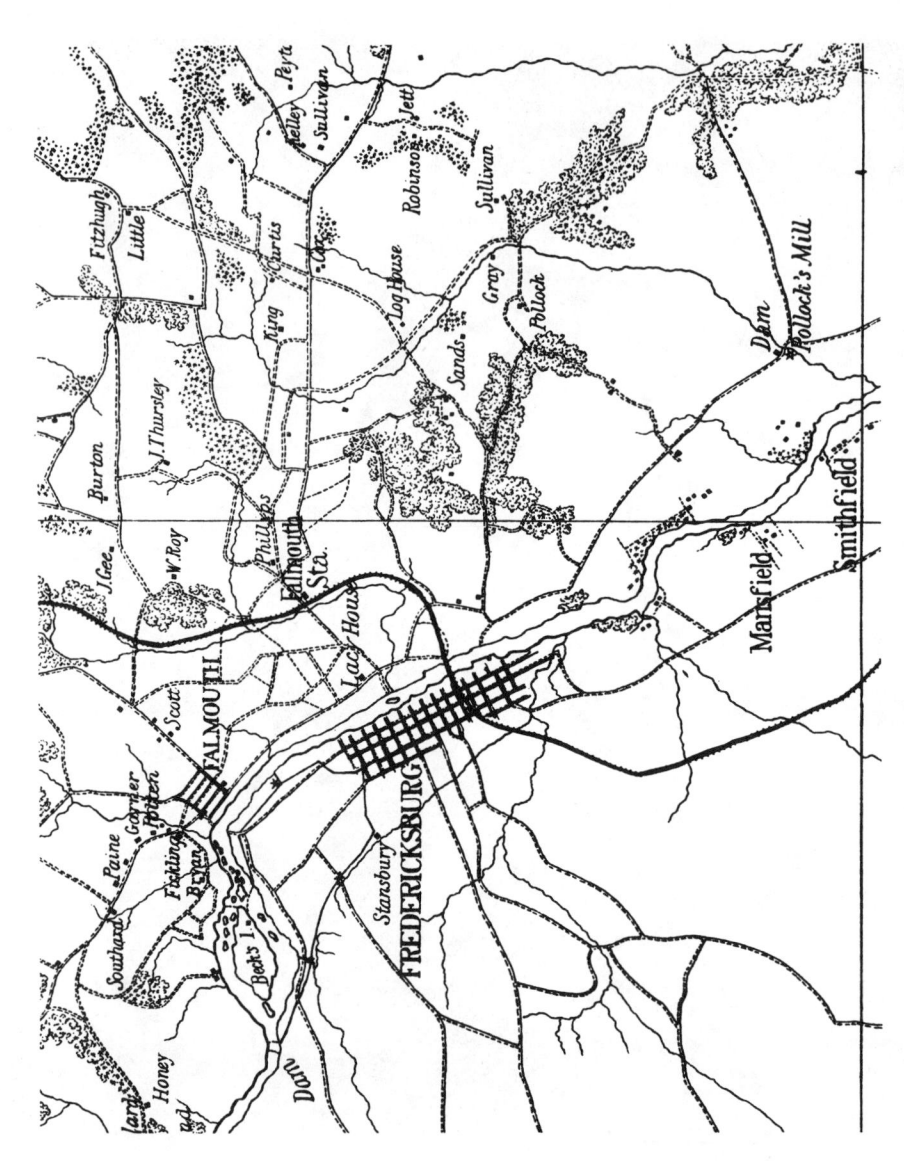

Fig. 2. Map of the Fredericksburg area. (A section of a contemporary map in the possession of the author.)

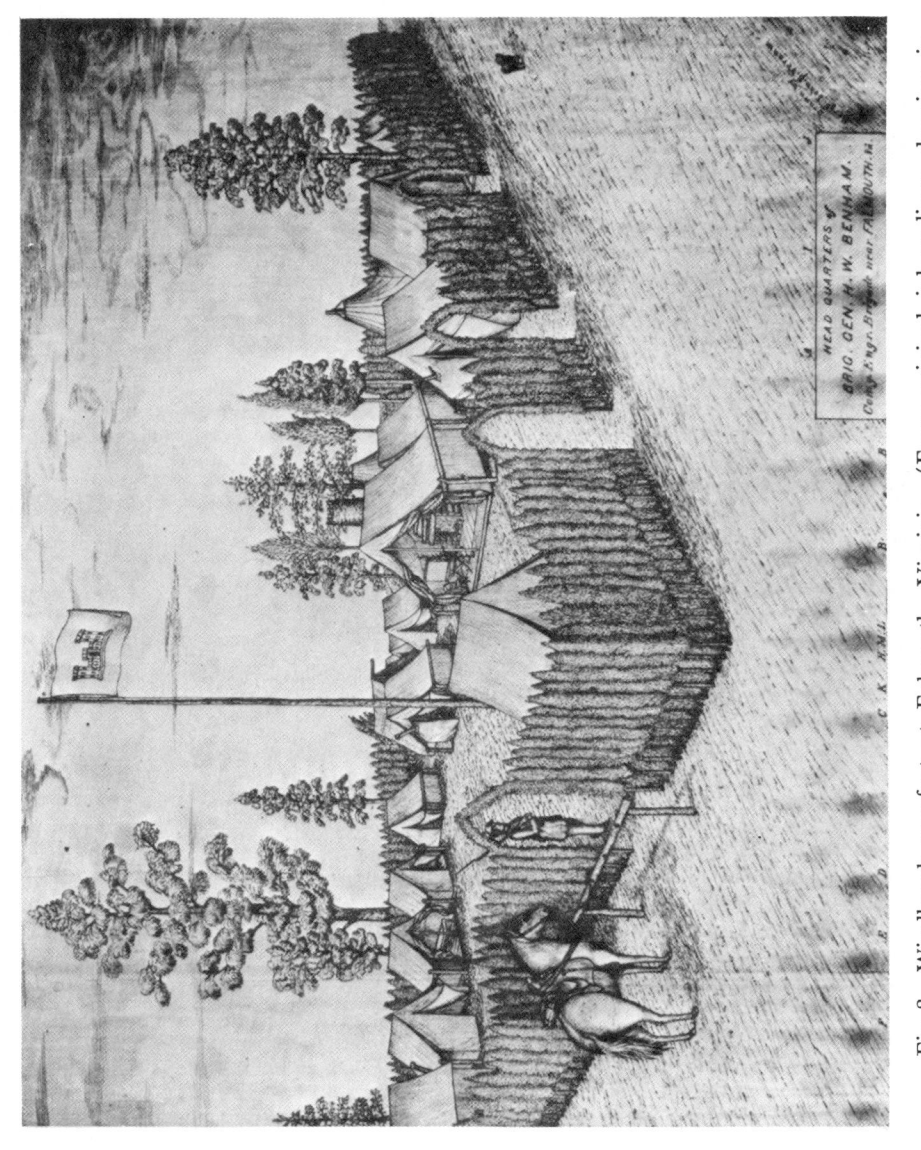

Fig. 3. Windbreak comfort at Falmouth, Virginia. (From original ink-on-linen drawing in the possession of the author.)

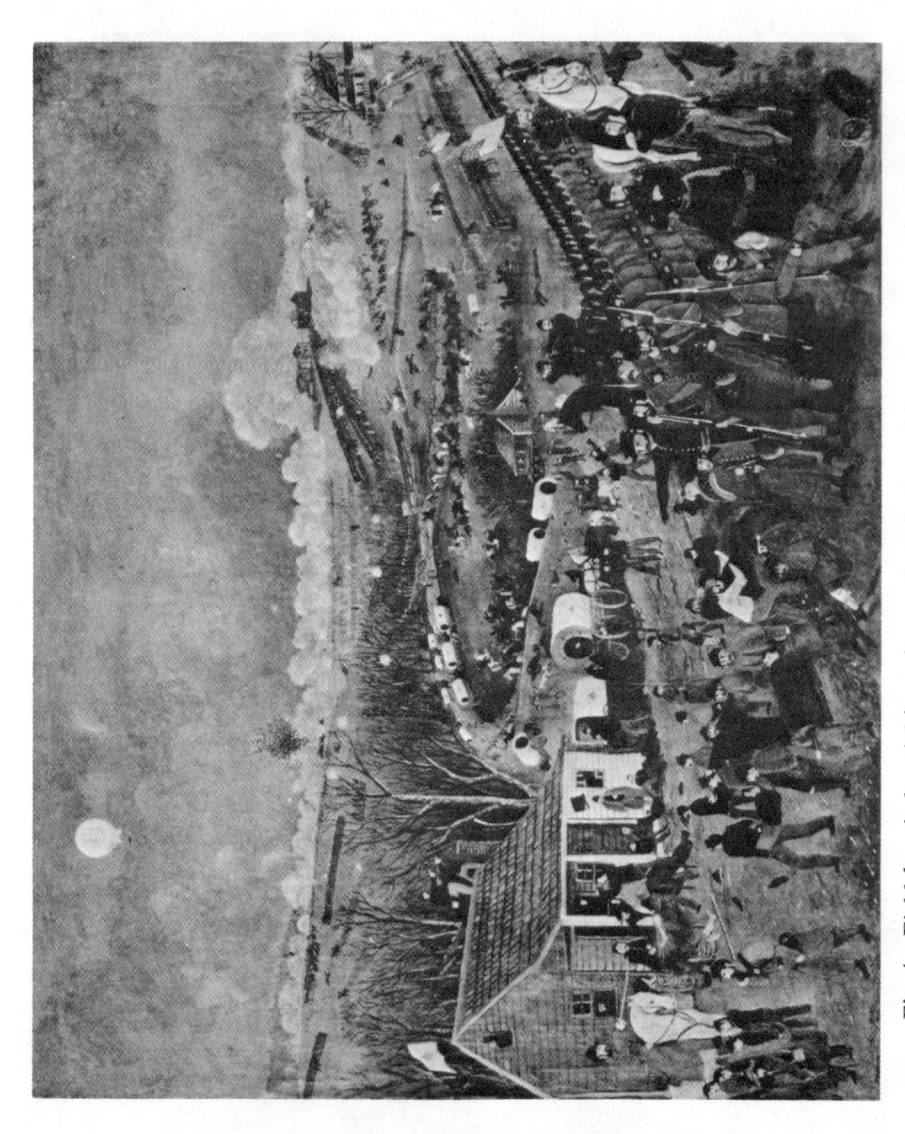

Fig. 4. Field hospital activities going on in full view of nervous reserves at the Battle of Fredericksburg. (From a private collection, New York.)

medical practice, but the hygiene of the Union troops was probably about average for the century. Some regiments were so well policed, and thus healthy, as to win the praise of foreign observers. Others were filthy. Typhoid and dysentery were common. Some regiments had an enormous percentage of sick, either in quarters or in the little regimental hospitals (division hospitals were, in Letterman's scheme, for battle emergency only). Assistant Surgeon Steinach of the 103rd New York reported that usually he had six or eight men in his hospital and from six to eighteen sick in quarters, but only three or four cases of typhoid. Of his sick, one man died of dysentery and one man shot himself shortly before the battle.[8] In contrast, Surgeon Church of the 141st Pennsylvania sent the amazing total of 169 men to a general hospital before the battle.[9] This was in obedience to the quite sensible order that all really sick men be sent off before the fight. However, many surgeons, perhaps on orders from their colonels, did not obey. More than one typhoid fever patient had his feet frost-bitten as he lay negelcted while the army was away fighting.

"Quarters" for the 120,000 Union soldiers meant tents. These were comfortable enough. Some units further protected themselves by erecting barricades of cedar boughs (see Fig. 3). In theory, the men were well fed. In fact, they were often fortunate if they had enough hard army bread (hard tack). Moving supplies by rail through an area which had to be guarded against guerrillas and then by wagon over miles of dirt roads was a great problem. Munitions came first, comfort second.

This problem of supply was one reason for Burnside's move to Falmouth. He gained easier access to his main base of supply; bulk transport by water was cheap and easy. Aquia Landing on the Potomac, only a few miles by rail from Falmouth and convenient to Washington, soon became a vast depot of munitions. Here also the medical director created a reserve of hospital supplies and medicines. However, Letterman evidently tried to handle too many details personally. He had no commissary of supply.[10] There may have been some order in his depot, but there were

---

[8] U.S. Surgeon-General's Office. *The medical and surgical history of the War of the Rebellion.* Washington, D. C. 1870-1888 (hereafter cited as *M.S.H.*) Medical volume, pt. 1, Appendix, p. 134 (hereafter cited as *M.S.H.* Appendix).
[9] Fatout, Paul, Ed. *Letters of a civil war surgeon.* West Lafayette, Indiana, 1961, p. 40. Some of these men were sent to Washington, some to what were called "corps general hospitals" at Brooke and Aquia Landing, Virginia.
[10] According to Perley who is quoted below. Apparently as a kind of rebuttal Letterman reported his satisfaction with Assistant Surgeon McMillin and his efforts as medical purveyor at Fredericksburg. *M.S.H.* Appendix, p. 103.

also confusion and error. For instance, 500 extra hospital tents were stored there, but I find no mention of cots. There were many coal stoves to heat the tents but they were too large and too hard to handle.[11] They also overheated, and surgeons later complained more of the heat than of the bitter cold on the Fredericksburg plain. There was a serious shortage of warm woolen clothing for the wounded after the battle. This lack was remedied only by the Sanitary Commission.[12] These and other shortages and mistakes were partly due to a very human underestimate of the casualty toll. Furthermore, Letterman had evidently planned for transshipment of wounded to Washington, if his own "general" hospitals at Brooke and Aquia did not suffice.

However, Letterman's fame does not rest on his abilities as a commissary officer but rather on his reorganization of the medical personnel and his over-all direction of his medical chain of command. His officers made much more elaborate preparations for the Battle of Fredericksburg than did the Confederates.

As soon as the Union army had managed, on 12 December, to seize the deserted and damaged city and drive away the snipers, it was deployed in a remarkably leisurely manner. It became a "grand military spectacle" to the Confederates who watched from the hilltops about the town. But the medical officers took advantage of this delay and busily selected sites for their division field hospitals. Since the 254 Federal Regiments were divided among 18 divisions, there were necessarily 18 such field hospitals. It may be of interest to discuss a few of them briefly.

In the area which was occupied by the Federal left wing, down river from Fredericksburg, there were two fine mansions. One of these, Smithfield, became the field hospital of the First Division of the First Corps. It was very comfortable, even hot, according to J. T. Heard, the medical officer in charge. In a deep ravine just riverward from this mansion the Third Division established a tent hospital which was quite well protected from enemy fire despite the fact that the Confederate cannon were hardly more than 3,600 yards away. These two division hospitals were so close to the front that stretcher bearers were able to bring in the wounded directly from the firing line.[13]

[11] *O.R.*, ser. I, vol. 21, pp. 957-959.
[12] Stillé, C. J. *History of the United States sanitary commission.* Philadelphia, 1866, pp. 368ff.
[13] *M.S.H.* Appendix, p. 131.

It suited General Franklin to take the other big house, Mansfield, later destroyed, as headquarters and thus keep it out of medical hands. As a result, the hospital for his other division had to be established on the opposite side of the river almost directly north of Smithfield, at the Pollock house. This necessitated more handling of the wounded of that division: men on stretchers were taken to an ambulance station behind Mansfield, transferred, and carried by ambulance by a roundabout route over the pontoon bridge to the hospital.

In Fredericksburg proper there were many deserted buildings suitable for hospital use, despite the fighting and shelling prior to the occupation. In fact, Dr. Brinton was surprised at how little really serious damage had been done to the town beyond a few shell holes in walls and some rooms full of fallen plaster. As soon as Fredericksburg was secure, Letterman hurried over and inspected these buildings. He was especially pleased by the convenient cluster made by the Courthouse and the nearby churches. Furniture was moved, and straw was probably placed over the floors to receive the wounded. Operating rooms were quickly selected and furnished. One of these was the still-used courtroom. It saw great activity for more than fifty hours, with twelve doctors working at three tables. It was then abandoned, and just in time. Minutes after the last patients and the last Yankee doctors, among them Brinton, had left, a Confederate shell burst in the courtroom. The safety of this hospital group had been jeopardized by the use of the St. George's steeple as a signal and observation post. This activity had drawn enemy fire. Such disregard of the army command for the safety of the hospital group is striking.[14]

Other buildings in the center of the town used as hospitals were hit by shells, but no casualties resulted. Still others were in more protected spots. The desire for shelter made it occasionally necessary to permit hospital activities to be carried on in full view of nervous reserves (see Fig. 4). Field hospitals for the right wing were also set up in tents or buildings on the Falmouth side of the river. One was behind Burnside's headquarters at the Phillips house. Another was at famous Chatham, as we shall see. These Falmouth hospitals became overcrowded when Fredericksburg was evacuated. Perhaps Letterman had not calculated on defeat.

[14] Brinton, J. H. *Personal memoirs.* New York, 1914, pp. 213ff. I have made no attempt to list all the hospital sites in Fredericksburg. Probably every habitable house was used for this purpose or for billeting troops. Documentary proof is lacking for many of the traditional hospital sites.

"Vast" medical stores were brought to all these hospitals. Medical officers later reported pleasure, even amazement, at the abundance of these supplies—an abundance they had not seen before during the war.

The 88,000 Confederates were probably less well off physically than the Federals. Sanitation was no better. So far as diet was concerned, only flour, unsmoked bacon, and occasionally beef were issued. No vegetables were available. Lafayette Guild, Letterman's Confederate counterpart, worried over the tendency to "scorbutus" and begged for potatoes. He reported the usual dysentery, upper respiratory infections, and some smallpox during the winter.[15] Letterman, with too much to do, might well have envied Guild, for the comparative ease of his problem.

Guild's arrangements for the battle were simple. A surgeon and litter-bearer were ordered to the front with each regiment. After receiving first aid the wounded were sent back to "field infirmaries" which were little more than collecting stations. Very few "capital" operations were done on the field. At these infirmaries they were loaded on ambulances, of which the Confederates had remarkably few, and were carried along the good military road behind the lines to a rail depot. There the volunteer Richmond Ambulance Corps took over, loaded the wounded on cars, and took them by the easy rail haul through friendly territory to Richmond and its general hospitals.[16] A field hospital set-up like Letterman's was not practical. All barns and buildings south of Fredericksburg were filled with civilian refugees and Guild had very few tents for hospital purposes. After the battle several Confederate generals praised their medical officers for the speed with which they got the wounded out of the way. Richmond took the whole burden at once, Washington only after weeks. Letterman had aimed to help the seriously wounded immediately and not move them any more than necessary to get them out of danger.

As the Union soldiers advanced into battle on December 13th, their medical officers also went along, established themselves in the rear of their respective brigades or regiments in the most sheltered but accessible positions, and sent the stretcher men ahead for the wounded.[17] The wounded at these stations, after emergency

---

[15] *O.R.*, ser. I, vol. 21, pp. 1084-1085.

[16] *Ibid.*, p. 557.

[17] Be it noted that apparently the first true field first-aid stations were the invention of Baron Larrey during the Napoleonic wars.

attention, were sent back to the field hospital of the division for surgery.

The Battle of Fredericksburg was remarkable for the high proportion of injuries to the extremities. For example, in the Second Corps there were 900 wounds of the upper extremity, 825 of the lower, 250 of the head, but only 130 of the chest and abdomen.[18] One surgeon reported a larger number of excisions of elbow and shoulder joints than in any other engagement of the Army of the Potomac. There were many amputations. In the hospitals of the First Corps alone there were over a hundred during the first 48 hours.[19] Operations aside from orthopedic procedures and arterial ligations, were few. Abdominal wounds were untreated except for the removal of easily found foreign bodies. Since even a minor wound in the Civil War often meant death, it was a noteworthy advance that men could now receive definite medical attention only a few hundred yards behind the front.

The fighting, wounding, dying, and mending went on all day on December 13th. Wounded men lying on the field before the murderous Confederate guns suffered agonies of thirst and pain. No one could live who went to succor those who had charged the farthest. Yankee stretcher bearers had to await nightfall and stumble without lanterns over the field looking for the wounded; a flicker of light brought a Confederate bullet. The night was cold and bitter for the suffering men. Oozing wounds became frosted and frozen. Many recieved no relief before they died except from such a gallant foe as Sergeant Kirkland of South Carolina, who, after wringing reluctant consent from his commander, gave water to the delirious, thirsty, dying men in his front.[20] There were other instances of kindness. One middle-aged Confederate was never forgotten by a group of wounded who had to lie in the cold for fifty hours before they were rescued under a flag of truce. This man had moved about with friendly words, a few biscuits, and doses of whiskey and water.[21]

All night the Federal surgeons continued their work as the wounded were brought in. Blankets were nailed over windows so as not to attract Confederate marksmen, and the operations went

[18] Letterman, *op. cit.*, p. 79. See also the *Manuscript report of the medical director of the Army of the Potomac for 1862* in the National Archives.
[19] *M.S.H.* Appendix, p. 130.
[20] Kershaw, General J. B. "Richard Kirkland, the humane hero of Fredericksburg." *Southern Historical Society Papers*, vol. VIII, Richmond, 1880, pp. 186-188.
[21] Whitman, Walt. *The wound dresser*. R. M. Bucke, Ed. Boston, 1898, p. 27.

on by candle and lamplight.[22] By evening of the next day, December 14th, few major operations remained to be done, so long and fast had the surgeons worked on the nine thousand wounded. During the day, the Confederates on Marye's Heights had watched with "awed fascination" as the long lines of stretcher bearers wound across the field toward the division field hospitals and as the multitude of ambulances, their yellow flags flying, transferred patients over the pontoons. On that day five thousand wounded of the First and Sixth Corps alone were moved to hospital tents and requisitioned buildings on the Falmouth side of the river. The rest of the wounded were transported the following day. The medical officers then checked every hospital for forgotten men. Under a flag of truce more were sought on the field. There were many burials by details during this search although an English observer maintained that the Federals left most of their dead for the Confederates to bury. Certainly an afternoon is too short a time to bury 1,339 dead. The entire Federal army stole away that night across their pontoons, not to return until the next year.[23]

The multitude of wounded piled up in the division hospitals about Falmouth and in the regimental quarters. Care from this time onward was possibly better than it had been after other battles, but to us it would have seemed primitive. Of this period we have the eye-witness reports of the poet Walt Whitman. He visited the Falmouth camps and hospitals as a freelance reporter and philanthropist; he let the world know what he saw and did his best to help the sufferers. He was far from impressed by the comfort and care of the men even when they were housed in such fine buildings as Chatham, the Lacy house. That splendid brick mansion was filled to overflowing with 1,200 unwashed men lying on blankets in their dirty, bloody uniforms. Many were dying. At the foot of a tree on the lawn there was a heap of arms, legs, hands, all callously unburied. Nearby were several corpses covered with blankets. The men in the tent hospitals were no better

---

[22] This necessity to operate in the light of an open flame was a major reason for the almost universal use as an anesthetic of non-flammable chloroform rather than ether during the Civil War. The quick induction with chloroform was another advantage when there was a great backlog of surgery to be done. The mortality from its use was surprisingly low. It was positively stated that no deaths attributable to chloroform occurred at Fredericksburg, and this happy war experience prolonged its use. The consensus of the profession had been running heavily in favor of ether just before the war. See, for instance, "Ether and chloroform compared as anaesthetics" translated and reprinted from *Gaz. méd.* in *Boston med. surg. J.*, 1859, *61*, 129-135, and the editorial in the same issue, pp. 145-147.

[23] *Battle-fields of the South, from Bull Run to Fredericksburg*. By an English Combatant. New York, 1864, pp. 511-516. Also *M.S.H.* Appendix, p. 103.

situated. They too were crowded, and there were no cots. The men lay on blankets spread over pine boughs and leaves or even on the bare cold ground.[24]

This congestion was relieved as rapidly as possible by sending the wounded on to the Washington hospitals. Those injured least were sent away first. Such was the Union medical custom during the Civil War: leave to the last those who are least able to endure transhipment. Letterman, at Falmouth, did not want to move the serious cases at all. He dreaded exposing them to a long cold trip in the dead of winter. He pleaded with General Burnside, asserting that the men were surely as safe in Falmouth as in Washington. Burnside was adamant; the wounded had to be "cleaned out." A feeling of mercy toward the wounded was not noticeable among Civil War generals. This was one of the liabilities of the Medical Bureau. Letterman did manage to keep the severely wounded cases about two weeks, but, late in December, they too were moved. The patients were taken by ambulance to the railroad cars and then transferred to the bare boards of river steamers after a rough ride. Finally ambulances in Washington distributed them to the various hospitals. There were few, if any, officially reported fatalities on the way, but suffering was intense. Healthy medical officers reported that the weather was fine and warm for the season, but the helpless, roughly handled wounded did not agree. Many of the cars were mere platforms "such as hogs are transported on." The cold boat trip was a nightmare. All this Letterman had anticipated in his protests to Burnside. He did his best: he supplied the men with surgeons and sent along large quantities of the favorite stimulants of the day—whiskey and brandy.[25]

Walt Whitman claimed that he saw men die on the way. He saw feeble men neglected and even callously pushed about. And when the men joined the other fifty thousand wounded and sick in Washington, this most compassionate of men continued to snoop, befriend, and finally to labor long hours for the wounded. He was outraged when crude wardmasters roughly ordered men nearly dead from typhoid or wounds to care for themselves. He was disgusted by the military ritual, etiquette, and red tape which surely should have been abandoned among the sick.

However, most of the official reports of affairs at Fredericksburg, written by army surgeons, contradict Whitman. There is exultation over the treatment of the wounded. Brinton praised.

[24] Whitman, *op. cit.*, pp. 22-24.
[25] *Ibid.*, p. 5, p. 24. Also *M.S.H.* Appendix, p. 104.

Even Stillé of the Sanitary Commission was not very critical. Only by the strictest attention to the wording of some of these reports do we infer that all was not well. It is Whitman's evidence that first makes us suspicious. Whitman, be it emphasized, did not see the medical department in action during the battle.

Moreover, among all the professional praise, we find one harsh dissent, that contained in the report of Colonel Thomas F. Perley, the medical inspector general. It seems a little strange that this man should have attained such a high rank because his service records show that he had something of a reputation as a trouble maker. Early in the war he had been under arrest for some undisclosed reason. Perhaps it had to do with his anonymous letter blasting conditions in the Mound City, Ohio military hospital. He had denied this letter, but a court of inquiry, on which the ubiquitous Dr. Brinton had sat, had proved his authorship. On at least one other occasion he had made bitter comments about medical conditions in army hospitals. After the Battle of Fredericksburg, Letterman found him an unendurable gad fly and complained that Perley had high-handedly discharged men from service without proper formalities. Finally Surgeon General Hammond himself penciled a long letter to the Secretary of War recommending that the President dismiss Perley. Perley did resign as medical inspector on 10 August 1863. He was immediately reinstated as Surgeon of Volunteers. He apparently raised no further storms during the war.[26]

This was the one physician who criticized Letterman. Some days after the battle, while the wounded were still being transferred to Washington, Perley made a tour of inspection of the camps and hospitals in the Falmouth-Aquia region. He did not like what he saw. In a report which was little short of venomous he informed Surgeon General Hammond that not much had been right medically at Fredericksburg. He complained of the lack of such medical supplies as hospital clothing (a lack confirmed by Stillé). He was critical of the big stoves. "The right kind of stoves for the hospital tents should have been on hand when the battle started," he wrote. We can certainly agree that there had been enough time. Burnside had dallied at Falmouth for nearly a month before the battle, using as an excuse the absence of his promised pontoons. For this he blamed headquarters at

[26] See Perley's service records in the National Archives.

Washington. Perhaps Letterman's shortages were the fault of Washington, too.

Perley had yet harsher things to say. He claimed that he had never seen such misery, that the wounded were without food, except hard tack and what food private individuals brought them, for days after the battle. On 15 December many men were lying without shelter in the heavy rain. For a week after the battle there was no heat in the tent hospitals despite the very cold weather. It seems he even disagreed with other medical men about the weather. Further, Perley raged at the neglect on the transports between Aquia and Washington. He asserted that many men froze during the 17-hour trip. Without mentioning a name, he concluded his report by saying: "The principal medical officer of the Army of the Potomac is incompetent."[27] This, despite the fact that he, like Whitman, did not see what went on during the actual battle.

What is the truth? Letterman was proud of his reorganization and of the effective way it worked at Fredericksburg. There was general agreement; no one found fault with what happened during the battle and the withdrawal. But was there a breakdown afterwards? The answer, according to the old memoirs, not only of Whitman but of many nurses and doctors, is a qualified yes. And, however biased, Perley was certainly a witness. If we study Letterman's report, we perhaps detect a somewhat defensive attitude about this period in his career. Evidently, however, even here conditions, though not good, were better than before. Such a conclusion is justified by a study of the many favorable reports written by medical officers. These physicians were veterans; they had seen other battles. The aftermath of Fredericksburg was Whitman's first experience on the field. It was Perley's first, and only, tour as an inspector. Letterman's fame has remained secure. His contemporaries realized that he could hardly be blamed for the multitude of commissions or omissions of his subordinates while they cared for the sudden influx of thousands of badly hurt men. It was to these subordinates that Perley's criticism probably should have been directed. Bitterness, jealousy, or spite may have caused him to heap all the blame for the suffering after Fredericksburg on one overworked medical official. He was unnecessarily harsh; his comments thus had little influence at the time. From our twentieth century point of view his general observations,

[27] O.R., ser. I, vol. 21, pp. 957-959.

shorn of their harsh overtones, were probably correct. It was a terrible experience to be ill or wounded and friendless during the Civil War. Surely, adequate care of and mercy toward the wounded did not need to end with the battle. The ideas of Perley (both here and at Mound City) and of Whitman with their emphasis on mercy seem to have been in advance of their times. To be fair, however, we must also recall Letterman's efforts to change the often callous attitude of higher officers toward the wounded.[28]

Everything considered, Letterman's Fredericksburg accomplishment may be termed a nineteenth century military-medical classic. Supplies for the battle were adequate. The ambulance service worked well. Thousands of wounded received definitive treatment with dispatch. Evacuation over the potential bottle necks at the pontoon bridges was uneventful. A similar success was not soon repeated. It is possible that part of Letterman's good fortune at Fredericksburg was due to the fact, surprising to many, that Lee did not counterattack the morning of 14 December. At Chancellorsville in May of 1863 Lee's unexpected advance placed Letterman's field hospitals within cannon range. Confusion, even panic, resulted. Satisfactory results at Gettysburg were prevented by a lack of supplies, through no fault of his own, though there were enough ambulances and enough hospitals in a friendly countryside. At Wilderness and Spotsylvania in May of 1864 (Letterman had resigned before those battles), there were too few ambulances and much confusion due to Grant's abrupt change of base while the casualties were mounting rapidly. A truly efficient medical campaign, in the East at least, did not occur again until Letterman's pupil, James T. Ghiselin, became Sheridan's medical director in the Shenandoah in the fall of 1864. He followed Letterman's policy carefully and successfully. Letterman had taught well: he had proven his methods the one essential time.

---

[28] Letterman's report in *M.S.H.* Appendix, especially on pp. 103 and 104, seems to be in answer to Perley. Certainly affairs could not have been as favorable as Letterman claimed. Rife misery is hinted at or declared in Fatout (*op. cit.*, pp. 37-43), S. Emma E. Edmonds' *Nurse and spy in the union army* (Hartford, Connecticut, 1865, p. 309), and in other instances besides the statements of Perley and Whitman. Perley, incidentally, had a fine reputation late in December 1862 (*Amer. med. Times*, 27 Dec. 1862, p. 351). Surgeon General Hammond seemed to agree with Perley's remarks about the need for commissary officers: in his report for 1862 he asked for more medical storekeepers to relieve the medical purveyors (*Amer. med. Times*, 20 Dec. 1862, p. 345).

Surgical Anesthesia, 1846-1946

JOSIAH CHARLES TRENT*

IN THIS year we celebrate the centenary of the discovery of surgical anesthesia. For only one hundred years has man known the benefit of painless surgery, yet the concept has become so firmly established in our minds that we now think of anesthesia not as a refinement in surgery, but as the indispensable accompaniment of even the most minor surgical operation. Few, even among surgeons themselves, are able to conceive of operating without the use of anesthetics: we are bred to the practice as to the aseptic technique, and only the most extraordinary circumstances could bring us to dispense with either. In order to appreciate fully the tremendous significance of the introduction of anesthesia, we must for a moment abandon our modern attitude of taking anesthesia for granted, and attempt to visualize the conditions which existed in operating rooms before its introduction.

The spectacle cannot be regarded without emotion. The patients were few in number, for the fear of pain was a deterrent equally as strong as the fear of possible accidents or of fatal errors by the surgeon; many preferred to die rather than endure the exquisite agony which was in store for them. Once brought to the table, they responded to the ordeal in various ways: some struggled and screamed without remission, begging the surgeon to leave off or to make haste; some, usually the feeblest, fell into a trance-like state, which favored the progress of the operation but gave little promise of survival; some bravely made no sign of suffering at all. Some cursed, some prayed, few wept or fainted:

I asked a man once after an amputation if he felt faint during the operation. His reply was very curious and characteristic. "Did I feel faint? What a question to ask! Did I feel faint? Why of course I didn't. Neither would you if you had the same reason to keep you from fainting. It was a good deal too bad for that."[1]

For all patients the experience entailed severe nervous shock and a long period of depression to follow, conditions which interfered seriously with the healing of operative wounds and greatly protracted convalescence. Sir Benjamin Richardson wrote: "I have heard many express that if they

---

* Department of Thoracic Surgery, University of Michigan Hospital.
[1] Sir Benjamin Ward Richardson, *Vita Medica: Chapters of Medical Life and Work* (London 1897) 82.

had known beforehand what the suffering was, and the effects subsequently endured, they would rather have faced death than such a fearful struggle for continued existence."[2]

While we pity the patients of the days before anesthesia, we must not forget that for surgeons also operating was a terrible ordeal. As students they had to learn to harden themselves to the spectacle of pain. The lesson was a difficult one: it is told of Sir James Young Simpson that "after seeing the terrible agony of a poor Highland woman under amputation of the breast, he left the class-room and went to the Parliament House to seek work as a writer's clerk."[3] Callousness did not always come with years of experience; for many accomplished surgeons the morning of operating-day regularly brought anxiety and dread. The necessity for inflicting such pain seemed hard indeed to humane men; there was always the chance, too, that the agonized writhing of the patient might lead to some fatal slip. Valentine Mott wrote:

How often, when operating in some deep, dark wound, along the course of some great vein, with thin walls, alternately distended and flaccid with the vital current —how often have I dreaded that some unfortunate struggle of the patient would deviate the knife a little from its proper course, and that I, who fain would be the deliverer, should involuntarily become the executioner, seeing my patient perish in my hands by the most appalling form of death![4]

The presence of pain was, moreover, an insuperable barrier to the development of surgery as a science. Time was at a premium for the operator; he must have accurate anatomical knowledge, to be sure, and coolness and presence of mind, but, most of all, to be successful he must have great manual dexterity. The operations devised, the techniques employed, must fit with the requirement of speed. Operations were few in number and limited in kind, partly because of the reluctance of the patients, partly because surgeons themselves considered the knife their last resort, to be employed only after the most detailed conservative measures had failed. During the five years preceding the introduction of anesthesia, only 184 operations—three per month—were performed at the Massachusetts General Hospital; these were chiefly confined to the surface of the body, including excision of tumors, amputation of limbs and breasts, various plastic operations, and herniotomy.[5] Conditions were similar elsewhere: in 1844–1845, the British surgeon Robert Liston operated in "five

[2] *Ibid.*
[3] J. Duns, *Memoir of Sir James Y. Simpson, Bart* (Edinburgh 1873) 27.
[4] Valentine Mott, *Pain and Anæsthetics* (2nd ed., Washington 1863) 11.
[5] J. Collins Warren, *The Influence of Anæsthesia on the Surgery of the Nineteenth Century* (Boston 1906) 26.

cases of lithotomy, four of herniotomy, and one of perineal section for laceration of the urethra" and in several cases of phimosis, fistula *in ano*, and extravasation of urine; he excised tumors in 22 cases, including a large ovarian tumor; he performed ten amputations, one excision of a joint, one ligation for aneurism of the femoral artery, three subcutaneous and a number of plastic operations.[6] A limited program, certainly, for one of the most popular and skillful surgeons of the day, yet, save for a few established operations, Liston had no precedent for invading the three internal cavities. Trephining of the skull is a practice older than history; drainage for empyema is mentioned by Hippocrates; lithotomy, herniotomy, ovariotomy, and reparatory measures in cases of traumatism were the sole accepted excuses for entry into the abdominal cavity. Surgical diagnosis was severely hampered, since the barbarity of an exploratory incision was unthinkable. Great operations were planned and executed upon cadavers, but pain forbade their use in actual practice.

With pain thus standing inexorably in their path, it is not surprising that surgeons through the centuries should have endeavored to find some means of alleviation.[7] The story of anesthesia has a long foreground, beginning in prehistoric and classical times with the use of various drugs to induce sleep and deaden pain. Other methods were attempted: the compression of nerves and vessels adjacent to the operating field, the application of cold, intoxication of the patient, mesmerism, bleeding to the point of syncope. The true thread of the story appears in 1772 with Priestley's discovery of nitrous oxide gas. The effect of this gas in producing insensibility and its possible value in surgical operations was first pointed out in 1800 by Humphry Davy. Next Michael Faraday, in 1818, noted the soporific effects of the vapor of sulphuric ether. Six years later, Henry Hill Hickman conducted a series of experiments with carbon dioxide gas on animals, proving the feasibility of abolishing surgical pain by the prior administration of a gas. In January 1842, an American dentist, Elijah Pope, painlessly extracted a tooth from the jaw of a patient to whom ether had been administered by William E. Clarke. Two months later, Crawford W. Long, a Georgia physician, began the practice of administering ether before performing the minor surgical operations which came his way. In 1844, Horace Wells, a dentist of Hartford, Connecticut, employed nitrous oxide gas in tooth-extraction and vainly endeavored to

[6] J. Marshall, "A Forty Years' Retrospect," *Brit. Med. Jour.* 2 (1885) 238.
[7] For many of the facts included in the following paragraph, I am indebted to Thomas E. Keys, *The History of Surgical Anesthesia* (New York 1945) 3-27.

convince surgeons of its value. And finally, on the sixteenth of October, 1846, in the operating room of the Massachusetts General Hospital, the time, the place, and the men conjoined. From the jaw of Gilbert Abbott, unconscious after inhaling ether administered to him by William T. G. Morton, Dr. John C. Warren excised a tumor "without any expression of pain on the part of the patient." The news of this event and of the subsequent painless operations performed at the same hospital spread to all parts of the world, and surgical anesthesia became an accomplished fact.

The hypotheses and experiments of many men preceded Morton's demonstration. It is but just to admit that others anticipated his discovery of the principle of anesthesia; some—Hickman, Wells, and Long—realized fully its significance for surgery. Most great innovations are similarly anticipated: our world is conservative and discourages new beginnings. False starts and fruitless efforts cumulate through the years. Then the appointed hour comes and with it a man eager and able to drive the new truth home to the unwilling minds of men. Such was Morton's accomplishment.

Many words have been wasted upon the ether controversy during the past hundred years. Of late, however, some historians have come to disregard the vexed question of priority and to interest themselves rather in the development of anesthesia: its introduction into various countries, its influence upon surgical practice, the emergence of its various branches. The articles in the present issue of the JOURNAL are principally concerned with aspects of these topics, which may well be briefly surveyed here.

The first official account of Morton's etherization experiments to reach the public was a memoir read by Henry Jacob Bigelow before the American Academy of Arts and Sciences on the third of November, 1846. On November 7, Dr. George Hayward successfully amputated the limb of an etherized patient, and Bigelow

incorporated this confirmatory evidence into a second paper read before the Medical Improvement Society of [Boston on November 9]. This paper, afterwards published in [the *Boston Medical and Surgical Journal*], was the first upon the subject, and was, I believe, that which carried the news to the South and across the Atlantic.[8]

The article to which Bigelow here refers, his "Insensibility During Surgical Operations Produced by Inhalation," was published in the *Boston Medical and Surgical Journal* of November 18, 1846 (Fig. 1). By this time

[8] Henry Jacob Bigelow, *Surgical Anæsthesia: Addresses and Other Papers* (Boston 1894) 31.

THE
BOSTON MEDICAL AND SURGICAL
JOURNAL.

EDITED BY

J. V. C. SMITH, M.D.

Whole No. 979.   WEDNESDAY, NOVEMBER 18, 1846.   Vol. XXXV. No. 16.

CONTENTS.

ORIGINAL COMMUNICATIONS.

Insensibility during Surgical Operations produced by Inhalation. Read before the Boston Society of Medical Improvement, Nov. 9th, 1846, an Abstract having previously been read before the Am. Acad. of Arts and Sciences, Nov. 3d, 1846. By Henry J. Bigelow, M.D., one of the Surgeons of the Massachusetts General Hospital - - - 309
The Fevers of the Champlain Valley. An Essay read before the Vermont Medical Society, Oct. 14th, 1846. By Charles Hall, M.D., Burlington, Vt. - - 317
The Past and the Present - - - 322

EDITORIAL, AND MED. INTELLIGENCE.

Surgical Operations without Pain - 324
Fusible Gold for Filling Teeth - - 324
Hydropathy in Parturition - - - 324
Pharmaceutic Poetry - - - - 324
The Medical Schools of New York - 325
New York Correspondence: Hydropathy, Two Cases in which its moderate Use proved beneficial - - - - 325
Weekly Report of Deaths in Boston - 327
Effects of Galvanism on the Heart - 328
Composition of Patent Medicines in the State of Maine - - - - 328
Sulphuric Acid in Aphtha - - - 328
Medical Miscellany - - - - 328

Published every Wednesday——each Number containing one sheet, subject to newspaper postage only.—Price $3 a year, in advance.

BOSTON:
DAVID CLAPP, PRINTER AND PUBLISHER,
191 Washington St., corner of Franklin St.

FIG. 1. The title-page of the *Boston Medical and Surgical Journal* for November 18, 1846, containing the first published report on Morton's ether demonstration.

Boston surgeons were more or less thoroughly convinced of the utility and efficacy of etherization. New York was not far behind. On the twentieth of November, Dr. Horace Kimball, a New York dentist, gave Dr. A. L. Cox a copy of the Boston journal containing Bigelow's report.[9] Cox arranged to have Kimball etherize a patient on whom he was to operate the next day; unfortunately Kimball was unable to secure for the occasion the only ether-inhalation apparatus then available in New York. On the fourth of December Kimball, having become the agent of the patentees for New York and having secured the necessary apparatus, demonstrated its use in the case of "a young lady from Brooklyn," whose enlarged tonsils were then removed by Dr. Cox with little or no pain to the patient. Dr. Cox was equally successful in several other minor operations, but the true acceptance of etherization in New York City apparently came on the eighth of December, when the distinguished Dr. Valentine Mott removed a cluster of tumefied glands from the right axilla of a patient, whose sufferings were "in part averted entirely, while the rest was greatly mitigated" by etherization.

Quite different from the willing reception of ether in New York was that accorded by Philadelphia. The immediate response of the profession in the latter city to Bigelow's article was highly critical, accusing Boston physicians of sponsoring charlatanry; acceptance of anesthesia was slow and grudging. As late as 1850 it was possible for a writer in the *Medical News and Library* to remark, with misguided pride, of the Pennsylvania Hospital: "anæsthetic *agents have never been used at a single surgical operation in that* institution."[10] Apparently, however, half-hearted tests of etherization had been conducted. An amusing anecdote concerning one such fiasco has been preserved. Shortly after Morton's discovery, Dr. George W. Norris, prior to amputating a crushed leg, asked a resident physician, James Darrach, to get some ether and administer it to the patient. Darrach complied and was horrified to see the man lose consciousness. "He called to Dr. Norris: 'Sir the man is unconscious!' and Dr. Norris yelled to him: 'Take that damned stuff away, Darrach.'"[11] It is recorded that in May, 1847, Dr. William Gibson, then Professor of Surgery at the University of Pennsylvania Medical School, amputated the finger of a medical student under ether.[12]

[9] A. L. Cox, "Experiments with the Letheon in New York," *Boston Med. Surg. Jour.* 35 (1846) 456–59.
[10] *Med. News and Libr.*, Phila., 8 (May 1850) 38.
[11] Francis R. Packard, *Some Account of the Pennsylvania Hospital from Its First Rise to the Beginning of the Year 1938* (Philadelphia 1938) 43–44.
[12] Richard Manning Hodges, *A Narrative*

The Cunard steamer *Acadia*, sailing from Boston on the third of December, 1846, carried a letter from Dr. Jacob Bigelow to Dr. Francis Boott of Gower Street, Bedford Square, London. In his letter Bigelow announced the discovery of etherization and remarked briefly on its significance, enclosing a *Boston Daily Advertiser* containing extracts from his son's article.[13] The *Acadia* had reached Liverpool by the sixteenth of the month, and Boott received the letter in due course. He promptly made arrangements with a neighboring dentist, James Robinson, to test the powers of ether. On Saturday, December 19, at Boott's house Robinson successfully administered ether to a Miss Lonsdale and extracted a molar tooth from her jaw. Several subsequent trials were made, apparently on the same day, all proving unsuccessful because of a defect in the valve of the apparatus employed. Robert Liston attended one of these attempts and immediately set about securing a more efficient inhaler; with the help of William Squire, Liston's assistant, and Peter Squire, the chemist, a suitable apparatus was devised.[14] On Monday, December 21, at the University College Hospital Liston operated on two etherized patients, performing evulsion of a great toenail and amputation of a thigh. The entire success of these trials was sufficient to secure anesthesia a fair hearing in England, where the practice spread rapidly.

In France the introduction of ether occurred under less propitious circumstances. Dr. Francis Willis Fisher of Boston, then studying in Paris, was informed of the discovery in December.[15] After failing in an initial attempt to persuade Velpeau to try etherization on his operative cases, Fisher experimented on himself without success. On December 15, he gave ether at the St. Louis Hospital to a patient of Jobert de Lamballe, also unsuccessfully. By January 12, 1847, however, Malgaigne had performed at the same hospital four operations on patients under ether; on January 23, Fisher, using a "Boston Inhaler" successfully administered ether for an operation by Roux, while on the same day Velpeau operated

---

of Events Connected with the Introduction of Sulphuric Ether into Surgical Use (Boston 1891) 60.

[13] Francis Boott, "Surgical Operations Performed during Insensibility, Produced by the Inhalation of Sulphuric Ether," *Lancet* 1 (1847) 5–8.

Francis Boott (1792–1863) was born in Boston and educated at Harvard University; he spent several years thereafter in travelling between England and America, making life-long friendships in both countries. He took his M.D. at Edinburgh in 1824, practiced successfully in London for about seven years, then retired and devoted himself to literary and scientific studies (*D.N.B.* 2. 855).

[14] William Squire, "The First Operation under Ether in Great Britain" *Brit. Med. Jour.* 2 (1896) 1143.

[15] F. Willis Fisher, "The Ether Inhalation in Paris," *Boston Med. Jour.* 36 (March 1847) [109]–113. See also below, p. 607.

on an etherized patient at La Charité. In May of that year Henry Bryant remarked in a letter from Paris that during his month's stay there he had heard no allusion to the discovery of ether anesthesia: "It has taken its rank among medical agents, and is as quietly and firmly established as if it had been known for centuries."[16]

Thus the practice spread, with almost universal acclaim. The most immediate effect of the introduction of ether anesthesia was a change in the attitudes of both surgeons and patients toward operating: anesthesia brought not only abolition of pain, but also greater safety during the operation, greater readiness in healing. As a result, there was a rapid increase in the number of operations performed. As early as April of 1847, an editorial in *The Lancet* remarked: "the number of surgical operations in some of our hospitals has been more than *doubled* since the introduction into practice of the use of ETHER-VAPOUR."[17] During the five years following the Morton demonstration, the number of operations at the Massachusetts General Hospital increased to 487 as against 184 of the preceding five years.[18] The vast increase in the number of cases seen at the operating table facilitated the development of surgical diagnosis and favored the growth of the surgical specialties, plastic surgery, ophthalmology, and urology, in particular. For some years surgeons confined themselves to established techniques; then, gradually, new occasions for surgical intervention were found, and the thorax, abdomen, and skull were more and more freely invaded. Although surgery could not achieve its full triumph until Lister's establishment of the antiseptic principle, the science made greater strides in the twenty years after anesthesia than in the twenty centuries before.

Not only the nature of surgery, but also the qualifications for its practice changed. Manual dexterity and speed ceased to be prime desiderata in surgeons, deliberate and careful techniques took their place, and many able men rose to eminence despite their lack of mere mechanical talents. As Lawson Tait remarked of Syme: "He never could have been the surgeon he was without the encouraging influence of an anæsthetic."[19]

While working these many changes in surgery, anesthesia itself was far from static. Once its practicability had been demonstrated, attention was turned to the discovery of new drugs with anesthetic properties, for ether although effective was malodorous and irritant. In November 1847, just

[16] Henry Bryant, "Inhalation of Ether in Paris," *Boston Med. and Surg. Jour.* 36 (1847) [389].
[17] *Lancet* 1 (1847) 392.
[18] J. Collins Warren, *loc. cit.* (see note 5).
[19] Lawson Tait, "Surgical Training, Surgical Practice, Surgical Results," *Brit. Med. Jour.* 2 (1890) 270.

one year after the first report of ether anesthesia, Sir James Y. Simpson announced the introduction of a new drug, chloroform, thought to possess all the advantages and none of the disadvantages of ether. This was but the first of hundreds of anesthetic agents which have been introduced during the past century. Among the most important of these are morphine (Sertürner, 1808; Lafargue, 1836), cocaine (Gaedicke, 1855; Niemann, 1860; Bennett, 1873), procaine and its compounds (Einhorn, 1904), the barbiturates (Fischer, 1902), ethylene (Nunneley, 1849; Luckhardt and Carter, 1923), avertin (Eichholz, 1917; Butzengeiger, 1926), and cyclopropane (Freund, 1882; Lucas and Henderson, 1928; Waters and colleagues, 1934).

Early in the history of surgical anesthesia the emphasis was upon the open administration of ether and chloroform, but as other drugs with special properties became available special techniques were of necessity developed. In 1884 Carl Koller of Vienna first used cocaine topically in the eye. In 1885 James Leonard Corning injected cocaine in or around the spinal canal, producing "spinal" anesthesia.[20] Halsted (1885) and Cushing (1902) developed infiltration and nerve-block anesthesia. Intravenous anesthesia has of late become clinically important through the use of two rapidly acting barbiturates, evipal and pentothal. Rectal anesthesia came to the fore with the introduction of avertin in 1926. The youngest of the surgical specialties, thoracic surgery, has actually been made possible by the development of endotracheal "positive pressure" anesthesia.

The anesthetist's armamentarium now includes complex apparatus and numerous accessory drugs, which are used to facilitate smooth and effective anesthesia. Increasing knowledge of the physiology of respiration has led to the invention of elaborate machines to permit a "closed" system, in which the gases are conserved and the exhaled carbon dioxide is absorbed. Morphine and many of the barbiturates are no longer used to induce anesthesia but are valuable as sedatives preoperatively. Even curare, once considered a deadly poison, has been used as an aid to relaxation during anesthesia.

The literature of anesthesia has become so vast and specialized that many journals devoted entirely to this subject have appeared. The science of anesthesia has progressed to such a point that its proper application demands the services of trained anesthesiologists. To meet this need, more and more residencies in anesthesia are being made available. In 1937, in

[20] This has culminated in the recently perfected practices of continuous spinal and continuous caudal anesthesia.

the United States, a board of anesthesiology was established as an affiliate of the American Board of Surgery; in 1941 an independent board was instituted to pass upon the qualifications of persons trained in the field. All these developments give promise that the future of anesthesia will bring achievements even greater than the tremendous advances of the past one hundred years.

Development and Use of the Rubber Glove in Surgery and Gynecology

CURT PROSKAUER*

ON 10 January 1834 a young physician named Richard F. Cooke, who had "dropped anchor" in Hoboken, New Jersey, sent off a manuscript on medical ethics with an accompanying letter[1] to his former teacher, "Valentine Mott M.D. Professor of Surgical Anatomy &c. Park Place, New York," who taught surgery at the College of Physicians and Surgeons, Columbia University.

Cooke, whose life and work are relatively unknown, would have been surprised had anyone told him that a few lines of his letter to Mott would prove more important in the development of medicine than all 38 quarto pages of his manuscript put together. In this letter, for the first time, we find not only the statement that "a pair of India rubber gloves would be perfectly impenetrable to the most malignant virus" (Fig. 1c), but also reference to "a very nice solution of Caioutchiouc, dissolved in Guthries spiritus of Terpentine," a sample of which he sent along with his letter (Fig. 1a).

Hardly three years before, on 8 May 1831, the chemist, inventor, and physician Samuel Guthrie of Sackett's Harbor, New York, had informed the famous Connecticut chemist Benjamin Silliman, founder and editor of the *American Journal of Science and Arts*, of his experiments on the purification of oil of turpentine, a process he had discovered a year earlier.[2] "It is, as I think, an article of considerable importance. It dissolves caoutchouc, and the solution dries rapidly, and does not continue sticky like the solution made with common oil of turpentine." In another communication to Silliman, Guthrie wrote: "Few things that have engaged my attention, have cost me so much trouble as divesting spirits, or rather oil of turpentine, of the last particle of its resin. ... My first object was to obtain a perfect and clean solvent for caoutchouc.... The oil of turpentine thus prepared, with *warmth*

---

* Consultant to the Library of The New York Academy of Medicine and Curator of the Charles H. Land Museum, School of Dental and Oral Surgery of the Faculty of Medicine, Columbia University.
[1] Now in the manuscript collection of the Rare Book Room of The New York Academy of Medicine (sign: MS 560).
[2] *Amer. J. Sci.*, 1832, *21*, 93: Art. XI.

and strong solar light, is, as I believe, a *perfect solvent of caoutchouc."*[3]

The results of Guthrie's experiments appear to have impressed Richard F. Cooke so much that he repeats Guthrie's instructions for dissolving caoutchouc. In his letter to Mott he writes: "I take the liberty of leaving with this also a very nice solution of Caioutchiouc. I dissolve it in Guthrie's spt. [spiritus] of terpentine highly rectified by the acid of sulph-acid and add a few drops of ol. of wintergreen or any other essential oil, and in certain cases ol. of Tar.—" (Fig. 1a).

And now comes his splendid suggestion:

This if I mistake not, will become a useful material in the surgeon's hand. I have used it in phlegmonous and erysipelatous inflam[mations] with great benefit, also in sprains and bruises. . . . (Fig. 1a). When applied to a part by means of a brush or the finger the Terpentine evaporates and leaves an application, firmly and nicely applied to the most irregular surfaces. . . . (Fig. 1b) I would further add that this is convenient to use in dissecting rooms and in vaginal examinations. By lubricating the hands with it you have an insoluble pair of India rubber gloves—perfectly impenetrable to the most malignant virus. The Terpentine gives no inconvenience as it immediately evaporates. It may afterwards be completely removed, by bringing the hands together smoothly, or rubbing them with some granular substance as hair powder or Indian meal (Fig. 1c).

Here we have the first known mention of rubber gloves "in the surgeon's hand" to prevent infection by "the most malignant virus . . . in dissection rooms and in vaginal examinations."

About a decennium later, Thomas Watson (1792-1882), "Fellow of the Royal College of Physicians, Late physician to the Middlesex Hospital, and formerly Fellow of St. John's College, Cambridge," suggests gloves for antisepsis:[4] "In these days of ready invention, a glove, I think, might be devised, which should be impervious to fluids, and yet so thin and pliant as not to interfere materially with the delicate sense of touch required in these manipulations [gynecological examinations and child-birth]. One such glove, if such shall ever be fabricated and adopted, might well be sacrificed to the safety of the mother, in every labor." Watson recommended these gloves—and he may have meant rubber gloves—because of his

---

[3] Article VI. Remarks on various Chemical Preparations; in a letter from S. Guthrie to the Editor, dated Sacket's Harbor, N. Y. Sept. 12, 1831. *Amer. J. Sci. Art.,* 1832, *21,* 291-2.

[4] Watson, Thomas. *Lectures on the principles and practice of physic; Delivered at King's College, London.* London, John W. Parker, 1845, vol. II, p. 349. First published in the *Med. Times and Gazette,* 1840-1842.

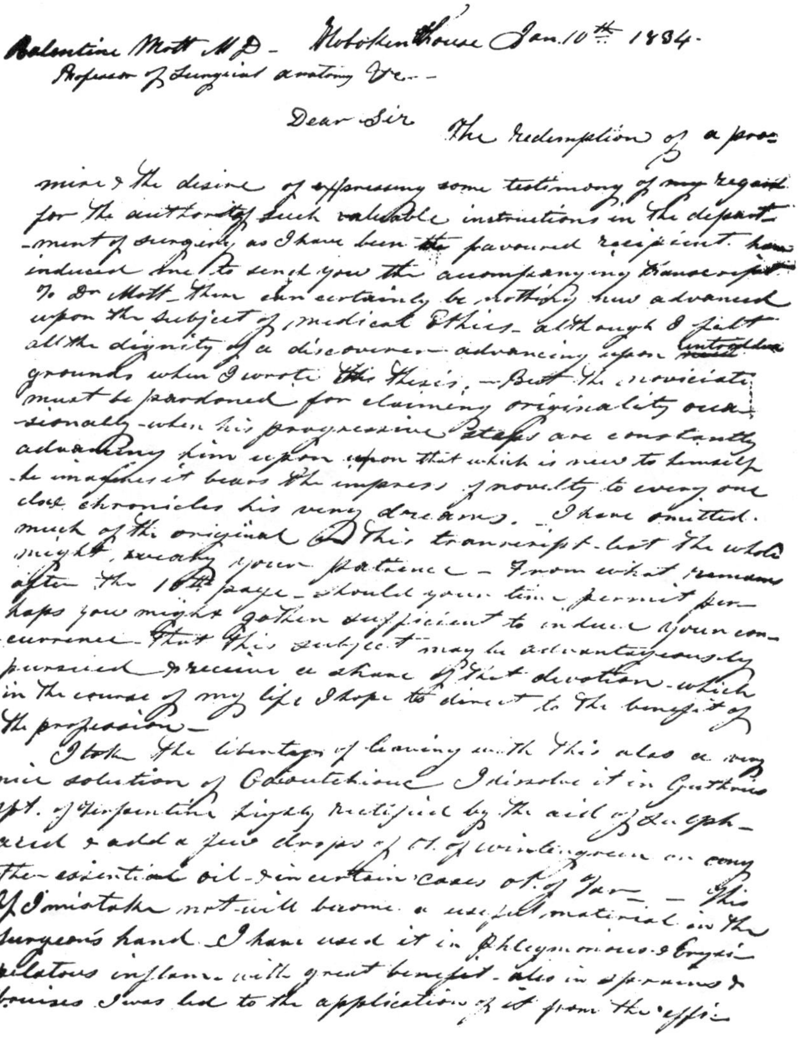

FIG. 1a. Page 1 of the letter from Richard F. Cooke to Valentine Mott. The paragraph at the bottom of the page contains the phrases quoted in the paper.

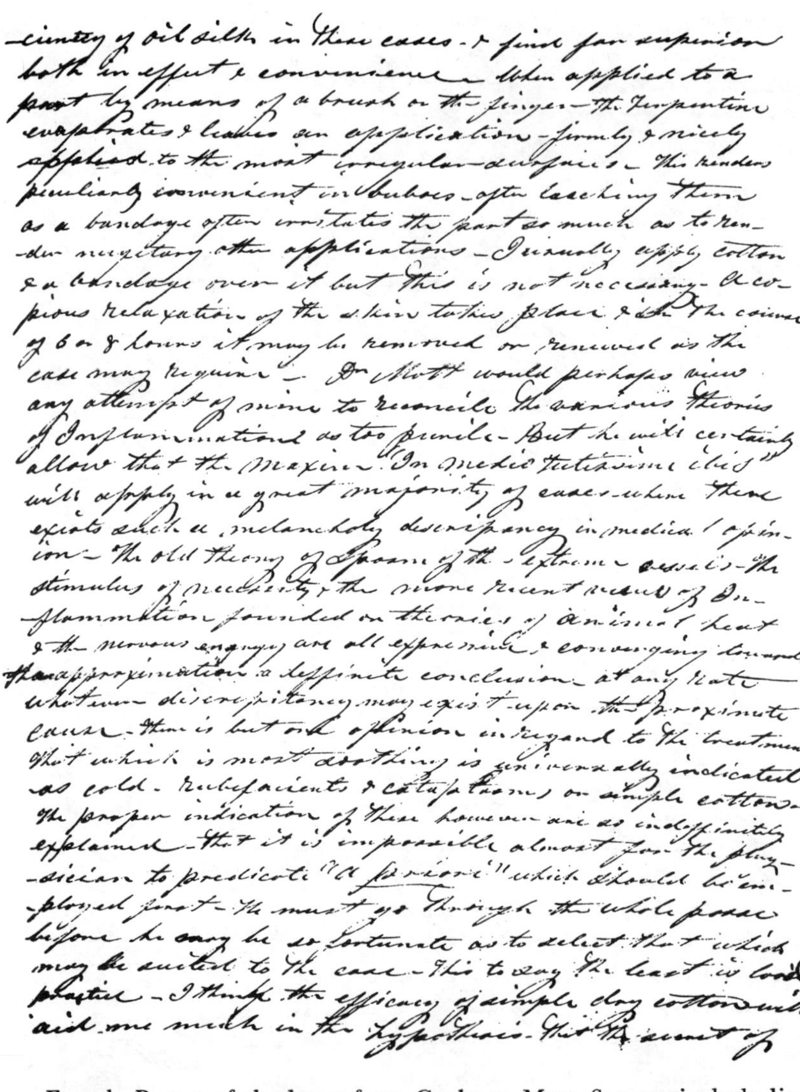

FIG. 1b. Page 2 of the letter from Cooke to Mott. See particularly lines 2 to 4.

all these remedies either directly or indirectly consist in arresting insensible transpiration from the surface the first two accomplish this when inflammation is deeply seated - the latter when approximating the surface they all accomplish this but in different ways - As the latter - viz Cataplasms & Cotton - being best suited to my present purpose - I will only detain you sir by stating - that they are simple non conductors of heat - by means of the air entangled in the fibres of the cotton & the warmth & moisture of the Cataplasms - Instead of increasing perspiration they retard it - they retard that insensible transpiration which is increased in the ratio that heat is radiated & when thus retarded it assumes the form of sweat upon the surface which has given rise to the delusion that poultices cause a part to perspire - I could prove this to your entire satisfaction by a number of experiments & observations I have already instituted but my account of these might weary you - So I must beg leave merely to state that this solution is an absolute Electric & as such a perfect non conductor & as such answers better than any rubefacient I am conscious of in incipient inflammation & better than any poultice the "Feces Boviles" which your lecture justly estimates not excepted in the suppurative stage — — Should this subject be sufficiently interesting to warrant the pains of your perusal I will be happy to give in form the history of several cases in which I have applied it & its results - I would further add that this is convenient to use in dissecting rooms & in vaginal examinations. By lubricating the hands with it you have an insoluble pair of India rubber gloves - perfectly impenetrable to the most malignant virus - the Turpentine gives no inconvenience as it immediately evaporates - It

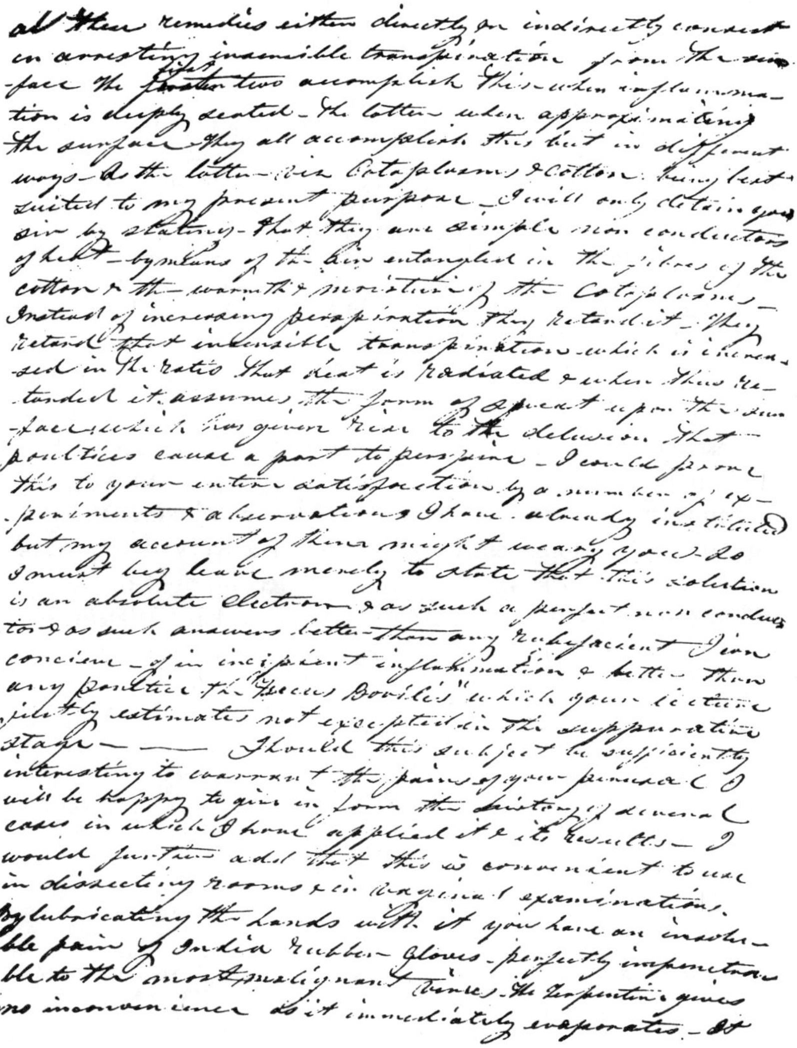

FIG. 1C. Page 3 of the letter from Cooke to Mott. See the last several lines for quotations in the text.

dreadful suspicion that the hand [of the physician] which is relied upon for succour in the painful and perilous hour of child-birth, and which is intended to secure the safety of both mother and child, but especially of the mother, may literally become the innocent cause of her destruction; innocent no longer, however, if, after warning and knowledge of the risk, suitable means are not used to avert a catastrophe so shocking. I need scarcely point to the practical lesson which these facts inculcate. Whenever puerperal fever is rife, or when a practitioner has attended any one instance of it, he should use most diligent ablution; he should even wash his hands with some disinfecting fluid, a weak solution of chlorine for instance: he should avoid going in the same dress to any other of his midwifery patients: in short, he should take all those precautions which, when the danger is understood, common sense will suggest, against his clothes or his body becoming a vehicle of contagion and death between one patient and another. And this is a duty so solemn and binding, that I have thought it right to bring it distinctly before you.[5]

These remarkable lines appeared about five years before the Viennese obstetrician Ignaz Philipp Semmelweis published his "Höchst wichtige Erfahrungen über die Aetiologie der in Gebäranstalten epidemischen Puerperalfieber" (Highly important observations on the etiology of puerperal fever epidemic in lying-in hospitals), 1847-1848,[6] setting forth his discovery that puerperal fever was in most cases transmitted by "decomposed organic matter" on the hands of physicians and students. Like Watson before him, Semmelweis recommended rigorous hand-washing in a cal-

[5] Rubber gloves are spoken of elsewhere, for instance by Warner Wells in "Surgical practice in North Carolina. A historical commentary." *(N. C. med. J.*, 1954, *15*, 281-7). The reference by Dr. Wells is to be found in the *North Carolina Medical Journal* [old ser.] March, 1878, *1*, 168-9: Our New York Letter. New York, February 26, 1878 by [M. J.] DeR.[osset] " . . . Your correspondent witnessed a late case of ovariotomy by Dr. [F. Wood] Thomas. The practical details in the procedure may be useful to those who are interested in that line. It was at the Woman's Hospital, not in the main building, however, but in a small frame cottage on the grounds, to diminish the danger of septic influences. . . . Six assistants, one for the ether, two for manipulating the abdomen and body, one having charge of the instruments, two for the carbolic sprays—besides two nurses for handing warm water to the operator to keep his hands clean. The instruments were scalpel, grooved-director, scissors, sounds, trocars, . . . *all kept in a shallow pan of carbolized water, in charge of an assistant who wore rubber gloves to preserve his hands from the caustic effects of the acid. . . .*" See also Miss Miriam Tucker. Men of medicine. The reluctant surgeon. *Postgraduate Medicine*, 1951, *9*, 74-81. "After his graduation from St. Louis Medical School in 1846, Dr. [Timothy Loisel] Papin went to Paris to study. . . . On his return to St. Louis, Dr. Papin brought the French knowledge of the use of the obstetric forceps, and early attracted much attention and some criticism. He wrote very few papers. . . . Back in the eighties Dr. Papin was already using rubber gloves when attending infected cases of parturition to, as he expressed it, 'prevent carrying the disease to other women.'" I am indebted to Dr. Martha Gnudi, Webster Library, Columbia University, for this reference. Miss Della O. Cooper, Saint Louis, informs me that she "checked with the various members of Dr. Blair's family, who do not remember hearing anything about their great grandfather's [Papin] using rubber gloves. Mrs. Richard Boyle, Dr. Blair's sister, does remember quite well that she and the other children amused themselves by making balloons out of their grandfather's rubber glove fingers." Dr. Papin, who "did not [do] much writing," published nothing about rubber gloves; the above-mentioned rubber fingers that he used were perhaps transformed by report into *gloves.*

[6] *Ges. Aerzte Wien*, 1847-48, *4*, pt. 2, 242-4; 1849, *5*, 64-5.

cium chloride solution before vaginal examination and medical care in connection with pregnancy and labor, although he did not know what transmitting agent he was destroying. It is quite possible that Semmelweis had read the famous lectures of Watson, the leading clinician of his day, which had been published not only in the journal *Medical Times and Gazette,* but also in book form; these were the most important and most popular clinical medical treatises to appear in Semmelweis's time.

Nevertheless, it took exactly half a century for Watson's dream to be realized—a practical glove "which should be impervious to fluids, and yet so thin and pliant as not to interfere materially with the delicate sense of touch required in these manipulations."

While Cook had hoped to make a glove which should protect the surgeon's hands against "the most malignant virus," and Watson wanted one to protect the patient against infection from the surgeon's hands, actual use of rubber gloves in surgical operations in fact resulted from a surgeon's compassion for the sensitive skin of his nurse's hands. Dr. William Stewart Halsted, graduate of the College of Physicians and Surgeons of Columbia University, and first Professor of Surgery at the newly founded (1889) Johns Hopkins Medical School in Baltimore, tells the story.[7] We learn that he was the man who actually introduced the use of rubber gloves in surgical operations: "In the winter of 1889 and 1890— I cannot recall the month—the nurse in charge of my operating-room complained that the solutions of mercuric chloroid produced a dermatitis of her arms and hands. As she was an unusually efficient woman, I gave the matter my consideration and one day in New York requested the Goodyear Rubber Company[8] to make as an experiment two pair of thin rubber gloves with gauntlets. On trial these proved to be so satisfactory that additional gloves were ordered. In the autumn, on my return to town, the assistant who passed the instruments and threaded the needles was also provided with rubber gloves to wear at the operations. . . . This assistant was given the gloves to protect his hands from the solution of phenol (carbolic acid) in which the instruments were submerged rather than to eliminate him as a source of infection." According to Halsted, the assistants in time became "so accus-

[7] *J. Amer. med. Ass.,* 1913, 60, 1123-4.
[8] The Goodyear Glove Rubber Division of the United States Rubber Company has informed the writer that they cannot find any photographs or drawings of the first rubber gloves manufactured for Professor Halsted. "Evidently through the years this material was lost or disposed of. . . ."

tomed to working in gloves that they also wore them as operators[9] and would remark that they seemed to be less expert with the bare hand than with the gloved hands." Dr. Joseph Colt Bloodgood, Halsted's house surgeon[10] called by the staff "Bloodclot,"[11] who first made this comment ". . . was the first to wear them, invariably, when operating." (Fig. 2)

In Dr. Bloodgood's report on hernia operations[12] in the Johns Hopkins Hospital (1899), his chapter on "the wearing of rubber gloves by the operator and assistants" gives these figures:[13]

The following study of the suppuration of the wound after operation for inguinal hernia is chiefly of historical interest, to the operator as well as all assistants, because since . . . the use of rubber gloves, the suppuration of the wound has been almost eliminated. Between February, 1897, and January, 1899, 1 year and 11 months, there have been 181 operations for inguinal herniae with only one case of suppuration[14] [whereas when gloves were not worn, in 1891-1892], there were 26 operations for hernia with 9 suppurations (29 per cent), 5 acute infections, 3 late infections, and 1 secondary stitch abscess.

These gloves have been worn by the operator with very few exceptions, and by all the assistants without an exception (Fig. 3) from February, 1897, to the present time, June 1899. . . . The writer was the first as operator to wear gloves as a routine practice in practically all clean operations. . . . The importance of wearing gloves, especially by all the assistants, and even by the operator, can easily be appreciated. The assistants come from the ward visit, where they may have handled all sorts of infections, directly to the operating-room. It is impossible in a large surgical clinic to isolate or to have dressed by assistants who do not come to the operating-room all cases of granulating and infected wounds. Many of these assistants operate on infected cases in the out-patient department; some assist at autopsies and work in pathology and bacteriology. Their hands and fingernails must always contain all sorts of bacteria, and now and then perhaps very virulent streptococci and staphylococci. It is perhaps impossible to sterilize such hands. The wearing of rubber gloves, which are sterilized by boiling, absolutely excludes hand infection. The writer was led to wear gloves when

---

[9] Dr. James F. Mitchell (now in Washington, D. C.), at that time anesthetist in Dr. Halsted's operating room, took a photograph of the first surgical operation for which the operator wore rubber gloves (1893). This photograph he reproduced in his excellent article entitled "The introduction of rubber gloves for use in surgical operations." (*Ann. Surg.*, 1945, *122*, 902-04). Dr. Mitchell has been so kind as to send me the negatives of this as well as the other photograph taken by him at the same time. I wish to express my deep appreciation for his generosity.

[10] In the photograph, from left to right, according to Dr. Mitchell: Chauncey Pelton Smith, James F. Mitchell, Joseph Colt Bloodgood, Harold C. Parsons, John (orderly), Sidney Cone.

[11] Blumer, George. Reminiscences of an old-time doctor. *Yale J. Biol. Med.*, 1955, *28*, 9.

[12] Bloodgood, J. C. Operations on 459 cases of hernia in the Johns Hopkins Hospital from June, 1889, to January, 1899. The special consideration of 268 cases operated on by the Halsted method, and the transplantation of the rectus muscle in certain cases of inguinal hernia in which the conjoined tendon is obliterated. *J. Hopk. Hosp. Rep.*, 1899, *7*, 223-562.

[13] *Ibid.*, pp. 304-6.

[14] *Ibid.*, p. 292, footnote.

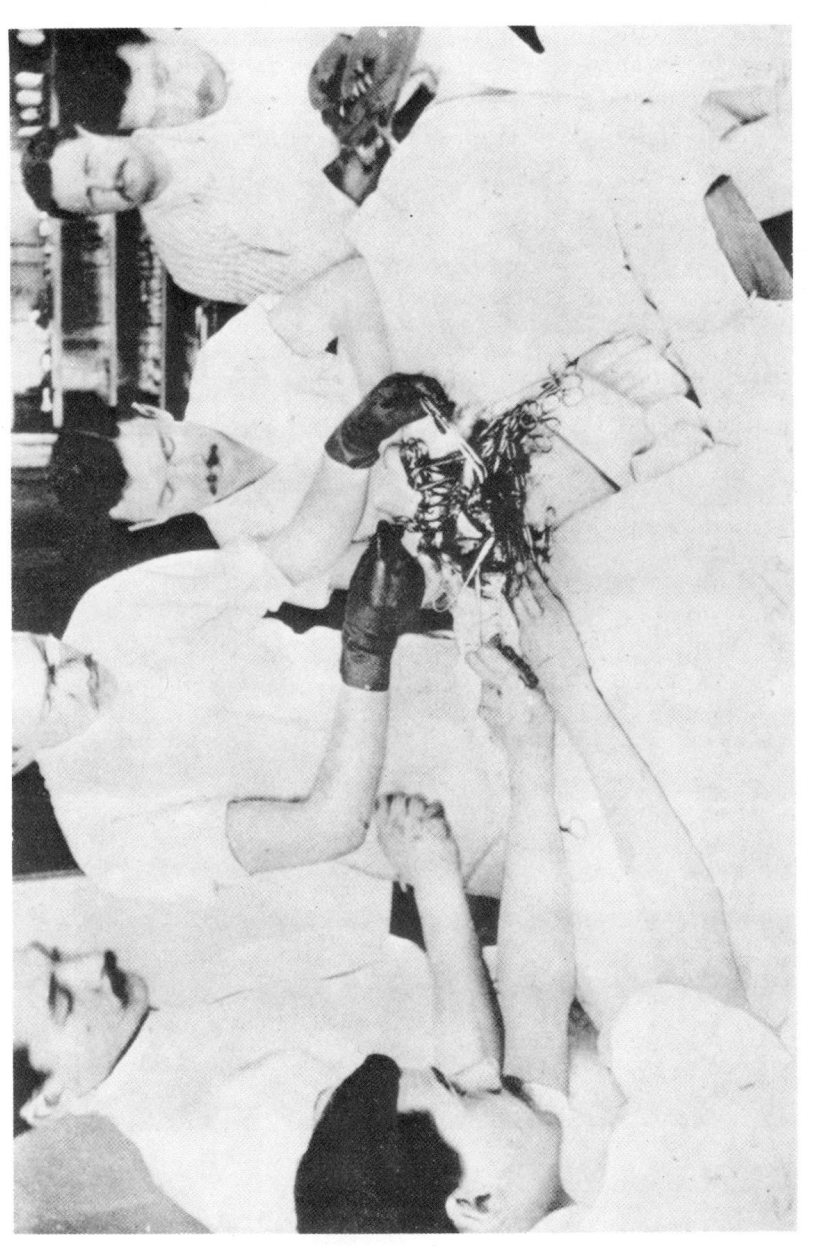

FIG. 2. A photograph of the first surgical operation in which the operator wore rubber gloves. (Reproduced from a photograph made in 1893 by Dr. James F. Mitchell)

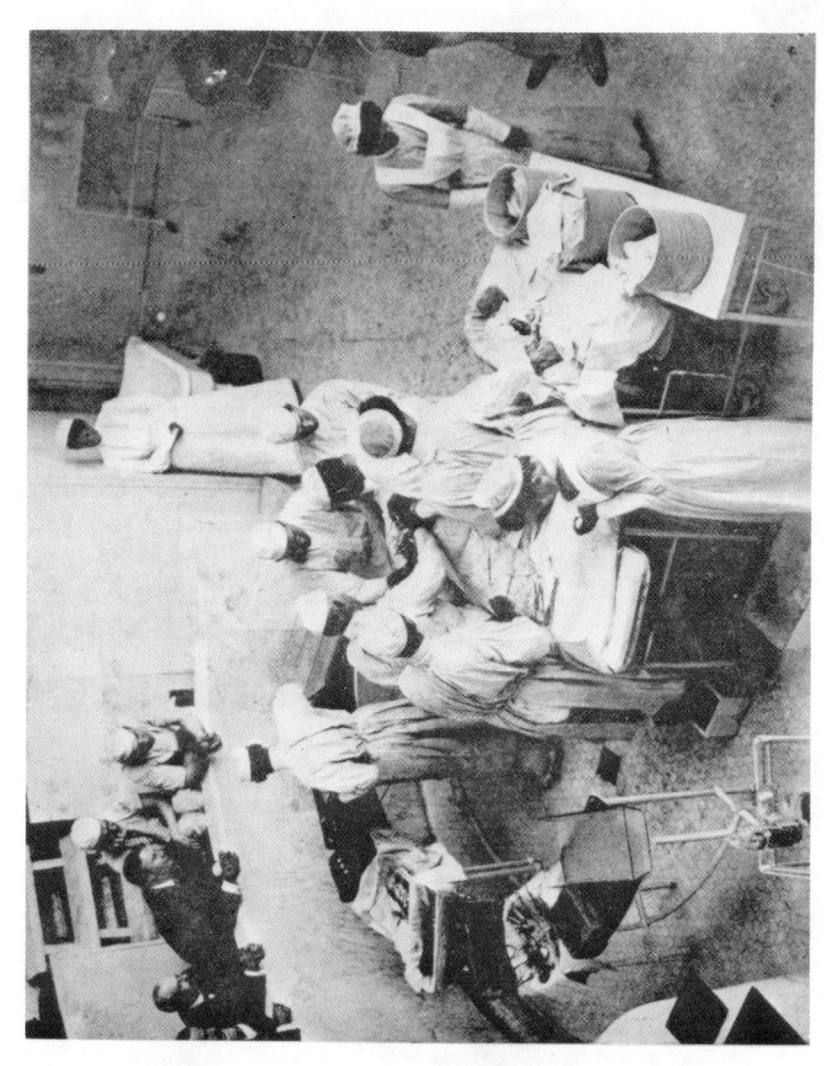

FIG. 3. A photograph of the first surgical operation in which the operator and assistants wore rubber gloves. (Courtesy of Dr. James F. Mitchell)

he operated because as resident surgeon he assisted Prof. Halsted at all of his operations, and was furthermore compelled to handle all sorts of infected cases, to make rectal examinations, and to operate on badly infected cases. He could not feel justified to operate without this protection. . . . The wearing of gloves practically excludes the danger of hand infection and leaves only one likely source of infection during operation—the skin of the patient. One can school himself to use gloves in almost any operation, and after a time forgets that he is using them.[15]

Dr. Mitchell introduced the method of anointing the hands with a sterilized boric ointment before the gloves are pulled on; it has proved most helpful. The gloves slip on more easily and are less likely to tear.

Observations on the impressive reduction of suppuration after introduction of rubber gloves conclusively proved their importance for the operating surgeon. Yet Halsted, who was responsible for this valuable innovation, remarks with admirable humility and frankness:

Thus the operating in gloves was an evolution rather than an inspiration or happy thought, and it is remarkable that during the four or five years when as operator I wore them only occasionally, we could have been so blind as not to have perceived the necessity for wearing them invariably at the operating-table. It is also noteworthy that none of the many surgeons, foreign and American, who visited our clinic in those years should have recognized the desirability of eliminating the hands as a source of infection, by the wearing of gloves.[16]

---

[15] *Ibid.*, pp. 304-5.
[16] *J. Amer. med. Ass.*, 1913, 60, 1124.

Evarts A. Graham, The American College of Surgeons, and the American Board of Surgery

PETER D. OLCH

AT the turn of the century and for some years thereafter surgery was a part-time specialty. Most surgeons were general practitioners who devoted more time to surgery only as they gained experience and a sufficient reputation to make such a practice economically feasible. The license granted by the state medical examining and licensing boards entitled the physician to practice medicine and surgery. There were no special certifying bodies to examine the competence and qualifications of the surgeon. Graduate surgical training was generally obtained by apprenticeship to a practicing surgeon, for the residency system as applied to surgery by Halsted at the Johns Hopkins had not developed in many other parts of the country.

Surgical instruction and practice continued to stress the importance of a knowledge of anatomy and surgical technique rather than the possession of surgical judgment. Dexterity and rapidity in operating continued to be tha hallmarks of greatness. A sea of surgical mediocrity was rising unchecked until 1913 and the founding of the American College of Surgeons (ACS). This organization, an outgrowth of the Clinical Congress of Surgeons of North America, was spearheaded by the dynamic, egotistical, and controversial Franklin H. Martin of Chicago. Its goals as stated in the by-laws were 'to elevate the standard of surgery, to provide a method of granting fellowship in the organization, and to educate the public and the profession to understand that the surgeon elected to fellowship in the College has had such training and is properly qualified to practice surgery.'

This paper was presented as the Sixteenth Annual Samuel Clark Harvey Lecture in the History of Surgery at the Yale University School of Medicine on 22 February 1971. The author is indebted to the late Dr. Helen T. Graham for permission to review her husband's papers, and wishes to thank Dr. Estelle Brodman and the staff of the Washington University School of Medicine Library for their assistance and hospitality while reviewing the Graham Papers. Appreciation is also expressed to Drs. C. Rollins Hanlon and George W. Stephenson of the American College of Surgeons for their assistance while working in the College archives.

This was difficult to accomplish in 1913. Franklin Martin, John B. Murphy, George Crile, Charles Mayo, and their colleagues adopted the basic tenet that the College was not to be an honorary society limited to men who had made their mark in the surgical world. Rather it was to be a forum for practicing surgeons to provide them with a means for self-improvement. The College attempted to upgrade surgery by opening its doors to vast numbers of individuals who practiced surgery and exposing them to operative clinics, dry clinics, and presentations conducted by leading surgeons of the day. It was therefore necessary to set rather low standards for membership in spite of the goals set forth in the bylaws.

Each candidate for Fellowship had to be a graduate of a medical school approved by the College and a licensed physician. He had to provide evidence of one year's internship in a creditable hospital and two years as a surgical assistant or provide evidence of an apprenticeship of equivalent value. He had to have been in practice for at least seven years with 50% to 80% of his work (depending on the size of the community) devoted to surgery. He had to be morally, ethically, and professionally acceptable as judged by the Credentials Committee of his own community and had to sign a pledge not to split fees. In place of an examination, the candidate had to submit a hundred case records or major operative procedures he had performed, fifty in complete detail and fifty in abstract. Although the absence of organized, progressive surgical residencies was bound to affect the standard of surgical education and therefore necessitated less rigorous membership requirements, there remained a major flaw in the philosophy behind these requirements. This was the stress on the applicant's ability to perform operations with only token concern for the basic medical knowledge supporting his surgical judgment.

The College came under attack from several different segments of the medical profession. The most publicized and abusive attacks were those representing the interests of the general practitioner and indirectly the American Medical Association. The *Journal* of the AMA carefully controlled its editorial comments. However, numerous state medical journals lambasted J. B. Murphy, Franklin Martin, and the College with bitter personal attacks and attempts to ridicule the concept of a college of surgeons.[1] The Surgical Section of the AMA, in existence since 1860, had made no effort to upgrade the standards of surgery. In 1914 the Illinois delegation introduced a resolution deprecating the founding of the Ameri-

---

1. See for example, editorials by Dr. P. M. Jones, Secretary of the California State Medical Society, in *Calif. state J. Med.*, 1913, *11*, 5, 175, and subsequent issues.

can College of Surgeons, but the House of Delegates tabled this and a substitute resolution.

The initial guarded and divided response from surgical academicians can best be described as a wait-and-see attitude. The venerable American Surgical Association (ASA), founded in 1880 with a strictly limited membership, contained the upper crust of American surgery and prided itself on being composed chiefly of teachers of surgery. It was in fact an honorary social club and as yet had made no active move to become involved as an organization in working for the improvement of surgical standards. Some individual members of the ASA had also joined the College of Surgeons and were involved in its policy-making bodies. A number of ASA members, particularly from the east coast, declined to support the ACS. Apparently a geographical bias—that not uncharacteristic feeling of the eastern medical centers from Boston to Baltimore that nothing worthwhile could originate in the Middle West—was coupled with a frank dislike of Franklin H. Martin and a critical view of George Crile and the Mayo brothers who, these members felt, were using the College of Surgeons to advertise their clinics.[2] In 1915 the College asked the ASA to appoint three members to stand for election to their Board of Governors. The ASA was to be one of fifteen surgical societies to have representation on the Board of Governors but it declined the invitation, stating that their organization had no precedent for appointing officers in other societies.[3]

The College meanwhile continued to grow and was the major national surgical organization attempting to elevate the standards of surgery in North America. One major thrust after several years was through the Hospital Standardization Program. In brief, this program developed a set of minimum standards covering the organization and activities of the medical staff, diagnostic and therapeutic facilities, and the accuracy and completeness of medical records. Of 692 hospitals with 100 beds and over surveyed in 1918, only 13% could meet the minimum requirements. This program accomplished a great deal more than merely upgrading the facilities for the practice and teaching of surgery.

By 1924, with the College membership nearly 7,000 and growing rapidly, the academic segment of the profession began to express some alarm. That year the ACS received petitions from both the Society of Clinical

---

2. Interviews conducted by Miss Eleanor K. Grimm, October 1953. MS in American College of Surgeons archives.

3. American Surgical Association. *Minutes of the Thirty-sixth Meeting . . . held at Rochester, Minnesota, June 9, 10, and 11, 1915* [n.p., n.d.].

Surgery and the Eclat Club, two rather exclusive societies made up of surgeons of renown, mostly academicians and members of the American Surgical Association. Both petitions commended the College for its original aims but pointed out what were considered serious shortcomings. Both expressed alarm over the large number and frequently poor quality of Fellows admitted each year. They asked for more rigid tests of character, training, and intelligence. The Eclat Club petition went further and accused Franklin Martin of dictatorial policies and questioned the College's financial policies.[4] In a sense the academicians had flung down the gauntlet and the town and gown split over the College was beginning to surface. J. M. T. Finney in his 1922 presidential address before the ASA gave the American College of Surgeons credit for making a beginning in the elevation of the standards of surgery among its Fellows and stressed the need for all surgical societies to join together in an organized effort to devise means by which prospective surgeons would receive adequate training and be properly certified before beginning to practice. The American Surgical Association as an organization nevertheless continued to lie dormant. The more concerned among the academicians in the ASA apparently channeled their protests through groups such as the Eclat Club and the Society for Clinical Surgery or spoke out as individuals.

Dr. Evarts A. Graham, Professor of Surgery at Washington University in St. Louis, for example, in an address entitled 'What is Surgery?' delivered before the Southern Medical Association in 1925, decried the overemphasis on the purely operative aspect of the surgeon's work. He stressed that standards based on the deftness of the operator, the number of operations performed, and even the income of the operator too often led to unwise operating and commercialism, with its attendant evils of fee-splitting and near fee-splitting. In his view original contributions to the science and art of surgery were the real measure of accomplishment, and the basis of surgical training should be to give the individual the maximum opportunity to prepare his mind for the reception of ideas while developing manual skills. He emphasized the need for an understanding of pathology and physiology and for individual research experience.[5]

Graham is well known to historians of surgery as the first surgeon to perform a successful total pneumonectomy for carcinoma of the lung in 1933. This achievement, together with his basic experimental studies as a

---

4. Loyal Davis, *Fellowship of surgeons: A history of the American College of Surgeons* (Springfield, Ill., 1960), pp. 492–494.

5. E. A. Graham, 'What is Surgery?' *Sth. med. J.* (*Nashville*), 1925, *18*, 864–867.

member of the Empyema Commission (1918–19) and his development of the technique of cholecystography with Warren Cole and Glover Copher (1924), has been the major source of his fame and recognition. Less well known today is Dr. Graham's important influence as an unyielding opponent of surgical mediocrity. He served as the prime mover in the uprising of academic surgeons against the American College of Surgeons in the early 1930s and also in the founding of the American Board of Surgery in 1937.

Evarts Ambrose Graham was born the son of Dr. David W. Graham and Ida Barnet Graham on 19 March 1883 in Chicago, Illinois. Following attendance at public schools and the Lewis Institute of Chicago he entered Princeton University in 1900 and Rush Medical College, Chicago, in 1904. After completing an internship at the Chicago Presbyterian Hospital in 1908 he devoted the next six or seven years to the nonclinical sciences of pathology and chemistry, chiefly the latter. He totally withdrew from the practice of surgery until 1915, when he entered private practice in Mason City, Iowa, for two years. Here he had his first exposure to fee-splitting and began a local campaign against it which was to be a continuous battle throughout his surgical career. His army career in 1918 and 1919 was highlighted by service on the Empyema Commission. In 1919 he was approached by Philip Shaffer, Canby Robinson, and Eugene Opie to join the faculty of Washington University in St. Louis as professor of surgery.

Graham was a forceful, outspoken individual who never minced words and would never sidestep an issue or confrontation if he felt that action was needed. In 1932 Dr. Graham first approached the officers of the ACS to express his displeasure and concern over the directions of the College. A Fellow since 1914, he had grown increasingly disenchanted with the organization. When elected vice-president in 1932 without his prior knowledge or consent, he objected strenuously and this led to a meeting with Franklin H. Martin. Subsequent correspondence indicates that Graham took this opportunity to speak forcefully and critically. His major complaint was that the younger men who had attained positions of leadership and who held the most important chairs of surgery in the country lacked representation on the Board of Regents. Martin either did not get the point or chose to ignore it. He sent Graham a list of young men who had been elected to the Board from 1916 until 1932, but the majority were private practitioners rather than university professors. Graham was invited to attend the next meeting of the Board of Regents in October 1933 and to participate in their deliberation and express his views.

In preparation for this meeting Graham wrote to twenty surgeons whom he considered leaders in American surgery, pointing out that he had certain serious criticisms to make of the College and had been invited to express his views to the Board of Regents. He asked the twenty for their candid views on the policies of the College and any constructive ideas they might have.[6]

Of this group fifteen were chairmen of departments of surgery and three were in private practice. Eighteen were members of the ASA and sixteen were also members of the ACS. Their responses were frank and critical of the College with few exceptions. They were heavily weighted with the academician's point of view. There was universal concern for the low standards of admission, which indicated greater interest in quantity than quality. As John J. Morton of Rochester, New York, said, 'There is about as much distinction in being a member of the American College of Surgeons as in belonging to the mob in Grand Central Station, New York City.'[7] Samuel C. Harvey of Yale wrote: 'As compared with the analagous organization in Great Britain, the American College of Surgeons has about the relative standards of a 5 and 10 cent store as compared with any first class department store.'[8]

The twenty expressed a common feeling that the College and its policies were dominated by a small group and particularly by one individual, Martin. It was stated frequently that the ruling body of the College was out of touch with reality and that the time had come for the younger generation of current leaders in surgery to be heard and represented on the Board of Regents. Elliott Cutler, who was a particularly outspoken individual, stated that 'University surgeons who on the whole are probably more interested in surgery than local surgeons, have always been poorly represented, and that surgeons who do surgery chiefly to make a living have largely controlled the destinies of this Institution.'[9] Continued fee-splitting by members of the ACS and the lack of adequate financial statements were also criticized.

Two of the twenty letters stand out, written, interestingly enough, by

6. The twenty surgeons with whom Graham corresponded were Barney Brooks, Edward D. Churchill, Frederick A. Coller, Elliott C. Cutler, Samuel C. Harvey, Carl A. Hedblom, George J. Heuer, Emile Holman, E. Starr Judd, Frank H. Lahey, Edwin P. Lehman, Dean D. Lewis, John J. Morton, George P. Muller, Howard C. Naffziger, Alton Ochsner, Dallas B. Phemister, Mont R. Reid, Erwin R. Schmidt, and Allen O. Whipple. This correspondence is in the Graham Papers at the Washington University School of Medicine Library.
7. J. J. Morton to Graham, 30 Aug. 1933.
8. S. C. Harvey to Graham, 16 Sept. 1933.
9. E. C. Cutler to Graham, 8 July 1933.

nonuniversity surgeons. Dr. George P. Muller of Philadelphia, a member of both the ACS and the ASA, added a further perspective to the town and gown aspect of this controversy.[10]

> ... from my contact with the small surgeons generally, particularly in towns and not cities, I have come to the conclusion that the American College of Surgeons has done a splendid thing for surgery. The title of F.R.C.S. usually comes as a reward for work done, but the title of F.A.C.S. signifies an inducement to do good work. I have an idea that things surgical would have been very chaotic in this country had it not been for the College. . . .
>
> I do not know whether or not you realize that the majority of surgeons are a bit impatient with the group that belongs to the American Surgical Association. They feel that we high hat them and yet except for a wearisome grind with papers read at the annual meeting the American Surgical Association is a club, a mutual admiration society, and has done nothing of a constructive nature since the Committee on Fractures years ago did its piece of work which was highly meritorious.

Muller wrote that he too felt the government of the College should be more in touch with the men of his own and Graham's generation who had become leaders in surgery, but he cautioned,

> However, if we examine this matter of leadership carefully, we will find that the control in the surgical societies is getting more and more into the hands of those men who are what are commonly called 'full-time research surgeons.' You and Dean Lewis represent the proper type but I doubt if Heuer or Cutler is very sympathetic towards the general surgeon in the sticks.

Muller's letter and the concern expressed by Dr. Frank Lahey for polarization in surgical societies between teachers and clinicians regrettably were the only expressions of a need for resolving differences between town and gown.[11]

Armed with letters from the twenty respondents Graham met with the Board of Regents of the College on 10 October 1933. He listed the criticisms received and elaborated upon them at some length. He suggested that the Board of Regents appoint a committee to confer with a selected group of the leading surgeons of his generation to discuss each criticism in depth and attempt to arrive at some solutions. He further suggested that the leadership in surgery had now passed to other hands than those who had run the College during the previous thirty years.

10. G. P. Muller to Graham, 22 July 1933.
11. F. H. Lahey to Graham, 18 July 1933.

After the meeting Graham prepared a letter to the twenty surgeons summarizing the proceedings. He was not optimistic about the results. At this point Graham hesitated, apparently wondering if mailing the summary would do more harm than good. Therefore he sent a copy to Dr. J. M. T. Finney, the first President of the College, with a covering letter giving him the full background. He asked Finney whether he thought the letter of summary should be mailed and whether Franklin Martin should receive a copy.

Finney's response must have bolstered Graham's determination. He was in complete sympathy with Graham's position and commended him for bringing into the open 'a very disagreeable but very menacing state of affairs.' He was convinced of the potential of the College but felt depressed that it was not being properly utilized. He believed that much of the trouble could not be remedied while Franklin Martin was in control, since Martin looked upon the College as his baby and acted as if he owned it. 'Martin is and always has been a great ballyhoo artist—quantity rather than quality appeals to him, and he gathered around him a group of men thoroughly imbued with the same ideas.' Finney further stated that his attempts to get through to George Crile and the Mayos, the powers behind the throne, never got anywhere. His attempts to put younger men on the Board of Regents had always failed. Everyone who got on the Board, according to Finney, was hand-picked by Martin. The policy makers were the Mayos and Crile, the other men, figureheads doing as they were told. He concluded, nevertheless, that a change in the policies of the College could best be accomplished through evolution rather than revolution and wished Graham well in his efforts.[12]

With Finney's blessing in hand, Graham mailed twenty-one copies of the letter. Martin acknowledged receipt and said a detailed response would follow. He also informed Graham that he had just had his annual physical and was pronounced 'o.k.' for the next fifty years which, he added, 'will be disturbing to some of my friends.'[13] In mid-November 1933 the Executive Committee of the Board of Regents met and prepared a ten-page single-spaced document responding to each criticism in turn and essentially justifying the status quo.

In acknowledging receipt of the statement, Graham expressed his disappointment that his argument for satisfactory representation of men of his generation had gone unheeded and that his request for a meeting of the

12. J. M. T. Finney to Graham, 31 Oct. 1933.
13. F. H. Martin to Graham, 16 Nov. 1933, in Graham Papers.

Board with representatives of the Young Turks had seemingly been ignored. He could not have been aware of the differences of opinion among Board members on this latter point. Martin apparently was in favor of a meeting of the full Board with its critics in Chicago where all records would be available. Others, such as Allen Kanavel, shared his view. The latter wrote Martin that he felt that Graham's letter was a logical yet restrained presentation and that it stated the case as fairly as anyone could who was not familiar with the workings of the College. Urging that a meeting be set up with the critics, Kanavel concluded, 'Graham is worth winning since he will probably be the strongest man in surgery ten years from now.'[14]

Will Mayo on the other hand summed up the situation by saying, 'A group of men who thought they had this College killed years ago, suddenly found it had become a great institution and they would like to take over the running of it. . . . Personally I think the treatment they have had for all these years, letting them holler, has been successful and should be continued.'[15] The cooler heads prevailed, and on 10 June 1934 the Board of Regents met with a group of the Young Turks including Graham and Samuel Harvey. The visitors and the Board had a free discussion. Graham repeated his argument for adding to the Board three or four men who were young surgical department heads. In the fall Samuel Harvey was elected; the young academicians were at last making inroads into the administration of the College.

Meanwhile, Drs. Elliott Cutler, George Heuer, and Allen Whipple had been appointed members of a committee by the Regents of the College in 1931 to study undergraduate, graduate, and postgraduate teaching of surgery. Each was scheduled to give a portion of this report at the October 1933 meeting, but for some reason they were refused the floor. The three, shocked and angered, threatened to resign from the College, apparently feeling that lack of interest in or support for the subject was responsible for the last minute cancellation. In a letter to Graham in January 1934 Cutler suggested that the presentation be given at a meeting of the American Surgical Association with a preamble stating that this was the only surgical organization of great size and high position before which such a paper could be given, since the College of Surgeons refused such papers and therefore was not interested in the education of the surgeon. The 1935 meeting was held in Boston and Cutler, as program chairman, planned a

14. Allen Kanavel to F. H. Martin, quoted in Davis (n. 4), p. 299.
15. William Mayo to F. H. Martin, *ibid.*, p. 299.

symposium on surgical education featuring the three papers by himself, Heuer, and Whipple covering undergraduate surgical education, graduate surgical training in university hospitals, and graduate training in non-university hospitals. These three papers, preceded by Edward W. Archibald's presidential address on 'Higher Degrees in the Profession of Surgery,' set the stage for some vigorous discussion.[16] The members generally agreed that the private practice of surgery, where there existed only 'a sprinkling of surgeons' but a 'deluge of operators,'[17] urgently needed improvement. They disagreed on the best means of obtaining the necessary graduate training, whether by apprenticeship or by the residency system developed by Halsted and described by Heuer.

Archibald, in his address, after comparing the certification of surgeons in the United States, Canada, England, Australia, France, and Germany, pointed out the weaknesses in the requirements for admission to the American College of Surgeons and suggested the establishment of a Board of Examiners which would demand a stricter examination in the fundamental principles and practice of surgery. Thirteen years before, J. M. T. Finney had made a similar suggestion before this same group. The difference in response was noteworthy. Evarts Graham boldly suggested that the ASA as *the* group of teachers in surgery had the duty and the responsibility to take an active part in improving the training of surgeons and proposed that President Archibald appoint a standing committee of the ASA to report the following year on their continuing deliberations on proper qualifications.

Archibald appointed a six-member Committee on the Elevation of Surgical Standards with Graham as chairman.[18] He wasted no time. Ten days after the meeting, he wrote the five other members: 'You are of course familiar with the general dissatisfaction which exists with the existing qualification of Fellows of the American College of Surgeons. The ASA feels that there is an urgent need for the creation of some mechanism by which properly qualified surgeons can be certified to the public.' His letter contained a series of key questions and a statement of his views. At this point he apparently had a relatively open mind toward the role of the College in his plans *if* the College had a radical change in its administra-

16. E. W. Archibald, 'Higher degrees in the profession of surgery,' *Trans. Amer. surg. Ass.*, 1935, 53, 1–15.
17. T. G. Orr, discussion of paper on graduate teaching of surgery, *Trans. Amer. surg. Ass.*, 1935, 53, 44.
18. The committee members were Edward W. Archibald, Arthur W. Elting, Thomas M. Joyce, Thomas G. Orr, Allen O. Whipple, and Evarts A. Graham.

tion. Even though Franklin Martin had died four months earlier, he did not want the authority for certification placed in the hands of a group beholden to one individual, such as the Director General of the College, whoever that might be. The Committee agreed that a more representative body should receive this authority and recommended that other surgical societies be enlisted in the movement to organize the qualifying board and be represented in its final makeup.

Dr. George Crile, Chairman of the Executive Committee of the ACS, visited Graham and urged that the College assume the functions of the proposed independent certifying board. Dr. Graham firmly opposed this suggestion and warned Crile that the annual meeting of the ACS would be little more than a surgical circus if the College did not participate with the other surgical organizations in the founding of the independent board.[19] The result of this conversation was an agreement to hold a meeting in Chicago at the headquarters of the College in October 1935 with the ASA Committee, the representatives of the Surgical Section of the AMA, and representatives of the ACS.

The ASA Committee arrived at this meeting with a resolution proposing the formation of the National Committee for the Elevation of the Standards of Surgery to be composed of six members each from the American College of Surgeons, the American Medical Association, and the American Surgical Association and two each from the Western Surgical Association, the Southern Surgical Association, and the Pacific Coast Surgical Association.

At the meeting it was Graham and his allies (the representatives of the AMA were all on his side on this issue) confronting the American College of Surgeons. The discussion was prolonged and at times acrimonious. J. Bentley Squier of the College accused the ASA Committee of some ulterior motive in not stating clearly in the draft resolution everything they had in mind for the future.[20] Some ACS representatives stated bluntly that the proposal was unnecessary, since the College had long been interested in surgical standards. They reminded the group that theirs had been the only surgical organization with an interest in the problem for years and now was being asked to step aside. After much discussion the College

---

19. Personal communication from Dr. Nathan Womack, 27 May 1971.
20. The acrimony and heated nature of some of the discussion is not obvious in the official minutes of the joint session. However, a set of minutes recorded by Dr. Graham for the ASA Committee on the Elevation of Surgical Standards and subsequent correspondence between members of the ASA Committee leave little doubt that certain representatives of the College were angry and resented the involvement of the American Surgical Association. Both sets of minutes are in the Graham Papers.

representatives did agree to recommend that the College appoint six members to serve on the proposed national committee.

One week later this recommendation was approved by the Board of Regents, but further concern was expressed by several members of the Board over the possibility of lessening the influence of the College upon the elevation of the practice of surgery. Some individuals were frankly suspicious of the motives of Graham and his colleagues who, as members of the Society of Clinical Surgery and the Eclat Club, were felt to be hostile critics of the College. There also was the ever-present division along the lines of town and gown, the private practitioner versus the academician.

With the College participation assured, Graham called the National Committee for the Elevation of the Standards of Surgery together to meet in Chicago on 15 and 16 February 1936. In his opening remarks he certainly did nothing to endear himself to his critics from the College of Surgeons. He categorically stated that even though the ACS had improved ordinary hospital internships through its Hospital Standardization Program, none of the medical organizations in the country had taken on the task of developing increased opportunities for capable young men to get properly supervised experience in the handling of surgical cases. He pointed out that there was little use in establishing a scheme for the qualification and certification of properly trained surgeons until such training opportunities existed. He referred to the shortcomings of Fellowship in the ACS. Noting that the College probably felt that the qualification of surgeons was its special province, he bluntly asked of his colleagues, 'Is it not the feeling of this group that this movement is of such importance that it transcends the desires of any particular surgical organization?' He further suggested that such matters as training and certification would best be controlled by a Board of Surgery composed of representative surgical organizations with a limited term of service for each member rather than having the control in the hands of a single organization which might be dominated by a small group reelecting itself to office. He closed with the statement, issued as a warning, that he felt this movement should proceed even if an existing surgical organization should attempt to throttle it.[21]

Following the election of officers, including Graham as chairman, the group broke up into two subcommittees, one on organization and the other devoted to the problem of increasing facilities for the training of surgeons. The first subcommittee proposed the establishment of a Board

21. MS in Graham Papers.

of Surgery following in general the organizational scheme of other specialty boards except that responsibility for the ABS would rest with the large national and regional surgical associations. The Board was to consist of three men each from the national organizations—the ASA, ACS, and AMA—and one man each from the Southern, Western, Pacific Coast, and New England Surgical Associations. Each member would serve for six years except the original members, who would serve two, four, or six years in order to assure continuity.

The subcommittee on organization decided that the Board should qualify a Founders group without examination. This group included the active and senior members of all the surgical organizations represented on the Board with the exception of the American College of Surgeons. This portion of the plan was of some concern to Graham and several others, but the importance of support of the regional surgical societies outweighed the problem of a small number of unqualified individuals certified as Founders. Surgeons with a rank of associate professor or above in Class A medical schools in the United States and Canada, and assistant professors of five years' standing, were also eligible. A private practitioner could be a Founder member if he had limited his practice to surgery for fifteen years and was approved by the Board on direct application.

Other candidates for certification by the Board were expected to present themselves for examination after fulfilling certain requirements. The most important was for special training consisting of at least three years of graduate study beyond the internship in a recognized graduate school of medicine or in a hospital or under a sponsor accredited by the Board. The training had to include sufficient graduate work in anatomy, physiology, pathology, and other basic medical sciences for a proper understanding of the practice of surgery, as well as adequate operative experience. Beyond this, two additional years of study or practice were required. The examinations were to be in two parts, one written and the other oral or practical.

The subcommittee on increasing facilities for the training of surgeons had recommended that the ACS and AMA jointly organize and carry out a program for the training of surgeons in qualified hospitals, setting up such standards as would meet the requirements of the Board. This proposal would prove difficult to implement.[22] Within two days the reports

22. The AMA and ACS had ongoing programs of hospital inspection and agreed to participate in a joint venture. However, there was much foot-dragging by the AMA, which finally disavowed any intention to work with the College on this particular problem. The tortuous path which led to the establishment of the Conference Committee on Graduate Training in Surgery in 1950 with equal representation from the ABS, ACS, and AMA is described with differing perspectives in W. M. Firor,

of both subcommittees had been approved by the parent committee and the proposed American Board of Surgery had been approved by the Executive Committee of the Advisory Board for Medical Specialties. When the American Board of Surgery held its first meeting in January 1937, it was the twelfth approved specialty Board.[23]

The founding of the American Board of Surgery in 1937 was an important step in upgrading the quality of surgical training. Though born in conflict and immediately under fire from those who felt that such specialty boards led to overstandardization and regimentation or were formed primarily to limit the number of specialists for economic reasons, the American Board of Surgery soon became the most powerful force on the surgical scene. Though the Board specifically denied any intent to define requirements for membership on hospital staffs, it soon became obvious that diplomates received preferential treatment. In World War II, Board-certified surgeons received higher rank and more responsible positions in the military services than surgeons without such certification. In civilian life some hospitals began limiting surgical privileges to Board-certified individuals.

The relationship of the College of Surgeons and the Board remained amicable though strained at times. Evarts Graham, after serving as chairman of the American Board of Surgery for its first four years, stepped down in 1941 and devoted his attention to the American College of Surgeons, first as president, then as a member of the Board of Regents, and finally as chairman of the Board from 1951 to 1954. The Young Turks had become Old Turks, and the next generation of surgeons was stirring for recognition. In 1953 Dr. Graham admitted that perhaps he and his colleagues had been a little too ambitious for recognition when they confronted the administration of the College in the early 1930s.[24] However, there is little doubt that his impatience and determination were factors in bringing about change and general improvement in the standards and the image of the American College of Surgeons.

'Residency training in surgery. Birth, decay, and recovery,' *Rev. Surg.*, 1965, 22, 153–157; and 'Conference committee on graduate education in surgery,' *Bull. Amer. Coll. Surg.*, 1971, 56, 39–46. The latter is in a special issue of the *Bulletin* entitled 'The American College of Surgeons and graduate education in surgery' written by Dr. George W. Stephenson, Assistant Director, Fellowship, American College of Surgeons.

23. The specialty Boards in operation prior to the American Board of Surgery were in the fields of ophthalmology (1917), otolaryngology (1924), obstetrics and gynecology (1930), dermatology (1932), pediatrics (1933), orthopedic surgery (1934), psychiatry and neurology (1934), radiology (1934), urology (1935), internal medicine (1936), and pathology (1936).

24. Eleanor K. Grimm (n. 2).

Although the purpose of this paper has been to describe the central role of Dr. Graham in the reform of the American College of Surgeons and the establishment of the American Board of Surgery, it would be an injustice to leave the subject without acknowledging the more recent and continuing efforts of the ACS in the area of graduate education in surgery. The College is now an effective part of a triad of organizations involved in graduate surgical education along with the Council on Medical Education and Hospitals of the AMA and the surgical specialty Boards. The Boards, including the American Board of Surgery, and the College have now a closer and more effective relationship. Finally, it should be noted that in 1970 a joint ACS-ASA study was initiated on the delivery of surgical services in the United States. For the first time the two major surgical societies were sitting down together and attacking problems of mutual concern.[25]

National Library of Medicine
Bethesda, Maryland

---

25. 'The study on surgical services for the United States,' *Bull. Amer. Coll. Surg.*, 1971, 56, 14-21.

Class, Ethnicity, and Race in American Mental Hospitals, 1830–75

GERALD N. GROB

IN the decades following 1830 most states and a number of cities established public hospitals to provide care and treatment for the mentally ill. Reflecting both an emphasis on the curability of insanity and a desire to protect the community against ostensibly dangerous behavior, these institutions were also predicated on the assumption that all persons, irrespective of class, ethnicity, and color, should have equal access to public facilities. Indeed, the manner in which hospitals were financed embodied this assumption; the state provided funds for capital expenditures, while local communities assumed the responsibility of reimbursing hospitals for their poor and indigent residents who required institutionalization, but who lacked the means to pay for the costs of their upkeep.[1]

A theoretical framework, of course, rarely if ever corresponds precisely with reality, for few persons behave in ways that are completely consistent with their ideals. In many instances the situational choice faced by individuals is morally ambiguous; in others behavior reflects affective factors that are often at variance with supposedly rational principles. Whatever the case, most human institutions generally fall far short of ideal types precisely because individuals and groups—often without a clear recognition of the sources of their conduct—behave in ways that appear inconsistent or in direct conflict with the principles that stipulate the manner in which they *ought* to behave.

---

1. For much of the nineteenth century public mental hospitals were expected to be self-supporting insofar as operating expenditures were concerned. Their income was derived from three sources: families who paid for private patients; local communities which were responsible for poorer and indigent residents; and states, which paid for foreign-born poor and indigent patients or else provided a lump sum subsidy. The revenue derived from the labor of patients was negligible.

I am greatly indebted to the National Institute of Mental Health (HEW), which supported this study by Grant 17859.

The evolution of the mental hospital offers an unusually good illustration of how a social institution, established with the best and most honorable of intentions, was inadvertently transformed by the behavior of many individuals and groups. In theory hospital officials never discriminated against patients on any basis whatsoever; within the hospital all persons received identical care and treatment. In practice, however, patients were *not treated* equally. Some psychiatrists manifested unconscious hostility toward patients coming from backgrounds different from their own; some structured hospitals in ways that inadvertently promoted discriminatory treatment; and some shared many of the racial, ethnic, and class stereotypes of the larger society. Much the same was true of state legislators and public officials. And it was not at all uncommon for patients to behave in ways that ultimately defeated attempts to make certain that equal care and treatment would be made available for all Americans.

The pattern of differential care that ultimately prevailed at mental hospitals was a complex phenomenon, for the influence of class, ethnic, and racial factors were not equal, nor did they operate independently of each other. It is possible, however, to spell out with some degree of precision the relationships between class, ethnicity, and race on the one hand and the quality of care and treatment on the other hand. In general, the best care was given native-born paying patients. On a descending scale, they were followed by native-born poor and indigent patients, and below them were poor and indigent immigrants. At the bottom were blacks, who received the lowest quality of care.

The persistence of practices that resulted in less than equal treatment for some groups was to have profound implications for the institutional care of the mentally ill in the United States. For ultimately the mental hospital —precisely because it reflected some of the same class, ethnic, and racial antagonisms of the larger society in which it existed—found itself incapable of providing the therapeutic care for which it was established. As it lost its therapeutic character, it was converted into a broad welfare-type institution that provided inexpensive custodial care for a variety of groups, including those deemed dangerous to the security of the community, the aged, the poor, and those individuals seemingly incapable of surviving without a highly structured environment.

I

In most public mental hospitals native-born poor and indigent patients did not receive the same care as patients who paid for the costs of institutionalization. Yet the differences were contained within relatively narrow limits. In part this situation reflected the fact that superintendents and patients for the most part shared a common cultural and religious heritage. It should also be kept in mind that not all or even most of the mentally ill persons in hospitals and supported at public expense were paupers; in many cases the family income level simply did not allow for an illness that required protracted institutionalization (particularly if the person hospitalized were the principal wage earner). The values of superintendents, moreover, did not place a premium on wealth; most regarded acquisitiveness as a prime cause of disease. Consequently, there was no disposition to punish poor and indigent patients. The differential care that did exist arose largely out of two factors: a desire to maintain a heterogeneous patient body, which in turn helped to assure the broad community support such institutions required; and the more subtle differential care that followed a homogeneous ward structure.[2]

While overt discrimination between patients coming from different class backgrounds was not immediately visible, a careful analysis of the manner in which hospitals functioned reveals its presence, though in somewhat subtle ways. Inadvertent discrimination, for example, grew out of the manner in which hospitals were structured and administered. As hospital managers, superintendents had to organize their hospitals. Being physicians, they naturally thought in terms of the traditional divisions of general hospitals with their fairly elaborate system of wards to care for different types of cases (i.e., surgery, infectious diseases, pregnancy, etc.). So too mental hospitals were divided into wards. But upon what basis should wards be organized? One possibility was a series of wards corresponding to the diagnostic categories then in use. Most superintendents, however, were not especially impressed with the traditional division of insanity into mania, melancholia, and dementia, if only because the relationship of these categories to therapy was not at all clear. Another possibility was to assign patients to wards on the basis of their date of admission or even on a purely random basis. Neither of these alternatives were seri-

---

2. The available evidence offers fairly conclusive proof that differential patterns of *care* (better physical quarters, privileges, etc.) existed at most hospitals. Evidence about differential *treatment* is far more difficult to come by, if only because there are virtually no descriptions of treatment in terms of what psychiatrists actually did with patients. Aside from drugs and medication (which may or may not have been administered on a nondiscriminatory basis), I have assumed that differential care inevitably involved differential treatment. If the success of moral treatment rested on the creation of an internal therapeutic environment, it is difficult to see how patients would not react adversely to clear patterns of differential care and how this reaction would not impair the effectiveness of moral management.

ously considered because from a therapeutic viewpoint they appeared to be devoid of meaning.

Fortunately the principles of moral treatment offered to most superintendents a sure guide. This therapeutic system, which developed in England and France in the early nineteenth century, was based upon the belief that the creation of a new environment was crucial in the treatment of mental disease. It followed logically that the classification of wards was of vital importance because of the interaction of patients with each other. A rational system of classification thus became one of the cardinal tenets of moral therapy. In 1841 Luther V. Bell made classification one of his four indispensable principles of moral treatment (the other three being separation from the patient's previous environment, direction within the hospital, and occupational therapy), and Kirkbride in his classic work on hospital architecture also insisted on its importance.[3] Though there were minor disagreements on specifics, no superintendent was disposed to question the vital importance of proper classification.

If proper classification was an indispensable part of moral treatment, how could its effect be maximized? Obviously wards had to separate the sexes, given the fundamental differences between men and women and also the need to discourage illicit relationships. Beyond the separation of the sexes, there was general agreement that earlier practices both in the United States and abroad of separating patients on the basis of status or the amount paid for board was improper, for it brought together 'the violent maniac, the drivelling idiot, and the tranquil monomaniac, the outrageous, profane, and noisy, the convalescent, the timid, and the sensitive.'[4] The assignment of similar cases to the same ward (e.g., the violent with the violent), while better, still presented problems. The best and most rational system, in the words of Kirkbride, was 'to associate in the same ward those who are least likely to injure and most likely to benefit each other, no matter what may be the character or form of their disease, or whether supposed to be curable or incurable.'[5]

Such a system of classification appeared to provide all patients with an environment that promoted therapy and avoided any type of differential

---

3. McLean Asylum for the Insane, *Annu. Rep.*, 1841, *24*, in Mass. General Hospital, *Annu. Rep.* 1841, 22–23, 30–31; T. S. Kirkbride, *On the construction, organization and general arrangements of hospitals for the insane* (Philadelphia, 1854), p. 58. For examples of similar statements see Virginia Western Lunatic Asylum, *Annu. Rep.*, 1842, *15*, 34–35; New Jersey State Lunatic Asylum, *Annu. Rep.*, 1853, *7*, 14–15; Friends' Asylum for the Insane, *Annu. Rep.*, 1856, *39*, 15; Vermont Asylum for the Insane, *Ann. Rep.*, 1860, *24*, 12.

4. Worcester State Lunatic Hospital, *Annu. Rep.*, 1844, *12*, 89.

5. Kirkbride (n. 3), p. 58.

care. In practice, however, the system did not work out precisely in this manner. In deciding to bring together patients who could benefit each other, superintendents were in effect adopting a system based on socioeconomic characteristics, for they often employed educational, cultural, and religious criteria for classifying patients. They were especially concerned—to quote Samuel B. Woodward—'that no one shall associate with those particularly obnoxious to him.'[6] Another superintendent, though denying that he drew 'unnecessary distinctions' among his patients, nevertheless argued that a patient's previous environment had to be taken into account at the hospital if therapeutic aims were not to be subordinated. 'It is certainly exceedingly unpleasant,' he noted,

to be almost compelled to associate with those whose education, conduct and moral habits, are unlike and repugnant to us. Because persons are insane, we must not conclude that they always lose the power of appreciating suitable associates, or are insensible to the influence of improper communications. This is by no means true. It is among our greatest perplexities here, to know how to quiet the complaints of those whose delicacy is shocked, whose tempers are perturbed, and whose quietude is annoyed by improper and unwelcome associates.[7]

The assignment of similar types of patients to particular wards was an understandable practice, for most individuals moved in homogeneous circles. This procedure, however, set the stage for other inherently unequal practices. Most psychiatrists felt that the institutional environment should replicate as closely as possible those features of the patient's home environment that had not played a part in bringing on mental disease. Consequently, patients from middle-class backgrounds and private patients tended to be assigned to more luxurious accommodations and receive greater privileges. At the Worcester hospital such patients were permitted to keep their trunks in their own rooms and take charge of their own clothing, books, and work.[8] The situation was much the same elsewhere.

The fact that hospitals provided (within certain well-defined limits) differential care and treatment did not go unnoticed by the psychiatric profession. While recommending that more affluent patients be provided with luxuries if they so desired, one superintendent warned against the practice of drawing distinctions openly since it would destroy 'the contentment of the many ... for the indulgence of the few.' He recommended that complete separation between paying and nonpaying patients was the

6. Worcester State Lunatic Hospital, *Annu. Rep.*, 1844, *12*, 89.
7. Kentucky [Eastern] Lunatic Asylum, *Annu. Rep.*, 1845, *23*, 24.
8. Worcester State Lunatic Hospital, *Annu. Rep.*, 1839, *7*, 89.

only means of alleviating the problem and preventing it from interfering with the therapeutic process.[9] Another superintendent insisted that invidious distinctions could be abolished only if all patients—irrespective of their financial condition—were admitted on a nonpaying basis.[10] Nevertheless, to the majority of superintendents there seemed clear and compelling reasons for differential care. Isaac Ray—without doubt the most influential mid-nineteenth century psychiatrist—felt that patients from 'poor and laboring' classes required less attention than those from 'educated and affluent' backgrounds. The former were used to work and could be pleased by such simple things as a walk in the country or by some favorable employment. The latter, on the other hand, could only 'be satisfied by long and repeated interviews with the superintendent.' Each class, therefore, required different forms of therapy.[11] With some isolated exceptions, most psychiatrists saw no reason why hospitals should not continue to provide certain amenities to patients willing and able to pay for them.[12]

The argument most frequently employed by superintendents in defending—even urging—the admission of private patients was that their presence was essential if hospitals were to retain broad community support and avoid a process of deterioration. They were especially fearful of seeing their institutions converted into glorified poorhouses. Aside from detracting from their own professional status, such a process was clearly not in the interests of their patients. The best means of preventing mental hospitals from becoming pauper establishments was to attract a sufficiently large number of more affluent patients, who would then make the institution more attractive and also give it a strong base of support among articulate and influential groups. Though they recognized that a dual system of private and public hospitals was already in existence, they nevertheless felt that its further extension would be detrimental to the interests of the mentally ill.[13] Moreover, the group that would be hardest hit by the conver-

9. Kentucky [Eastern] Lunatic Asylum, *Annu. Rep.*, 1845, *23*, 24–25, 1846, *24*, 20.

10. Ohio Lunatic Asylum, *Annu. Rep.*, 1851, *13*, 20–23.

11. Isaac Ray, 'Observations on the principal hospitals for the insane in Great Britain, France and Germany,' *Amer. J. Insan.*, 1846, *2*, 387–388.

12. Cf. T. S. Kirkbride, 'Remarks on cottages for certain classes of patients, in connection with hospitals for the insane,' *Amer. J. Insan.*, 1851, *7*, 376; New Jersey State Lunatic Asylum, *Annu. Rep.*, 1850, *4*, 28; Maine Insane Hospital, *Annu. Rep.*, 1852, *12*, 34; Worcester State Lunatic Hospital, *Annu. Rep.*, 1857, *25*, 57; Kentucky Western Lunatic Asylum, *Annu. Rep.*, 1864, 14; Insane Asylum of Louisiana, *Annu. Rep.*, 1866, 6.

13. Superintendents of private hospitals, on the other hand, defended their institutions on the grounds that better facilities should be made available for more affluent patients. For typical statements see Connecticut Retreat for the Insane, *Annu. Rep.*, 1867, *43*, 33, 1869/1870, *45–46*, 21; McLean Asylum for the Insane, *Annu. Rep.*, 1839, *22*, 1840, *23*, 1841, *24*, 1851, *34*, 1868, *51*, all in Mass. Gen-

sion of the hospital into a pauper institution would be those independent families who were neither rich nor poor; they could not afford the costs of private hospitals nor would they be willing to commit relatives to public welfare hospitals. Justice and wisdom therefore required a proper mix at all public institutions. The directors of the Ohio Lunatic Asylum recognized some of these dangers when they took a somewhat novel step in 1851 by abolishing all charges for private patients. In defending their action, the superintendent recalled the results of requiring patients to pay the costs of institutionalization if they could so afford.

The distinction was invidious; its bad consequences were manifold, and far outweighed all pecuniary advantages. Often did our halls resound with the exclamation, '*You* are only a pauper, *I pay* for my board.' . . . But if she [Ohio] does not pursue the course she has commenced—if she does not speedily make ample and free provision for *all* those of her insane requiring constant care—private establishments, where the luxury indulged in by the patients is graduated by the scale of weekly payments, will spring into being, and the distinction, so invidious and pernicious among individuals in the same hospital, will exist equally invidiously and perniciously between public and private institutions. These latter will most certainly attract nearly all whose relatives are able to pay the sum demanded for their maintenance in them, and *State institutions will sink to the level of pauper establishments.*[14]

Moreover, many superintendents argued that a heterogeneous patient population had a beneficial therapeutic effect within mental hospitals. Although classification of patients usually resulted in homogeneous wards, it was virtually impossible to maintain a rigorous and unyielding system of internal segregation on the basis of class. Consequently, there was considerable interaction among patients, often with beneficial results for all concerned. The superintendent of the New Jersey asylum noted that many desirable behavioral traits could be secured 'by a proper association of different individuals.' And Francis T. Stribling of the Virginia Western Lunatic Asylum employed classification as an incentive for good behavior. Paying patients who misbehaved were removed 'to a circle better adapted' to

---

eral Hospital, *Annu. Rep.*, 1839, 16, 1840, 25–26, 1841, 20–21, 1851, 21–22, 1868, 34–37; Friends' Asylum for the Insane, *Annu. Rep.*, 1841, *24*, 5; Pennsylvania Hospital for the Insane, *Annu. Rep.*, 1848, *8*, 19–20; Butler Hospital for the Insane, *Annu. Rep.*, 1868, 22; John W. Sawyer to Dorothea L. Dix, 16 September 1870, Dix Papers, Houghton Library, Harvard University, Cambridge, Mass.; Isaac Ray to John W. Sawyer, 10 March 1872, Library of Butler Hospital, Providence, R.I.

14. Ohio Lunatic Asylum, *Annu. Rep.*, 1851, *13*, 22–23. For similar statements see Worcester State Lunatic Hospital, *Annu. Rep.*, 1845, *13*, 45, 1858, *26*, 10; New Jersey State Lunatic Asylum, *Annu. Rep.*, 1850, *4*, 28; Kentucky [Eastern] Lunatic Asylum, *Annu. Rep.*, 1845, *23*, 27.

their dispositions and habits. Such a system, he argued, induced patients 'to efforts of self-control and self-respect, for the purposes of retaining their place or ascending still higher in the scale of distinction.'[15]

Interestingly enough, superintendents in general evinced little overt hostility toward the native poor and indigent insane. While their theoretical discussions had indicated that mental disease was often self-inflicted by those who disobeyed the natural laws that governed their behavior and whose character was morally deficient, they did not necessarily draw the conclusion that poor and indigent persons who had become insane were therefore less deserving. As a matter of fact, they insisted that the state had a moral obligation to help such unfortunate persons in order that they might recover and become self-supporting; from a therapeutic point of view, no psychiatrist favored a policy that was basically penal in nature. Indeed, Ray maintained that the United States lacked a permanent pauper class such as existed in England. The British pauper, he wrote, 'is a being sui generis. . . . He is born of paupers, lives a pauper, dies a pauper, and leaves behind him a train of pauper successors.' The future for such persons promised no chance of improvement and hope was entirely absent; confinement in a mental hospital was a welcome relief from the vicissitudes of life. In America, on the other hand, poverty was 'a casual condition, a temporary misfortune, the result of accident, disease, or mischance, and dies out with its unfortunate subject.' Such differences made Americans far less deferential and far more independent; they simply would not observe the 'distinctions of rank' characteristic of English society.[16] If this were true, then it would be difficult, if not impossible, to provide openly discriminatory care within public hospitals.

II

While native poor and indigent patients at mental hospitals did not receive exactly the same care as private patients, their lot tended to be better than that of foreign-born patients (especially those coming from Ireland). To put it another way, ethnicity—particularly of non-Protestant groups—when combined with a lower-class background, increased somewhat the differential in care and treatment at many institutions (excluding private ones, which had almost no patients from minority ethnic groups). The

15. New Jersey State Lunatic Asylum, *Annu. Rep.*, 1853, *7*, 15; Virginia Western Lunatic Asylum, *Annu. Rep.*, 1841, *14*, 56. See also Worcester State Lunatic Hospital, *Annu. Rep.*, 1858, *26*, 56–57.

16. Ray, 'Observations on the principal hospitals for the insane in Great Britain, France and Germany,' *loc. cit.*, 344–347. For a similar analysis by Woodward see Worcester State Lunatic Hospital, *Annu. Rep.*, 1845, *13*, 22.

differential was greatest in New England hospitals and least in institutions located in areas with small numbers of foreign-born patients.

At precisely the same time that most states were establishing mental hospitals, the pace of immigration to the United States began to accelerate. Unlike the earlier waves of immigration during the seventeenth and eighteenth centuries, the individuals who flocked to American shores between 1840 and 1860 were far less likely to be of Protestant descent. About two-fifths of the nearly 2,750,000 immigrants who entered the United States between 1847 and 1854 were Irish Catholics who had fled their native land following the devastating famines of that period. Another third was from Germany, and the remainder from all other countries combined.

As a result of population growth from immigration and births, the number of institutionalized patients began to increase (reflecting also the establishment of new hospitals and expansion of older ones). The rise in patient populations at public mental hospitals was often accompanied by a disproportionately high number of lower-class patients from minority ethnic groups. At the New York City Lunatic Asylum on Blackwell's Island—to cite the most extreme example—8,620 out of 11,141 admissions between 1847 and 1870 were immigrants; of this number 5,219 were from Ireland and 2,056 from Germany. In the single year of 1850, 534 patients were foreign born and only 121 natives—this despite the fact that the foreign born constituted slightly less than half of the city's population. Similarly, at the Longview Asylum, which served Cincinnati, 68% of the resident patients in 1875 were foreign born, although this group constituted only 32% of the general population. Much the same held true throughout the Northeast, although (with some exceptions) the proportion of Irish patients was lower. Urban institutions in particular, including those in New York, Boston, Philadelphia, Cincinnati, and St. Louis, all had high percentages of foreign-born inmates, as did state institutions in Massachusetts. It is interesting to note that in states like New York, Ohio, Pennsylvania, and Missouri—all of which had urban-supported institutions—the percentage of foreign-born inmates at the state institutions remained lower. This reflected both location of state institutions and the tendency to permit large urban areas to handle their problems alone without any substantial state aid. Thus 77% of the patient population at the New York City Lunatic Asylum between 1847 and 1870 was foreign born, while at the Utica institution the comparable figure rarely exceeded one-third. Only in Massachusetts was the differential between state institutions and the Boston Lunatic Hospital narrower; and even in the Bay State the latter had a larger concentration of immigrants. Southern hospitals, on the other hand, had the smallest proportion of foreign-born patients, if only because that section received relatively small numbers of immigrants. Overall, nevertheless, the proportion of institutionalized immigrants was higher than their representation in the general population.[17]

The growing heterogeneity of patients in public mental hospitals was a factor of major importance, for it contributed to the decline in the therapeutic institution, which assumed a harmonious and trusting relationship between doctor and patient, and helped to hasten its transformation into a custodial welfare-type institution. So long as psychiatrists treated patients who came from a background similar to their own and who shared a common religion, values, and culture, no conflict ensued. But when these physicians began to deal with patients—especially impoverished immigrants—whose customs, language, culture, traditions, and values seemed to diverge sharply from their own, they found themselves unable to communicate in the familiar manner to which they had grown accustomed. Even those psychiatrists who genuinely sympathized with the plight of less fortunate individuals found themselves in a difficult situation, for they recognized their inability to create the type of therapeutic relationship that was essential to success. 'Our want of success in the treatment of their mental diseases,' observed Ray with chagrin and sympathy, 'is in some degree to be attributed, I imagine, to our inability to approach them in a proper way.... Modes of address like those used in our intercourse with our own people, generally fall upon their ears like an unknown tongue, or are comprehended just enough to render the whole misunderstood, and thereby excite feelings very different from such as were intended.'[18] 'We are not so successful in our treatment of them [the Irish] as with the native population of New England,' observed another superintendent. 'It is difficult to obtain their confidence, for they seem to be jealous of our motives; and the embarrassment they are under, from not clearly comprehending our language, is another obstacle in the way of their recovery.'[19]

The growing number of foreign-born patients in public institutions, which undoubtedly exacerbated internal problems of classification and management and rendered therapeutic relationships more difficult, led superintendents to examine carefully whether or not immigrants who be-

---

17. These figures and generalizations based on an analysis of admissions and nativity statistics to 1875 (when available), have been compiled from the annual reports of mental hospitals.
18. Butler Hospital for the Insane, *Annu. Rep.*, 1849, 32.
19. Worcester State Lunatic Hospital, *Annu. Rep.*, 1847, 15, 33.

came insane could be cured as easily as native Americans. Was it possible that innate differences between the two groups was responsible for the obvious differential recovery rates that clearly favored natives? Had a state of chronic poverty and deprivation so impaired the mental faculties of foreigners that chances for recovery were at best remote? Or was the problem simply one of developing appropriate approaches to immigrant patients, who would then respond in the same manner as natives? These were but some of the issues that faced superintendents who had to confront immigrants not on an abstract level (as did many public officials), but rather on an everyday basis.

In general, there was little unanimity among superintendents whose heterogeneous patient populations made it difficult for them to evade some of the problems involved. Those who had small numbers of foreign-born patients had little or nothing to say, if only because the questions appeared academic. Others who could not avoid the issue offered a variety of explanations. Some saw mental illness among immigrants as an outgrowth of the process whereby individuals uprooted themselves from a familiar environment and migrated to a new and strange country some three thousand or more miles away where they faced a multitude of problems and where their expectations far surpassed their actual achievements. Noting that over 70% of his patients were foreigners, one superintendent explained this fact in terms of circumstances rather than as a consequence of natural disposition toward mental disease. 'Regrets after parents, the absence of the cheering voice of friends, the cold indifference of strangers, difficulties, hardships, privations, and disappointments no doubt predispose many an immigrant to mental aberration, who, in the midst of relatives would never become the subject of insanity.'[20] This point of view was held in one form or another by a number of superintendents, who found no innate differences between immigrant and native patients.[21] Indeed, a few even felt that immigrants were far more amenable to moral treatment than natives. One superintendent found German patients among the easiest to care for; they possessed 'a healthy and elastic mental constitution' and were 'docile and affectionate under treatment, and grateful when they recover.'[22] The head of the New York City Lunatic Asylum was favorably disposed toward Irish inmates. Prior to their admission, he pointed out, they felt

20. Hamilton County Lunatic Asylum, *Annu. Rep.*, 1855, *2*, 10.
21. Cf. Utica State Lunatic Asylum, *Annu. Rep.*, 1854, *12*, 25; Longview Asylum, *Annu. Rep.*, 1861, *2*, 13, 1875, *16*, 6; Kansas Asylum for the Insane, *Annu. Rep.*, 1871, *7*, 5.
22. Illinois State Hospital for the Insane, *Bienn. Rep.*, 1853/1854, *4*, in *Reports of the Illinois State Hospital for the Insane 1847–1862* (Chicago, 1863), p. 159.

abandoned and friendless. But with sincere efforts by concerned physicians, 'their complete confidence will be gained, and the great change from a hopeless and forlorn condition, gives an influence of the strongest character.'[23]

Other superintendents, however, were less certain that lower-class immigrants became insane simply because of the trials and tribulations involved in the shock of moving to a strange and different land. Their contacts with such individuals had convinced them that more was involved, particularly in the case of the Irish, a group that provided not only a disproportionate number of admissions to mental hospitals, but also the lowest percentage of recoveries. Moreover, Irish patients presented more problems in hospitals and were less intelligent, independent, refined, and self-reliant than natives. From their observations and contacts with such individuals, some superintendents began to argue that perhaps a combination of ethnic characteristics and environmental influences was responsible for the high rate of therapeutic failures and the ensuing accumulation of incurable cases. Such explanations, of course, had significant implications for the manner in which such patients were cared for within institutions as well as for the broad framework of public policy.

Few superintendents ever adopted a purely genetic explanation of the seemingly high incidence of mental illness among the Irish. Nevertheless, they found far greater problems with Irish patients as compared with natives. At a discussion at the annual meeting of the Association of Medical Superintendents of American Institutions for the Insane (the professional organization of superintendents and later the American Psychiatric Association) in 1857 one superintendent found foreigners to be 'more noisy, destructive, and troublesome,' while another commented on the low curability rate of the Irish, which he attributed to their nativity.[24] 'It is the experience of all, I believe,' noted the superintendent of the Maine hospital, 'who have had the care of insane Irish in this country, that they, from some cause or another, seldom recover.' Ray observed that 'very ignorant, uncultivated people' often failed to have any insight into their delusions and could not distinguish the subjective from the objective in their mental experience. This trait was especially common 'among the lower class of the Irish.'[25] The ambivalence that was inherent in such views was well ex-

23. M. H. Ranney, 'On insane foreigners,' *Amer. J. Insan.*, 1850, 7, 56–57.
24. *Amer. J. Insan.*, 1857, 14, 79, 103.
25. Maine Insane Hospital, *Annu. Rep.*, 1852, 12, 19; Isaac Ray, 'Doubtful Recoveries,' *Amer. J. Insan.*, 1863, 20, 33.

pressed by Ralph L. Parsons, superintendent of the New York City asylum. In discussing the relative differentials in curability rates between Irish and native patients, he refused to draw any hard and fast conclusions because of the complex issues involved. Many of the Irish in mental hospitals were 'persons of exceptionally bad habits.' In a new and strange country they experienced 'many disappointments and hardships' while simultaneously separated from their families and friends. In addition, their health had been severely impaired by their indigent straits, poor diet, substandard living conditions, and intemperance. 'The majority of such patients,' continued Parsons, 'are of a low order of intelligence, and very many of them have imperfectly developed brains. When such persons become insane, I am inclined to think that the prognosis is peculiarly unfavorable.'[26]

Nowhere did the combined influence of class and ethnicity have as great an impact upon care and treatment as in Massachusetts. A state where anti-Catholicism had a long tradition, its citizens and public officials were beginning to find by the late 1840s and 1850s that the number of destitute Irish at public institutions was increasing rapidly. At the Boston Lunatic Hospital, a municipal institution opened in 1839, foreign-born inmates constituted by far the largest group. By 1846 no less than 90 of the 169 patients were immigrants; of this number 70 were from Ireland. Unhappy at this state of affairs, the Board of Visitors urged the state to relieve the city of the responsibility of caring for immigrant paupers.[27] Much the same was true at state institutions. In 1846 only 12 Irish patients had been admitted to the Worcester hospital; by 1854 this figure had risen to 96. Though initially its superintendent attempted to avoid differential care and treatment, the pressures on him began to mount, particularly since the increase in immigrant inmates (many of whom were chronic cases) meant that fewer spaces were available for native patients. The hospital's trustees were particularly distressed at the fact that foreigners were so numerous. 'Among the insane of this State,' they noted,

are wives and daughters, widows and orphans, of farmers, mechanics, ministers, schoolmasters, and the like. These women were taught in our public schools, trained up in our proverbially neat and orderly households, and accustomed to cultivated society; and, however ready and willing they might have been, when sane, to help the poor, and elevate the humble, of whatever race or color, they would have shrunk most sensitively from living next door even to a wretched

---

26. *Amer. J. Insan.*, 1870, *27*, 158–159.
27. Boston Lunatic Hospital, *Annu. Rep.*, 1846, *7*, 2–5, 10–13. See also ibid., 1843, *4*, 15–16, 1849, *10*, 10–11, 1850, *11*, 14–16.

hovel, and from intimate association with those who are accustomed to, and satisfied with filthy habitations and filthier habits. Now, they do not lose their sensibilities by becoming insane, and they ought not to have them wounded by being herded together in the same apartment with persons whose language, whose habits, and whose manners, offend and shock them. Besides, such associations do not promote the good of any patient, but may retard, and perhaps prevent, the cure of some.[28]

Similarly, in his famous study of insanity for the Massachusetts legislature in 1854, Edward Jarvis—noting that foreigners were enjoying the benefits of public hospitals to a far greater degree than natives—drew an unfavorable portrait of the Irish and recommended that they be sent to separate institutions. Coming from a different environment and holding dissimilar customs, attitudes, and religious beliefs, these aliens resembled the English poor rather than the native poor. The interests of all, claimed Jarvis, would best be served by keeping native and state paupers (Irish) apart.[29] And the most vehement denunciation of the situation at the Worcester hospital appeared in 1852 in the pages of the influential *Boston Medical and Surgical Journal*. 'Never was a sovereign State so grievously burdened,' it remarked on one occasion. 'The people bear the growing evil without a murmur, and it is therefore taken for granted that taxation for the support of the cast-off humanity of Europe is an agreeable exercise of their charity.'[30]

Although specific descriptions of care and treatment within mental hospitals are almost nonexistent for this period, there is circumstantial evidence that the relationships between physicians and especially Irish patients were hardly cordial, a fact that undoubtedly played a role in the effective-

28. Worcester State Lunatic Hospital, *Annu. Rep.*, 1854, *22*, 10–11. See also *ibid.*, 1846, *14*, 42, 1847, *15*, 3–4, 33, 1848, *16*, 33, 1850, *18*, 3, 1851, *19*, 8–9, 1852, *20*, 6–7, 39–40, 1853, *21*, 6–8, 52–54, 1854, *22*, 73, 1855, *23*, 36.

29. *Report on insanity and idiocy in Massachusetts, by the commission on lunacy*, Mass. House Document, No. 144 (1855) pp. 145–150. It should be noted that few of the more than 800 questionnaires received by Jarvis were anti-Catholic or anti-immigrant (all of the correspondents were given an opportunity to express their own opinions). The original returns can be found in 'Report of the physicians of Massachusetts, superintendents of hospitals. . . . Made to the commissioners on lunacy,' MS vol. in the Countway Library of Medicine, Harvard Medical School, Boston, Mass. In other words, Jarvis's hostility toward the Irish was seemingly not a product or reflection of the pressure of public opinion in any form (at least as regards the survey). See also Jarvis to Gov. John A. Andrew, 11 February 1861, Andrew Papers, Mass. Historical Society, Boston, Mass.

30. *Boston med. surg. J.*, 1852, *45*, 537. See also *ibid.*, 1850, *42*, 146, 1851, *44*, 467, 1852, *46*, 85. Luther V. Bell, superintendent of McLean (one of the nation's most exclusive mental hospitals in Boston), favored the establishment of a separate institution for Irish patients administered by an Irish superintendent and officers and subject to a board of trustees. See Mass. House Document No. *139*, 5 April 1848, 3, and Bell's article 'Considerations on a new state lunatic hospital,' *Boston med. surg. J.*, 1849, *41*, 349–355.

ness of therapy. The case histories at the Worcester hospital, for example, often included descriptions of patient behavior that revealed marked revulsion on the part of the physician. One Irish female, to cite one example out of many, was described in 1854 in the following terms: 'This girl is much of the time noisy and troublesome. Has nymphomania and exposes her person. . . . Is vulgar and obscene. . . . Is noisy destructive violent and vulgar.'[31] By 1858 the superintendent had even reorganized the wards in order to maintain 'a complete separation' of foreign and native patients. Such a policy, he maintained, was not in any way motivated by considerations of economy or a desire to discriminate; treatment, though separate, was in all respects equal.[32] The superintendent of the Taunton hospital was of the same persuasion. Though his buildings did not permit separation on the basis of ethnicity, he kept urging that new facilities be constructed so as to permit a segregated policy. In a like vein the head of the Northampton institution urged the state to consider some alternative policy so that hospitals would not become asylums for incurable foreign paupers.[33]

Though less pronounced and more subtle, the influence of ethnicity was especially evident in one form or another in most urban areas with large immigrant populations. The institutions in New York City, Philadelphia, Cincinnati, and St. Louis, all of which had as high or higher a proportion of foreign-born inmates than Massachusetts' hospitals, are a case in point. Like the Boston Lunatic Hospital, they were founded by municipal governments because state-supported institutions simply did not serve the needs of these populous areas. Yet they were, as contemporary observers were quick to recognize, among the worst in the nation.[34] At the New York City Lunatic Asylum, for example, convicts were employed as attendants, and—as its superintendent noted—its facilities were used by native and middle-class groups only infrequently precisely because of its character. Indeed, on a number of occasions its superintendent complained bitterly about the fact that the Commissioners of Emigration (a state body)

---

31. Case No. 4710, Case Book No. 28, p. 240, Record Storage Section, Worcester State Hospital, Worcester, Mass.
32. Worcester State Lunatic Hospital, *Annu. Rep.*, 1858, *26*, 56–57. See the critical comments in the *Amer. J. Insan.*, 1859, *16*, 106–107.
33. Taunton State Lunatic Hospital, *Annu. Rep.*, 1854, *1*, 8, 32–33, 1855, *2*, 26, 1856, *3*, 17–18, 25–26, 1857, *4*, 4–5, 14–15, 29, 1858, *5*, 27–28, 1859, *6*, 3–4, 1861, *8*, 12–13, 1864, *11*, 13–16, 1868, *15*, 14–15; Northampton State Lunatic Hospital, *Annu. Rep.*, 1862, *7*, 23–25, 1863, *8*, 9–11. The situation in Maine (which became separate from Massachusetts in the early nineteenth century) was similar. See Maine Insane Hospital, *Annu. Rep.*, 1849, *9*, 35–36, 1850, *10*, 31–32, 1852, *12*, 19, 1855, *15*, 15, 1859, *19*, 15.
34. See the description of urban institutions by the distinguished British alienist John C. Bucknill in his *Notes on asylums for the insane in America* (London, 1876).

accepted fiscal responsibility for immigrants for only five years after their arrival; thereafter such persons were thrust upon the city for support. Moreover, the city was in effect supporting the Utica State Lunatic Asylum through the taxes its citizens paid while deriving little or no benefit from this institution. Though he opposed differential care and insisted that all insane persons should have equal access to treatment, he noted that the crowded state of the institution 'destroys all efforts at classification, bringing in close proximity the violent, the filthy, the stupid, the sensitive, each mutually irritating the other.'[35]

The situation in New York City as well as in other urban areas rapidly gave rise to a widespread belief that municipal hospitals served as receptacles for large numbers of undesirable elements. 'The feeling is quite too common,' observed one such superintendent, 'that a lunatic asylum is a grand receptacle for all who are troublesome.'[36] Given the hostilities between natives and immigrants, it was not at all surprising that urban mental hospitals provided the lowest quality of care for patient populations composed largely of impoverished immigrants.

III

The most significant differentials in care and treatment during the nineteenth century were clearly related to color. Blacks who became mentally ill were either denied admission to hospitals or else were segregated within existing institutions (where the quality of care provided them was inferior to that accorded lower-class immigrants). Yet the differentials that existed were—with a few exceptions—not the product of a systematic body of racial theory that related race and mental illness. While the scientific community in the mid-nineteenth century was engaged in an extended debate about the relative mental capabilities and the unity or separate origins of diverse races, superintendents rarely discussed the issue in theoretical terms. As administrators, they were involved in managerial issues and spent little time in speculating over such abstract problems. Consequently, the treatment of black mentally ill persons was invariably a function of prevailing community attitudes and practices rather than a product of the application of a body of ostensibly scientific and objective knowledge.

Outside of the South the issue of mental illness among blacks did not arouse any sense of urgency either among hospital or welfare officials, if

---

35. New York City Lunatic Asylum, Blackwell's Island, *Annu. Rep.*, 1848, 27–28, 1849, 23–24, 1853, 6, 1855, 12–15, 1856, 5–6, 11–12, 1858, 11–17.
36. *Ibid.*, 1861, 18.

only because the proportion of blacks in the general population was low. The general practice in most areas was either to exclude blacks or else to provide separate facilities. In this respect the policies of public mental hospitals were not fundamentally dissimilar from those of other welfare and medical institutions. At the Massachusetts General Hospital, for example, the trustees were confronted with the 'painful necessity' of rejecting black applicants because of the 'unwillingness of the ward patients to admit among them individuals of that description.'[37] At the New York City Almshouse, on the other hand, a separate but clearly unequal building was set aside for black inmates.[38]

The availability of facilities for blacks tended to vary from state to state and institution to institution. In Massachusetts the new Worcester hospital faced the problem shortly after it opened in 1833. The trustees, including Horace Mann, were in agreement that 'Africans . . . ought not to mingle with the other female patients,' and they resolved the issue by constructing separate lodgings for the former in the brick shop.[39] Others also followed the practice of providing separate quarters. Such was the case at the Government Hospital for the Insane in Washington, D.C. In California the state asylum set aside a ward for blacks and Chinese patients. In Indiana, on the other hand, the state hospital rejected black applicants both on the grounds of chronicity and the fact that they were not considered to be citizens. This policy came under sharp attack by the superintendent. Recognizing the existence of deeply ingrained prejudices among whites, he nevertheless insisted that the state should construct separate quarters for black insane persons. Much the same situation existed at the Ohio state hospitals, while in Cincinnati the county jail served as the place of confinement.[40]

37. Massachusetts General Hospital, *Annu. Rep.*, 1836, 4.
38. See the description of the Almshouse in the *Report of the commissioners of the alms house, bridewell and penitentiary*, New York City Board of Aldermen, Document No. *32*, 1837, 204. See also Boston Prison Discipline Society, *Annu. Rep.*, 1834, *9*, 87–88; Pennsylvania Board of Commissioners of Public Charities, *Annu. Rep.*, 1872, *3*, xxxiv; Philadelphia Alms House [Hospital], 'Report of the Secretary of the Medical Board,' *Annual reports of the insane and hospital departments*, 1870, 1–2.
39. Bezaleel Taft, Jr., to Horace Mann, 14 April 1833, William B. Calhoun to Mann, 28 June 1833, Mann Papers, Mass. Historical Society, Boston, Mass.; Worcester State Lunatic Hospital, *Annu. Rep.*, 1869, *37*, 70.
40. *Report of the superintendent of the Government Hospital for the Insane* (Washington, D.C., 1855), pp. 3, 5; *Majority report of Assembly Committee on State Hospitals in relation to Assembly Bill No. 226* [California] (n.p., n.d., 1863?), p. 4; Indiana Hospital for the Insane, *Annu. Rep.*, 1854, 36–37; Richard Gundry to George T. Chapman, 10 September 1863, R. Hills to Chapman, 21 September 1863, American Freedmen's Inquiry Commission MSS, Houghton Library, Harvard University, Cambridge, Mass.; Longview Asylum, *Annu. Rep.*, 1860, *1*, 16; Central Ohio Lunatic Asylum, *Annu. Rep.*, 1867, *29*, 7–8.

Prior to 1875 the number of blacks in hospitals outside the South was never large. A survey undertaken in 1863 by the American Freedmen's Inquiry Commission provided some specific data. In Maine, Michigan, Illinois, Iowa, New Hampshire, Pennsylvania, and Vermont the number admitted from the time that their respective institutions had opened to 1863 was less than ten per hospital. At the time of the survey 3 out of 531 residents at the Utica hospital were black; the comparable figures at the New Jersey institution were 4 and 340. Of 8,411 admissions at the Northampton State Lunatic Hospital in Massachusetts 12 were black; the figures for the Boston Lunatic Hospital were 1,764 and 30, respectively. Private hospitals had virtually no black patients, a fact that reflected in part their high costs (as compared with public institutions).[41]

It is difficult, however, to draw precise conclusions from these statistics. The figures dealing with the incidence of mental illness among blacks prior to 1880 are notoriously inaccurate; statistically the numbers are too small; and it is not known whether blacks were discouraged from applying for admission to mental hospitals. Nevertheless, the number of admissions of black insane persons was not fundamentally different from their proportion in the general population. In New York City, for example, blacks constituted slightly more than 1.6% of the population as compared with 2.5% of the total admissions at the municipal lunatic hospital; comparable figures for Maine were .21% and .15%, for Boston 1.7% and 1.7%, for New Jersey 3.8% and 1.2%, and for Michigan .9% and 1%. The statistics in most other northern states were similar. This is not in any way to imply that black patients, once admitted to hospitals, received the same care as whites; in most institutions—if they were not excluded—they were cared for in separate facilities, which usually constituted de facto evidence of differential care because of their inferior quality.

Curiously enough, northern superintendents, though articulate on many issues, tended to ignore almost completely questions involving mental illness among blacks. Outside of an occasional reference on the subject, they neither argued that blacks were more or less prone to insanity than whites, nor did they attempt to defend the obvious differentials in care and treatment in racial terms. Like their fellow citizens, they accepted the prevailing belief that separate facilities were required for black and white, a view up-

---

41. Figures compiled from letters from virtually every mental hospital superintendent in the United States to George T. Chapman in the American Freedmen's Inquiry Commission MSS, Houghton Library, Harvard University, Cambridge, Mass.

held by Charles Nichols, a superintendent and president of the Association. 'I think yr views & mine,' he wrote to Kirkbride,

> in regard to what is a suitable provision for col'd insane agree, & that our views are that it *is the duty* of all State, County, & City Hospitals for Insane, situated in communities composed in any considerable part of blacks, whether slave or free, to receive col'd patients; that they sh'd be accommodated in special cottages or lodges situated near the main edifice for whites, but so entirely distinct from it that all desirable separation of the races may be maintained; that such an arrangement may be carried into effect without prejudice to either party, & that entirely separate Hospitals for col'd insane is not practicable nor even desirable.[42]

Unlike their northern brethren, southern superintendents were never able to ignore the problems posed by mental illness among both free and slave blacks. Though the incidence of mental illness among southern blacks seemed far lower than among southern whites before 1860,[43] most hospital officials in the South still had to contend with substantial numbers of applications for admission from either slave owners or free black families. Given the large black population, the fact that close contacts between black and white were unavoidable, and the belief that whites had an obligation toward blacks, it was understandable that there was more concern with the problem in the South than the North.

The pattern of institutional care for blacks in the South varied from state to state. The Maryland hospital did not segregate patients, for the superintendent saw no reason for such a policy.[44] The Kentucky Western Lunatic Asylum admitted limited numbers of slaves when the costs were borne by their owners and 'when there was accommodation for them such as would prevent indiscriminate mingling of white and black.' The Kentucky East-

---

42. C. H. Nichols to Kirkbride, 24 April 1855; see also Nichols to Kirkbride, 14 April 1855, Kirkbride Papers, Institute of the Pennsylvania Hospital, Philadelphia, Pa.

43. A number of explanations about the low rate of mental illness among slaves (none of which have either been proven or disproven) apply, assuming that the incidence *was indeed low*. First, Southerners believed that slaves were not prone to mental disease since they were not subject to the pressures of an advanced civilization; they also regarded bondsmen as possessing a childlike nature. Consequently, whites were less prone to see aberrant black behavior in terms of mental disease, since their perceptual framework told them that mental illness among blacks was an oddity. Moreover, childlike behavior, which might have led to a diagnosis of insanity among whites, was regarded by whites as closer to black normative behavior. Another operative factor may have been the unwillingness on the part of whites to commit their slaves to a hospital; not only would the labor of the slave be lost, but the owner would be financially liable for the costs of institutionalization. Finally, slavery was such a closed and authoritarian system that slaves who behaved in a deviant manner were treated so harshly that they were forced to conform. Evidence as to the validity of these explanations is presently lacking.

44. Maryland Hospital for the Insane, *Annu. Rep.*, 1851, 7–8. Charles H. Nichols regarded this practice as 'a sort of corollary of a low view of management generally.' Nichols to Kirkbride, 14 April 1855, Kirkbride Papers, Institute of the Pennsylvania Hospital, Philadelphia, Pa.

ern Lunatic Asylum, on the other hand, refused to accept slaves because the institution had no separate facilities and, as the superintendent remarked, 'it would be manifestly improper to mingle these persons with our own race.' He nevertheless urged the legislature to make some provision for such individuals. The costs of maintenance, he pointed out, were nonexistent, since slave owners would have to pay the full costs of institutionalization.[45]

Without doubt the most curious situation existed in Virginia, the first state to have more than one public hospital. When the Williamsburg institution opened in the late eighteenth century, the law stipulated that it would receive all 'persons,' but it made no mention of slaves. During its early history the institution accepted free blacks; if slaves were admitted it would have been an oddity and an exception. Under John M. Galt, who became superintendent in 1841, the hospital began to accept insane slave patients. Galt was firm in his belief that separate institutions for black and white were unfeasible and uneconomical; he was convinced that blacks could be cured either in a separate building or in a completely integrated one. At his hospital black females were housed in a separate structure, while black males were kept in integrated wards with whites. Since all of the hospital's servants were black slaves, noted Galt, white patients regarded black patients 'pretty much in the same light as they do the servants.' By 1856, however, the hospital no longer accepted slaves, and the following year Galt, probably under public pressure, retreated from the flexibility that he had shown in regard to the mixing of black and white.[46] At the Virginia Western Lunatic Asylum, by way of contrast, blacks were completely excluded. Its superintendent adamantly opposed integrated hospitals; his policies undoubtedly represented the feelings of Virginians residing in the western part of the state, since nearly 90% of the black population was located east of the Blue Ridge.[47]

Elsewhere in the South the pattern was equally mixed. Georgia made no provision for black insane persons, although its governor and those con-

---

45. Kentucky Western Lunatic Asylum, *Annu. Rep.*, 1865, 14; Kentucky Eastern Lunatic Asylum, *Bien. Rep.*, 1856/1857, *33–34*, 24.

46. Virginia Eastern Asylum, *Annu. Rep.*, 1848, 23–29, 1849, 5–6, 17; N. Dain, *Disordered minds: the first century of Eastern State Hospital in Williamsburg, Virginia 1766–1866* (Williamsburg, 1971), pp. 110–113.

47. *Report of the Court of Directors of the Western Lunatic Hospital, December, 1828*, document appended to the *Journal of the House of Delegates of the Commonwealth of Virginia, begun . . . the first day of December, one thousand eight hundred and twenty-eight* (Richmond, 1828), p. 5; Virginia Western Lunatic Asylum, *Annu. Rep.*, 1844, *17*, 26, 1845, *18*, 7–8, 29–31, 1848, *21*, 4–5, 32–34, *Bienn. Rep.*, 1867/1868–1868/1869, 6–7; C. H. Nichols to Kirkbride, 14 April 1855, Kirkbride Papers, Institute of the Pennsylvania Hospital, Philadelphia, Pa.

nected with the state asylum favored entirely separate buildings to care for the small number of such persons in the state. Much the same held true for Tennessee and Mississippi. Louisiana accepted free blacks and some slaves as patients. Similarly, the South Carolina legislature in 1848 authorized the state's hospital to accept black patients, and soon afterwards separate facilities (and inferior to those provided white inmates) were constructed. Nevertheless, the hospital by 1860 accepted only black females, since the removal of males from the older buildings had eliminated the quarters occupied by black males.[48]

After 1865 the South was confronted with far more serious problems regarding the care and treatment of black insane persons. Since blacks were —at least in theory if not in practice—entitled to the same rights and privileges as other citizens, most states were faced with a policy dilemma—a dilemma that was complicated by the fact some pressure was exerted by blacks and some whites for nondiscriminatory treatment. Moreover, white southerners had always viewed their relationships with blacks in benevolent and paternalistic terms, and even after the abolition of slavery this tradition continued to be of influence. Finally, there was some fear among officials that the incidence of mental illness among blacks would rise sharply and surpass that of whites. 'Unrestrained freedom,' noted a Maryland official, 'has had the effect of multiplying their [blacks] desires and wants, but together with them it has also multiplied greatly their disappointments, and in very many instances the price of liberty to them has been the prison, the almshouse and the insane asylum.'[49]

In general, a consensus among southern hospital superintendents emerged relatively early on the question of facilities for black insane persons. First, they insisted that the state had a legal and moral obligation to provide care and treatment for blacks as well as whites. Secondly, there was unanimous agreement that it was impossible to provide such care in integrated wards.[50]

48. Georgia State Lunatic Asylum, *Rep.*, 1858/1859, 15; Tennessee Hospital for the Insane, *Bienn. Rep.*, 1852/1853, 1, 21; Mississippi State Lunatic Asylum, *Annu. Rep.*, 1858, 4, 11–12, 1859, 5, 24; S. Chaillé, *A memoir of the insane asylum of the state of Louisiana, at Jackson* (New Orleans, 1858), pp. 8–9; Insane Asylum of Louisiana, *Annu. Rep.*, 1866, 6; South Carolina Lunatic Asylum, *Annu. Rep.*, 1844, 5, 1850, 12, 1851, 8–9, 1858, 12–13, 1860, 13.

49. *Report on the public charities, reformatories, prisons and almshouses, of the state of Maryland, by C. W. Chancellor, M.D., secretary of the State Board of Health, made to his excellency, John Lee Carroll, governor. July, 1877* (Frederick, Md., 1877), pp. 14–15.

50. For the consensus of views among southern superintendents, see the following: Kentucky Western Lunatic Asylum, *Annu. Rep.*, 1865, 14, 1866, 12–13; Insane Asylum of North Carolina, *Annu. Rep.*, 1865, 10, 2–3; Texas State Lunatic Asylum, *Annu. Rep.*, 1866, 10; Kentucky Eastern Lunatic Asylum, *Annu. Rep.*, 1866, 42, 17; Lunatic Asylum of the State of Georgia, *Rep.*, 1865, 7, 1867/1868, 10–11; Virginia Western Lunatic Asylum, *Annu. Rep.*, 1866, 11, *Bienn. Rep.*, 1867/1868–1868/1869, 37–45;

This broad consensus reflected to a considerable degree developments in most southern states after 1865. The majority of states set aside separate quarters for blacks either in the same building used by whites or in a separate one, although usually of inferior quality. Some states, including North Carolina, Mississippi, and West Virginia, were slower than others in authorizing segregated facilities. Others, like Kentucky, provided limited accommodations. The general policy, however, was clearly to move in the direction of segregated care. A few states carried this policy to its logical conclusion by founding entirely separate and distinct institutions for blacks. Tennessee, for example, opened a Hospital for the Colored Insane shortly after the end of the war. This facility, however, was located adjacent to the Tennessee Hospital for the Insane and remained under a common administration. Virginia, on the other hand, eventually converted a black general hospital founded by the Freedmen's Bureau into the first truly separate hospital for black insane persons. Whatever the individual policy, the facilities provided blacks rarely equalled those for whites.[51]

By the late nineteenth century, therefore, more hospital facilities were beginning to be made available to blacks, though in most areas these facilities were segregated and often below the quality of those that served poor and indigent whites as well as ethnic minorities. Like the overwhelming majority of white Americans, virtually no member of the psychiatric pro-

---

West Virginia Hospital for the Insane, *Annu. Rep.*, 1867, *4*, 24–25, 1872, *9*, 16; Missouri State Lunatic Asylum, *Bienn. Rep.*, 1867/1868, *8*, 15–16; St. Louis County Insane Asylum, *Ann. Rep.*, 1869/1870, *1*, 18; Tennessee Hospital for the Insane, *Bienn. Rep.*, 1868/1869, 24; South Carolina Lunatic Asylum, *Annu. Rep.*, 1869, 6, 1872, 24–26; Mississippi State Lunatic Asylum, *Annu. Rep.*, 1871, 20–21, 1872, 21; Alabama Insane Hospital, *Annu. Rep.*, 1875, *15*, 18.

51. Alabama Insane Hospital, *Annu. Rep.*, 1867, *7*, 8–9, 1869, *9*, 8, 1870, *10*, 11, 1872, *12*, 25–26, 1875, *15*, 18; Lunatic Asylum of the State of Georgia, *Rep.*, 1865/1866, 7, 1866/1867, 7–8, 1867/1868, 10–11; Kentucky Eastern Lunatic Asylum, *Annu. Rep.*, 1866, *42*, 17, 1868, *44*, 7–8, 1873, *49*, 14; Kentucky Western Lunatic Asylum, *Annu. Rep.*, 1865, 14–15, 1866, 12–13; Central Kentucky Lunatic Asylum, *Annu. Rep.*, 1874, *2*, 19, 1875, *3*, 9–11, 18; Mississippi State Lunatic Asylum, *Annu. Rep.*, 1871, 20–21, 1872, 15–23; Missouri State Lunatic Asylum, *Bienn. Rep.*, 1865/1866, 7 (in *Missouri Senate J.*, 24th General Assembly, 1867, Appendix), 443–444, 1867/1868, *8*, 15–16; Insane Asylum of North Carolina, *Annu. Rep.*, 1865, *10*, 2–3, 1866, *11*, 10, 1875, *20*, 3–18; South Carolina Lunatic Asylum, *Annu. Rep.*, 1868, 5–6, 1869, 6, 1871, 27, 1872, 24–25, 1873, 10, 1875, 13; Tennessee Hospital for the Insane, *Rep.*, 1865/1867, 15–17, *Annu. Rep.*, 1866, 6, *Bienn. Rep.*, 1868/1869, 7, 24, 1869/1871, *8*, 17; Texas State Lunatic Asylum, *Annu. Rep.*, 1866, 10–11, *Semi-Annu. Rep.*, August 1866/March 1867, *1*, 8–9; Virginia Western Lunatic Asylum, *Annu. Rep.*, 1866, 11, *Bienn. Rep.*, 1867/1868–1868/1869, 6–7, 34–35; Virginia Eastern Lunatic Asylum, *Annu. Rep.*, 1868, 4–6, 1870, 28, 1873, 18; Virginia Central Lunatic Asylum, *Annu. Rep.*, 1870, *1*, 4–10, 1871/1872, *2*, 6–13, 1872/1873, *3*, 13–26; West Virginia Hospital for the Insane, *Annu. Rep.*, 1867, *4*, 24–25, 1872, *9*, 16, 21, *Bienn. Rep.*, 1875/1876, *12*, 5, 34–35; *Amer. J. Insan.*, 1874, *31*, 155–157, 1878, *35*, 125–127, 129–130. It should be noted that northern areas with relatively large concentrations of blacks pursued policies not fundamentally different from those in the South.

fession was willing to challenge the dominant separate but equal doctrine that was the basis of public policy. Most psychiatrists not only accepted the assumptions underlying this policy, but they proved to be among its staunchest supporters. A few who might have opposed it took the position instead that their function was to provide care and treatment and not to educate the public on racial issues. Concerned also that integrated hospitals and wards might undermine the system of public hospitals that had been so laboriously constructed, they followed what appeared to be a logical and reasonable policy.

IV

In theory the public mental hospital was a beneficent medical institution that served all groups. In practice, however, the quality of care was partially dependent upon class, ethnic origin, and color, with the last playing a more important role than the other two. Ultimately all three, operating simultaneously and reinforcing each other, would have a significant influence over the entire system of public mental hospitals because in proportion as mental hospitals served predominantly lower-class, ethnic minority, and nonwhite groups their reputation, funding, and quality of care declined. It must also be emphasized that while class, ethnic group, and race played an important role in shaping the configuration of hospitals, few psychiatrists (or public officials for that matter) were completely cognizant of this fact. Policy issues tended to be defined within a narrow and limited range; often only immediate circumstances and factors were considered. An inability to appreciate the subtle influence of these three factors, therefore, tended to heighten their actual importance in shaping the care of the mentally ill in the United States.

Department of History
Rutgers University

Social Class and Medical Care in Nineteenth-Century America: The Rise and Fall of the Dispensary

CHARLES E. ROSENBERG

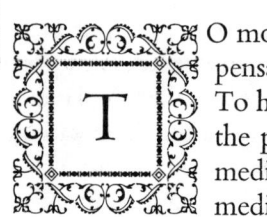

To most mid-twentieth-century physicians, the term 'dispensary' evokes the image of a hectic hospital pharmacy. To his mid-nineteenth-century counterpart, it was both the primary means for providing the urban poor with medical care and a vital link in the prevailing system of medical education. These institutions had an effective life-span of roughly a hundred years. Founded in the closing decades of the eighteenth century, American dispensaries increased in scale and number throughout the nineteenth century and remained significant providers of health care well into the twentieth century. By the 1920s, however, the dispensaries were on the road to extinction, increasingly submerged in the outpatient departments of urban hospitals. Historians have found the dispensary of little interest; even those contemporary medical activists seeking a usable past for experiments in the delivery of medical care, are hardly aware of their existence.[1] Yet a study of the dispensary illustrates not only an important aspect of medicine and philanthropy in the nineteenth-century city—but the social logic implicit in their rise and fall underlines permanently significant relationships between general social needs and values and the narrower world of medical men and ideas.

The dispensary was invented in late-eighteenth-century England; it was an autonomous, free-standing institution, created in the hope of providing an alternative to the hospital in providing medical care for the urban poor. Like most such benevolent innovations, it was soon copied by socially con-

1. The most valuable study of the dispensary is still that by Michael M. Davis, Jr. and Andrew R. Warner, *Dispensaries. Their Management and Development* (New York, 1918). The most useful account of the early years of any single dispensary is: [William Lawrence], *A History of the Boston Dispensary* (Boston, 1859). For an example of contemporary interest, see George Rosen, 'The First Neighborhood Health Center Movement—Its Rise and Fall,' *Am. J. publ. Hlth.*, 1971, 61, 1620–37.

scious Americans; dispensaries were established in 1786 at Philadelphia, 1791 at New York, 1796 at Boston, and at Baltimore in 1800. Their growth was at first very slow. No additional dispensaries were established until 1816, when the managers of the Philadelphia Dispensary helped establish two new dispensaries, the Northern and Southern, to serve their city's rapidly developing fringes.[2] New Yorkers established the Northern Dispensary in 1827, the Eastern in 1832, the DeMilt in 1851, and Northwestern in 1852. By 1874 there were twenty-nine dispensaries in New York, by 1877, thirty-three in Philadelphia. Their growth was equally impressive in terms of number of patients treated; in New York, for example, the city's dispensaries treated 134,069 patients in 1860, roughly 180,000 in 1866, 213,000 in 1874 and 876,000 in 1900.[3]

The dispensaries shared certain organizational characteristics. Almost all had a central building—with the prominent exception of Boston which had none until the 1850s—and usually employed one full-time employee, an apothecary or house-physician who acted as steward, performed minor surgery, often vaccinated and pulled teeth—as well as prescribing for some patients. (Though most dispensaries limited their aid to prescriptions written by their own staff physicians, a few would fill prescriptions for the indigent patients of any regular physician).[4] By mid-century the house-physicianship had in the larger dispensaries evolved into two separate positions, resident physician and druggist-apothecary. Most dispensaries also appointed younger physicians who visited patients too ill to attend the dispensary. Such 'district visiting' was the principal task of the Philadelphia Dispensary when founded in 1786, remained the sole activity of the Boston Dispensary until 1856—and was continued by almost all urban dispensaries until the end of the nineteenth century, though the treatment of ambulatory patients grew proportionately more prominent in all. The dispensaries also appointed attending and consulting staffs from among their community's established practitioners, the attending staff treating patients well

---

2. Philadelphia Dispensary, Minutebook, 18, 25 June 1816, Archives of the Pennsylvania Hospital, Philadelphia. (Hereafter APH). Cf: 'Brief History of the Southern Dispensary,' Southern Dispensary, *Eighty-first Annual Report* (Philadelphia, 1898), pp. 6–10.

3. Charles E. Rosenberg, 'The Practice of Medicine in New York a Century Ago,' *Bull. Hist. Med.*, 1967, *41*, 223–253, p. 236; F. B. Kirkbride, *The Dispensary Problem in Philadelphia. A Report made to the Hospital Association of Philadelphia, October 28, 1903* (Philadelphia, 1903). By 1900, Davis and Warner (*Dispensaries*, p. 10) estimated that there were roughly one hundred dispensaries in the United States, seventy-five general and twenty-five special.

4. As late as 1899, the City of Baltimore still compensated the Baltimore Dispensary when it filled prescriptions for the indigent patients of any legal practitioner. Baltimore General Dispensary, *Charter, By-Laws, &c. . . . Revised 1899* (Baltimore, 1899), p. 14.

enough to visit the dispensary, the consulting staff serving a largely honorary role.

The dispensaries were shoe-string operations. Most, with the exception of those in New York which enjoyed state and city subventions, were supported by private contributions and the often-voluntary services of local physicians.[5] As late as the 1870s and 1880s—when a dispensary might treat over 25,000 patients a year—budgets of four or five thousand dollars were still common and annual reports vied in reporting how little had been spent for prescriptions—an average of under five cents per prescription was common. The Boston Dispensary and Philadelphia Dispensary gradually accumulated some endowment funds, though most others remained financially marginal. All, however, were sensitive to cyclical economic shifts, for contributions declined in periods of depression while patient pressure increased proportionately. As a result of the economy's downturn in 1857, for example, New York's Eastern Dispensary reported an increase of twenty-two per cent in cases over 1858 and forty-two per cent over 1856.[6] A useful index to the shaky financial condition of many of the dispensaries was their frequent practice of renting a portion of their building to commercial tenants; such income often constituted a substantial portion of the institution's budget and could not be given up even when the dispensary needed room for expansion.[7]

Some of the dispensaries published detailed statistics of the numbers and kinds of ailments treated by their physicians; thus we can begin to reconstruct their everyday responsibilities. Most cases were, of course, relatively minor—for example, bronchitis, colds or dyspepsia—and rarely were the numbers of deaths equal to more than two or three per cent of the patients treated. Consistently enough, the number of female patients was always greater than that of males, in some instances as much as two to one; work-

5. New York's Eastern Dispensary reported in 1857 that the city's donation to the New York Dispensary had been set at $1000.00 in 1827. As other dispensaries were founded, these too received the same subvention. *23rd Annual Report, 1856* (New York, 1857), p. 19.

6. *25th Annual Report, 1858* (New York, 1859), pp. 16-17. The panics of 1857, 1873 and 1893 as well as the Civil War years all represented such periods of stress for the dispensaries. New York's Northeastern Dispensary, for example, was so pressed by the Panic of 1873 that it could not even publish annual reports in 1874 and 1875. *15th Annual Report, 1876* (New York, 1877), p. 6.

7. As late as 1891, Philadelphia's Northern Dispensary bemoaned the fact that they could still not afford to stop renting their second floor, despite their establishment of five new specialty clinics and consequent need for space. Northern Dispensary, *74th Annual Report, 1891* (Philadelphia, 1892), p. 9. As early as 1803, the Philadelphia Dispensary was happy to rent its basement to a commercial tenant. Minutes, 12 December 1803. The typical pattern was illustrated clearly by the New York Dispensary's decision in 1868 to build a four-story building, the basement, first, third, and fourth levels being rented, only the second used by the Dispensary itself. *77th Annual Report, 1868* (New York, 1869), p. 12.

ing men, that is, had necessarily to tolerate disease symptoms of far greater intensity before feeling able to consult a physician. In those cases serious enough to be treated at home by visiting physicians sex ratios tended to be more nearly equal. (It was not until the end of the century that dispensaries began to consider evening hours for workers.) Although the general level of mortality among all dispensary patients was low, mortality among patients treated in their homes approached the ten or eleven per cent normal for hospitals at the beginning of the century. Such death rates were particularly discouraging, for the district physician never treated many intractable cases. Chronic and degenerative ailments brought incapacity and eventual alms-house incarceration; these cases never found their way into the dispensary's mortality statistics. The dispensaries also performed minor surgery, treating fractures, contusions and lacerations—as well as casual if frequent dentistry, essentially the 'indiscriminate extirpation' of offending teeth.[8]

The dispensaries also played an important public health role in providing vaccination for the poor and vaccine matter for the use of private practitioners. From a purely demographic point of view, indeed, vaccination was the most important function performed by the dispensaries. The dispensaries not only made vaccination available without cost, but some mounted door-to-door vaccination programs in their city's tenement districts. In periods of intense demand, most frequently at the outset or threat of a smallpox epidemic, the dispensaries were able to supply large amounts of vaccine matter at short notice. In the opening months of the Civil War for example, the New York Dispensary provided vaccine matter for all the state's recruits.[9]

Despite ventures into surgery, dentistry, and vaccination, dispensary therapeutics were generally synonymous with the writing of prescriptions; dispensaries dispensed. Throughout the first three-quarters of the nineteenth century, the phrase 'prescribing for' was generally synonymous

8. Eastern Dispensary (New York), *23rd Annual Report, 1856* (New York, 1857), p. 22; S. L. Abbott to G. F. Thayer, 6 April 1844, Chronological File, Boston Dispensary Archives, New England Medical Center, Boston. (Hereinafter BDA.) The phrase describing the dispensary's casual dentistry is from New York Dispensary, *81st Annual Report, 1870* (New York, 1871), p. 17.

9. For a convenient summary of early vaccination work by the dispensaries, see: DeMilt Dispensary (New York), *25th Annual Report, 1875* (1876), pp. 20–22. For the role of the dispensaries in the Civil War, see: New York Dispensary, *72nd Annual Report, 1862* (New York, 1863), pp. 9–10; Eastern Dispensary (New York), *25th Annual Report, 1861* (New York, 1862), pp. 23–25. Though the poor were normally uninterested in vaccination, the threat of epidemics often created a sudden upsurge of interest; in one case, indeed, the New York Dispensary could refer to a 'vaccination riot' on their premises. *76th Annual Report, 1865* (New York, 1865), p. 20. Many of the dispensaries were financially dependent on their sale of vaccine matter.

with seeing a patient; busy dispensary physicians could hardly be expected to do more than compose hasty and routine prescriptions. (Dispensary managers tended by mid-century to demand the use of formularies limited in both cost and variety; later in the century some dispensaries were charged with filling prescriptions by number, the dispensing physician being constrained by an abbreviated list of numbered and pre-formulated prescriptions).[10] In this routine and exclusive dependence on drug therapy lay the principal difference between the care provided the urban poor and that paid for by the middle class. Physicians in private practice relied consistently in their therapeutics upon adjusting the regimen of their patients, especially in chronic ills; such injunctions were hardly appropriate in dispensary practice. The city poor could not well vary their diet, take up horse-back riding, visit the seaside, or voyage to the West Indies.

Not surprisingly, the dispensaries tended to develop ties both formal and informal with other urban charities—in New York, for example, with the Commissioners of Emigration, Association for Improving the Condition of the Poor, and Children's Aid Society; in Philadelphia with the Board of Guardians for the Poor.[11] Dispensary physicians were in this sense *de facto* social workers. In New York, for example, a note from the dispensary physician was necessary if the commissioners were to issue a ration of coal; thus a mid-century whimsy referred to 'coal fever'—an illness which struck suddenly during cold weather in the city's tenements.[12] In the post-Civil War decades, efforts to provide such physical amenities became somewhat more organized; dispensary physicians continued to work with existing philanthropic agencies and began as well to establish their own auxiliaries in hopes of providing food and nursing in deserving cases. In Philadelphia, the Lying-in and Nurse Charity, and the Lying-In Department of the Northern Dispensary had provided some nursing service since

10. George Gould, 'Abuse of a Great Charity,' *Med. News*, N.Y., 1890, 57, 535: p. 6; Medical College of the Pacific, Faculty Minutes, 29 January 1878, 22 July 1881, Lane Medical Library, Stanford University. New York's Eastern Dispensary was so lacking in funds that its patients were given neither bottles nor printed instructions: 'The patients universally bring a bottle or tea-cup to receive and hold the medicine.' *25th Annual Report, 1861* (New York, 1862), p. 14. There were only occasional conflicts between physicians and lay managers in regard to such cutting of corners. A revealing incident of this kind shook the Boston Dispensary in 1844 when the managers sought to compel their visiting physicians to employ scarification and bleeding instead of the far more expensive leeches. The physicians argued not only that the leeches had a different physiological effect—but that they had well-nigh banished more painful modes of blood-letting from private practice. G. T. Thayer to Visiting Physicians, 8 February 1844; S. L. Abbott *et al.* to Thayer, 6 April 1844; S. L. Abbott *et al.* to President and Managers [February, 1844], BDA.

11. For an example of such ties in a particular dispensary, see: DeMilt Dispensary, *2nd Annual Report, 1852–53* (New York, 1853), p. 12; *4th Annual Report, 1855* (New York, 1856), pp. 10–11.

12. Eastern Dispensary (New York), *32nd Annual Report, 1865* (New York, 1866), p. 14.

the 1830s, while others had paid occasionally for nursing in selected cases since the opening years of the century. In a more contemporary idiom, the Instructive Visiting Nurse Service of the Boston Dispensary began in the 1880s to aid the dispensary's district physicians in their work, not only nursing, but educating the poor in hygiene and diet. In Boston and New York, diet kitchen associations provided nourishing food for patients bearing a dispensary physician's requisition. By 1883, the New York Diet Kitchen Association operated three kitchens in cooperation with the dispensaries and had fed 7,699 patients, filling 53,893 separate requisitions from dispensary physicians during the year.[13]

Another trend marking the nineteenth-century evolution of the dispensaries, reflecting and paralleling a more general development within the medical profession, was their internal reorganization along specialty lines. As early as 1826, the New York Dispensary reorganized itself, dividing patients treated at the Dispensary into 'classes' according to the nature of their ailment. Pioneering dispensaries for diseases of the eye and ear had come into being as early as the 1820s. By mid-century, the need for specialty differentiation was unquestioned. When the Brooklyn Dispensary opened in 1847, for example, it announced that patients would be distributed among the following classes: women and children, heart, lungs and throat, skin and vaccination, head and digestive organs, eye and ear, surgery and unclassified diseases. In the second-half of the century, specialty designations became increasingly narrow and gradually closer to modern categories; nervous and genito-urinary diseases were, for example, among the most frequently created of such departments in the late 1870s and early 1880s. By 1905, the forward-looking Boston Dispensary boasted these impressively varied out-patient clinics: surgical, general medical, children, skin, nervous system, nose and throat, women, eye and ear, genito-urinary, and x-ray.[14] An important related late-nineteenth-century trend was the increasingly frequent establishment of specialized dispensaries, institutions that treated only particular ailments or ailments of particular organs.

---

13. New York Diet Kitchen Association, *11th Annual Report, 1883* (New York, 1884), p. 5. On nursing, see, for example, Philadelphia Dispensary, Minutes, 15 February 1853, 17 October 1854, APH.

14. Brooklyn Dispensary, *Trustees's Report. April, 1847* (New York, 1847), p. 8; Boston Dispensary, *108th Annual Report* (Boston, 1905), pp. 10–12. For the crediting of the New York Dispensary with this particular first, see: DeMilt Dispensary, *25th Annual Report, 1875* (New York, 1876), p. 19n.

These in brief outline were the chief characteristics which marked the growth of the dispensaries between the end of the eighteenth and last decades of the nineteenth century. Why did the founders and managers of our pioneer dispensaries find them so plausible a response to social need? What factors led to their initial adoption and subsequent growth?

In their appeals for public support, dispensary founders and supporters left abundant records of their conscious motives. Most prominent in the last years of the eighteenth and opening decades of the nineteenth century was a traditional sense of stewardship. 'It is enough for us,' as one physician-philanthropist put it, 'to be assured that the poor are always with us, and that they are exposed to disease.'

Benevolence [he continued] is not that passive feeling which can be satisfied with doing no injury to our neighbor, or rest contented with mere good wishes for his well-being when he needs our assistance.

The poor, as a prominent New York clergyman explained the need for supporting the dispensary's work, 'have feelings as well as we; they are bone of our bone and flesh of our flesh; men of like passions with ourselves.'[15] Such sentiments remained deeply felt and were explicitly articulated throughout the first half of the century.

Other, more mundane, motives always coexisted with such humanitarian appeals. One was the familiar mercantilist contention that maintaining the health of the poor would not only save the tax dollars implied by the almshouse or hospital care of chronically-ill workers, but would aid the economy more generally by helping maintain the labor force at optimum efficiency. (These appeals assumed, of course, the ability of the dispensary physicians to diagnose ills at a stage when they might still respond to available treatment.) A related argument urged the dispensaries' function as first-line of defense against epidemic disease; though such ills ordinarily began and reached epidemic proportions among the poor, once established they might attack even the comfortable and well-to-do. No household could feel immune when servants and artisans moved easily from the world of their betters to that of tenement-dwelling friends and families.[16]

15. John G. Coffin, *An Address delivered before the Contributors of the Boston Dispensary, . . . October 21, 1813* (Boston, 1813), pp. 6, 15; John B. Romeyn, *The Good Samaritan: A Sermon, delivered in the Presbyterian Church, in Cedar-street, New York, . . . for the Benefit of the New York Dispensary* (New York, 1810), p. 16.
16. 'Servants,' one board of managers argued at mid-century, 'who have relations and friends in the lower walks of life, and who are in the habit of visiting them, often in company with the children of their employers, would be subject to more danger than they are now exposed.' DeMilt Dispensary, *3rd Annual Report, 1853-54* (New York, 1854), p. 10.

These arguments soon hardened into rhetorical formulae and were ritually intoned throughout the first two-thirds of the century. Thus, for example, a mid-century dispensary spokesman could, in appealing for support, argue that:[17]

The political economist will find here cheapness and utility combined. The statesman will discover the greatest good of the greatest number combined promoted. The city official will find his sanitary police materially assisted. The heads of families will soon find how much the lives and health of their household are cared for and secured. The tax-payer will see his burthens diminished. The benevolent will have opened to his view in the Dispensary and its kindred and associated charities the widest field for the exercise of good will towards man; and the Christian will find a new proof of the truth that they do not love God less who love mankind more.

Finally, and matter-of-factly, their advocates always contended that dispensaries would serve as much-needed schools of clinical medicine.

But to catalogue the arguments of managers and fund-raisers is not precisely to explain the logic of their commitment. Why did the dispensaries grow so rapidly? Obviously because they worked, worked that is in terms of particular social realities and expectations. At least four such factors help explain the evolution of the dispensary in nineteenth-century America. First, they were entirely functional in terms of the internal organization of the medical profession. Second, they were entirely consistent with available therapeutic modalities. Third, they were effectively scaled to the needs of a small and comparatively homogeneous community; once established they became indispensable as urban growth dramatically increased their client constituency. Fourth, the dispensaries made sense in terms of their founders' expectations of the roles to be played both by government and private citizens.

Most fundamental was the relationship between the dispensary and the world of medical education and status. Without the initiative and voluntary support of the medical profession dispensaries would not have been created nor could they have survived. Physicians formed the core-group in the formation of almost every American dispensary from the end of the eighteenth to the beginning of the twentieth century.[18]

17. DeMilt Dispensary, *5th Annual Report, 1855–56* (New York, 1856), p. 11.
18. For typical examples later in the century, see: Central Dispensary and Emergency Hospital of the District of Columbia, *24th Annual Report . . . Including an Historical Sketch of the Institution* (Washington, 1894), pp. 8–10; Camden City Dispensary, *26th Annual Report, 1892–93* (Camden, N.J., 1893), pp. 6–9.

In the first third of the nineteenth century, when formal clinical training could not be said to exist outside that presumed in the preceptorial relationship, the dispensary helped fill an important pedagogical void. Not only could visiting and attending physicians themselves accumulate experience and reputation while more firmly establishing their private practice—but they could use their dispensary appointment as a means of providing case materials for their apprentices. Thus Benjamin Rush could recommend Drs. Wistar and Griffits as preceptors since both held dispensary positions, 'where a young man will see more practice in a month than with most private physicians in a year.' Almost from the first years of the dispensaries, indeed, critics often charged that students and apprentices were allowed to treat the poor. (In Philadelphia, for example, such complaints found their way into newspapers as early as 1791).[19] In the second quarter of the nineteenth century, as the preceptorial system grew less significant, the role of the dispensaries in clinical training grew even more prominent; mid-century medical schools vied actively in establishing dispensaries for the benefit of their students.

Most significantly, dispensary physicianships served as a step in the career pattern of elite physicians. Despite the complaints of articulate mid-century critics as to the wretched state of medical education and practice, even a cursory analysis of the profession's structure indicates the existence of a well-defined elite, largely urban, often European-trained, and almost always enjoying the benefits of hospital and dispensary experience. It was just such ambitious young practitioners who served as dispensary visiting and attending physicians while they accumulated experience and gradually made the contacts so important to later success—contacts, it should be emphasized, with older established physicians at least as much as with prospective patients.[20] (Prestigious and largely honorary consulting physician-

---

19. Rush to John Dickinson, 4 October 1791, *Letters of Benjamin Rush*, ed. by L. H. Butterfield (Princeton, N.J., 1951), I, 610; Philadelphia *Dunlap's American Daily Advertiser*, 16, 18, August 1791; Minutes, Philadelphia Dispensary, 26 August 1791. Cf. [William Lawrence], *History of Boston Dispensary*, pp. 90–91, 98–99. Another dispensary noted at the mid-century that they had 'often been accused, as being rather the schools, where the young and inexperienced might find patients to their hands, than benevolent institutions where sufferings might be allayed and diseases cured.' DeMilt Dispensary, *2nd Annual Report, 1852–53* (New York, 1853), p. 8.

20. Surviving archives of the Boston Dispensary, for example, indicate in letters of recommendation for district physicians the pattern we have suggested: The Bigelows, James Jackson, and Oliver Wendell Holmes recommend and are recommended. Successful candidates had frequently studied in Europe and the Tremont Medical School or served as house physicians at the Massachusetts General Hospital. Cf. James Jackson to Board of Managers, 3 August 1831; O. W. Holmes to William Gray, 3 September 1845, or see letters in 1836 file from John Collins Warren, Jacob Bigelow, and George Hayward recommending O. W. Holmes as a visiting physician. BDA.

ships were normally reserved, in dispensaries as in hospitals, for a community's most influential and respected physicians.) Contemporaries never questioned the dispensary's teaching function. The trustees of the New York Dispensary admitted, for example, in 1854 that their institution served as 'a practical school for physicians,' but, they contended, it was a perfectly defensible policy: 'for, by this system, these Physicians must become accomplished practitioners, by the time the growth of their private practice shall oblige them to resign their posts at the Dispensary.' With the growing importance of specialization as prerequisite to intellectual status and economic success after mid-century, the increasingly specialized dispensaries served as *de facto* residency programs, allowing ambitious—and often well-connected—young men to accumulate experience and reputation. Though formal statements by medical spokesmen uniformly disowned 'exclusive' specialism until long after the Civil War, devotion to a pragmatic specialism was established much earlier in America's cities. In 1839, for example, the editor of the *Boston Medical & Surgical Journal* remarked, in commenting on the specialty organization of New York's Northern Dispensary, that 'such is manifestly the tendency in our times, in the great cities, and it is the only way of becoming eminently qualified for rendering the best professional services—to learn to do one thing as well as it can be done.'[21]

If the dispensary made excellent sense in terms of the institutional needs of American medicine, it was equally consistent with the technological means available—both at the end of the eighteenth century, and through the first half of the nineteenth. Beyond the stethoscope—not routinely applied before mid-century—no special aids to diagnosis were available to any physician, no therapeutics beyond bleeding, cupping, and administration of drugs. Surgery was ordinarily limited, for rich and poor alike, to the treatment of lacerations and fractures, the reduction of occasional dislocations, the lancing of boils and abscesses. Dispensaries seemed, for many decades into the nineteenth century, fully able to provide both adequate care for the poor and adequate training for their attendants.

The dispensaries seemed equally appropriate to the needs of a small and relatively homogeneous community. The world of the late eighteenth century assumed—even if it did not necessarily practice—face-to-face in-

21. New York Dispensary, *Annual Report, 1854* (New York, 1855), p. 9. A year later, the same Dispensary contended that their staff members 'in a few years, hope to be the eminent physicians of New York, and it is their right to expect, and of the community to require, that the unequaled advantages, to be found here, should be freely offered them.' *Annual Report, 1855* (New York, 1856), p. 10. *Boston med. surg. J.*, 1839, *20*, 351.

teraction between members of different social classes, interactions structured by customary relations of deference and stewardship. This social world-view is concretely illustrated in the acceptance by the dispensaries' founding generation of the contributor recommendation as basis for patient referrals. A certificate of recommendation was necessary, that is, before the dispensary would undertake treatment of a particular patient. This followed English hospital and dispensary practice. As the century progressed, however, the dispensaries which maintained the practice sometimes found it a cause of conflict between medical staff and lay managers. By-laws specified the privileges of recommendation accompanying each contributing membership; a typical arrangement was that which in exchange for a five dollar annual subscription offered the right to recommend two patients at any one time during the year. A fifty dollar subscription typically brought the same privilege for life. Similarly, early dispensary by-laws indicate that members of the boards of managers were expected to play an active and often personal role; the New York Dispensary, for example, created a trustees' committee to accompany visiting physicians on their rounds once a month.[22]

Equally revelatory of the world-view shared by the pious and benevolent Americans who founded the dispensaries, was their assumption that a crucial difference separated the dispensary from the hospital patient; the dispensary patients would be drawn from among the worthy poor, hard-working and able to support themselves, except in periods of sickness or general unemployment. Such worthy poor might also include widows, orphans, and the handicapped. The lying-in department of Philadelphia's Northern Dispensary declared in 1835, for example, that it could aid only married women of respectable character, 'such as require no aid when in health.' Financial support for the dispensary would, the argument followed, keep such honest folk from alms-house residence and morally-contaminating contact with those abandoned souls who were its natural inmates. Dispensary spokesmen tirelessly repeated these stylized categories by way of argument even as experience indicated that this neat and comforting ideological distinction failed to reflect reality. In 1830, a physician

22. New York (City) Dispensary, *Charter and By-Laws* . . . (New York, 1814), p. 8. Another indication of the social assumptions of the generation which created the dispensaries was their concern over whether servants and apprentices were appropriate patients. John Bard argued in New York that servants should indeed be treated, but not at their place of work—which would have compelled 'gentlemen to visit the servants of families in which they had no acquaintance with the Masters or Mistresses.' *A Letter from Dr. John Bard . . . to the Author of Thoughts on the Dispensary* . . . (New York, 1791), p. 20. See the entry for 17 July 1786 in the Minutes of the Philadelphia Dispensary for the question of treating apprentices.

of the Boston Dispensary could complain indignantly that persons of the 'most depraved and abandoned character frequently apply who think they have a right of choice between the Alms-House and the Dispensary.' As late as 1869, the Philadelphia Dispensary could still explain that[23]

> The principal object of this institution is to afford medical relief to the worthy (not the lowest class of) poor, in those cases where removal to a hospital would for any approved reason be ineligible. . . . In a thrifty population like our own, it is the exception . . . where removal to a hospital should be considered eligible.

The dispensaries were founded and grew, finally, because they were entirely consistent with the assumptions of most Americans in regard to the responsibilities of government and appropriate forms and functions of the public institutions which embodied such responsibilities. The prostitute, the drunkard, the lunatic and cripple were the city's responsibility—social subject matter for the alms-house or city physician. The dispensary, on the other hand, represented an appropriate response of humane and thoughtful Americans to the needs of hard-working fellow citizens, a response demanded both by Christian benevolence and community-oriented prudence; it was a form of social intervention limited, conservative and spiritually rewarding. In the second third of the nineteenth century, as demographic realities shifted inexorably, this traditional view still served to justify the now-expanded work of the dispensaries—and at the same time to avoid systematic analysis of the changing nature and social condition of the constituency they served. It was only very slowly, and only in the minds of a minority of those associated with dispensary work, that it became clear that many of their city's honest and industrious laboring men were unable to pay for medical care even in times of prosperity.

The dispensary continued to change throughout the second half of the nineteenth century. We have already referred to their increase in numbers and degree of specialization. Equally significant was expansion of the dispensary form under new kinds of auspices. First, most urban—and even some small town—medical schools anxious to compete for students, established their own dispensaries so as to offer 'clinical material' for their em-

---

23. Philadelphia Northern Dispensary, Philadelphia Lying-In Hospital, 'Rules and Regulations, Adopted November 4, 1835,' Historical Collections, College of Physicians of Philadelphia; [?] to Board of Managers, 1 October 1830, BDA. *Rules of the Philadelphia Dispensary with the Annual Report for 1869* (Philadelphia, 1870), p. 10. As late as 1879, the organizers of a specialized New York dispensary contended that they appealed to those patients able to pay a small fee and thus 'saved the necessary associations of a public, free dispensary.' *Report of the East Side Infirmary for Fistula and other Diseases of the Rectum* (New York, 1879), p. 5. Cf. Pittsburgh Free Dispensary, *3rd Annual Report, 1875* (Pittsburgh, 1876), p. 9.

bryo physicians. Second, hospitals not only increased in number in the last third of the century, they also began to provide more outpatient care, in some localities duplicating services already offered by dispensaries. In Philadelphia with its flourishing medical schools the rivalry between hospitals and dispensaries emerged as early as 1845.[24] In certain areas outpatient facilities competed for patients, medical school clinics in particular advertising in newspapers and posting handbills. All these events were correlated, of course, with a growing demand within the medical profession for clinical training at every level, for the possession of attending and consulting physicianships, for the accumulation of specialty credentials. At the end of the century, finally, a growing public health movement used the by now familiar dispensary form to shape and deliver medical care and would-be prophylactic measures in slum areas—most conspicuously in the identification and treatment of tuberculosis.

Underlying these developments were a series of parallel changes, first in the scale of the human problems the dispensaries faced, second in the intellectual tools and social organization of the medical profession. First in time came an absolute increase in the numbers and shift in the social origins of those urban Americans calling upon the dispensary. Secondly, in terms of chronology if not significance, were shifts within the world of medicine which made the dispensary increasingly marginal in the priorities of medical men. One need hardly demonstrate the significance to medical practice of increasing specialization, the germ theory and antisepsis, the development of modern surgery, x-ray and clinical laboratory methods, the increasing centrality of the hospital; the way in which demographic and social changes reshaped the dispensaries is perhaps less familiar.

Whatever degree of reality there had been in the original vision of a community bound by common ties of assumption and identity, this unifying vision corresponded less and less to reality as the nineteenth century progressed. The accustomed social distance between physician and charity patient seemed increasingly unbridgeable. A practical measure of this increasing social distance—and one which correlates with population and immigration statistics—was the growing disquietude of dispensary physicians in contemplating their patients. As early as 1828, New York's Northern Dispensary asked contributors to sympathize with their staff physicians'

... great sacrifices of feeling and comfort, which they must necessarily make, by being forced into daily and hourly association with the miserable and degraded

---

24. Philadelphia Dispensary, Minutes, 26 December 1845, APH.

of our species, loathsome from disease, and often still more so by those disgusting habits which go to the utter extinction of decency in all its forms.

The traditional system in which dispensary patients or their messengers called first upon contributors seeking a recommendation and then upon visiting physicians at their regular homes or offices also showed signs of strain. In Boston, where the dispensary's lay managers had long opposed the establishment of a 'central office,' a major factor helping to overcome this reluctance in the 1850s was the unwillingness of district physicians to have their offices used by so 'ignorant and degraded a class.' 'It is undesirable,' as Henry J. Bigelow explained it, 'for most physicians to receive at their own apartments the class of applicants who now form the mass of dispensary patients.'[25]

The patients who seemed most familiar, closest to the physicians' own experience were those most capable of evoking sympathy and understanding; thus the plight of those fallen in fortune, of the genteel widow, of the orphaned child of good parents were those which touched visiting physicians most deeply.

It is not infrequently that we witness much feeling manifested by those who have been able to employ their own physicians and purchase their own medicines, when through reverses of fortune they have for the first time applied for assistance from the Institution; such constitute the most interesting portion of our patients.

Other patients were far less interesting.[26]

There were, of course, the venereal and alcoholic; but these had always existed and their existence had always implied a certain conflict between morals and medical care. Far more unsettling by the 1840s were the new immigrants who streamed into America's cities and soon constituted a disproportionate part of the dispensary's clientele. By the early 1850s it was not uncommon for an absolute majority of a particular institutions' pa-

25. Northern Dispensary (New York), *1st Annual Report, 1828* (New York, 1828), cont. p. 10; DeMilt Dispensary, *2nd Annual Report, 1853* (New York, 1853), p. 12; Bigelow to D. D. Slade, 22 August 1855, BDA. Cf. D. D. Slade to My Dear Sir [William Lawrence], 3 September 1855, BDA; [Lawrence,] *History of the Boston Dispensary*, pp. 178–80.

26. Northern Dispensary (Philadelphia), *Annual Report, 1847* (Philadelphia, 1848), p. 10. Such sentiments were familiar ones. A 'Contributor' to the Boston Dispensary explained in 1819 that its appropriate clients were those 'many persons . . . who have been reduced from a state of competence to one little short of poverty, who while blessed with health, can, by industry, support themselves, but when attacked by sickness, and laid upon a bed of illness, find it impossible to pay the physician and apothecary.' *New-England Palladium and Commercial Advertiser*, 12 January 1819. The earliest rules of both Philadelphia and Boston dispensaries emphasized their wish to comfort 'those who have seen better days . . . without being humiliated.' Boston Dispensary, *Institution of . . . 1817* (Boston, 1817), p. 7.

tients to have been born in Ireland; in the districts of individual visiting physicians over ninety per cent of those treated might be foreign born. Not surprisingly, the 1840s and 1850s saw dispensary administrators and trustees pointing again and again to the immigrant as they sought to explain the difficulties of their work and their ever increasing financial need.[27]

It was not only the numbers and poverty, but the alienness of the immigrants which intensified the differences between them and their would-be medical attendants. It must be recalled that the desirability of dispensary appointments guaranteed their being filled by young physicians of at least middle class background—thus insuring as well a maximum social distance between physician and patient. As early as 1831, for example, Boston Dispensary visiting physicians, dismayed by the conditions they encountered, elected to survey the economic and moral status of their patients. In that age of temperance and pietism, it was only to have been expected that the district physicians found intemperance to be the most important single cause of disease in their patients—and intemperance to be most common among the foreign born. The Irish seemed particularly undesirable, filthy, drunken, generally inhospitable to middle class standards of behavior. 'Upon their habits—their mode of life,' a dispensary physician explained in 1850, 'depend the frequency and violence of disease. This I am fearful will continue to be the case, since no form of legislation can reach them, or force them to change their habits for those more conducive to cleanliness and health.' 'Deserving American poor,' another Boston Dispensary physician complained, were 'often deterred from seeking aid because they shrink from seeming to place themselves on a level with the degraded classes among the Irish.'[28] The unfamiliar attitudes and habits of these patients often added to their troublesomeness; they ignored hygienic advice and often defied the physician's simplest requests. The Irish, for example, considered it dangerous to have lymph removed from the lesion of an individual vaccinated for smallpox; thus they refused to return to the

27. In the New York Dispensary, for example, in 1853, of 7,188 patients treated, 1,582 were born in the United States and 4,886 in Ireland. At the Philadelphia Dispensary in 1857, 1,906 were born in the United States, 3,649 in Ireland. New York Dispensary, *64th Annual Report, 1853* (New York, 1854), p. 12; Philadelphia Dispensary, *Rules . . . with Annual Report for 1857* (Philadelphia, 1858), p. 14. Some dispensaries would not allow venereal cases to be treated, some imposed a special fee, while still others allowed individual physicians to decide whether they would treat such errant souls.

28. Luther Parks, Jr. to Board of Managers, 10 June 1850, Boston Dispensary Archives. Referring to the Irish, another Dispensary physician explained: 'Upon their habits,—and mode of life, depend the frequency and violence of disease. This I am fearful will continue to be the case, since no form of legislation can reach them, or force them to change their habits for those more conducive to cleanliness and health.' Charles W. Moore to Board of Managers, 1 April 1857, BDA. On the temperance question, see, for example: J. B. S. Jackson to Board of Managers, 8 October 1853, BDA.

dispensary after the required week to have the lesion checked (and to supply the lymph so useful in helping balance the dispensary's budget).[29] Later immigrant groups brought their peculiar beliefs and problems of communication; Jews and Italians replaced the Irish as objects of the dispensary physician's frustration and disdain.

A good many dispensary physicians were, of course, sympathetic to their patients, and in some cases not only sympathetic but convinced that environmental causes contributed to their clients' chronic ill-health. Yet even those individual physicians whose personal convictions made them most sensitive to the deprivation of their city's slum-dwellers, shared the ambivalence and even hostility of their peers. The same mid-century physicians, that is, who denounced basement dwellings, exploitative landlords, rotting meat and adulterated milk—shared a distaste for the intemperance, imprudence, filth and apparent sexual immorality of those victimized by such conditions. One of the harsher dispensary critics of mid-century tenement conditions could, for example, contend that

... there is much squalor and other evidences of poverty which might be remedied had the patients more pride in cleanliness and more ambition to be doing well in the world.

As another mid-century physician explained, his patients' degradation and ignorance called 'not for pity alone, but for the greatest exercise of patience and forbearance.'[30]

A concern with social realities was, moreover, supported by and consistent with mid-nineteenth-century etiological assumptions. Both acute and constitutional ills were seen as related closely to an individual's powers of resistance—itself a product of interaction between constitution and environment. And the conditions encountered by dispensary physicians were exactly those which seemed to lower resistance and hence increase the incidence and virulence of disease. Thus a dispensary physician could note casually that scarlet fever was particularly virulent one year, since it proved as fatal to the rich as to the poor. Similarly, a pioneer ophthalmologist could urge the need for ophthalmological dispensaries because of the relationship between poverty and diseases of the eye:

---

29. New York Dispensary, *64th Annual Report, 1853* (New York, 1854), p. 10; New York Dispensary, *72nd Annual Report, 1862* (1863), p. 20. When, in an effort to solve this problem New York's dispensaries initiated a small deposit to be refunded when the patient returned to have the vaccination checked, these intractable—and seemingly ungrateful—patients chose to regard it as a payment absolving them of any responsibility to the institution.

30. J. Trenor, Jr., physician to middle district, Eastern Dispensary (New York), *25th Annual Report, 1858* (New York, 1859), p. 32; New York Dispensary, *Annual Report, 1837* (New York, 1838), p. 7.

The sickly hue, and the toil worn features of these poor people are but the results of constitutional derangements . . . and as clearly reveal the inseparable union between the health of the body and the health of the eye, as between poverty and disease.

Throughout the century articulate dispensary spokesmen were aware of the need to provide food and clothing for their patients, convinced that medicines could be of only marginal help when patients had to return to work before their complete recovery, while their homes had no adequate heat, their tables only impure and decaying food. 'No persons can more readily appreciate than we,' as one put it, 'the utter uselessness of drugs, if there is no possibility of nourishing and warming the patient.'[31]

The attitudes of mid and late nineteenth-century physicians can best be described in terms not of hostility, but of ambivalence—and perhaps most importantly an ambivalence characterized by a world-view which related disease and morals alike to general social conditions. Both morality and morbidity were seen as resultants of the interactions between environmental circumstance and culpable moral decisions. This mixture of social concern, moralism, meliorism and deep seated antipathy was clearly apparent by mid-century and marked the writings of most dispensary spokesmen until the end of the century; it could not prove the basis of a long-lived commitment to the dispensary and the necessity of its peculiar social function.

Nevertheless, a handful of articulate spokesmen for the dispensary did elaborate a characteristic point of view by the century's end, in which disease was seen not only as related inextricably to environment, but which emphasized the dispensary's capacity to reach out into the homes of the sick poor, so as to deal with problems more fundamental than the symptoms which brought the patient to their attention. The ability of the dispensary to relate to the community surrounding it became in the arguments of such dispensary defenders an indispensable aspect of a socially adequate medical care system. Visiting physicians and nurses could simply not be replaced by a hospital out-patient department. Advocates of this higher dispensary calling argued again and again that one could not simply treat a patient's symptoms and do nothing about an environment which had much to do with causing those very symptoms. Such ideas were im-

---

[31]. Edward Reynolds, *An Address at the Dedication of the New Building of the Massachusetts Eye and Ear Infirmary, July 3, 1850* (Boston, 1850), p. 15; Mission Hospital and Dispensary for Women and Children, *2nd Annual Report, 1876* (Philadelphia, 1877), p. 10. The scarlet fever reference was by William Bibbins, DeMilt Dispensary, *6th Annual Report, 1856-57* (New York, 1857), p. 17.

plemented perhaps most fully in the tuberculosis dispensaries created so widely in the first decade of the twentieth century.[32]

Such would-be rationalizers of American medicine as Edward Corwin, S. S. Goldwater, Richard Cabot and Michael Davis contended that the dispensary could, in addition to supplying primary treatment for the indigent, supplement the necessarily unfinished work of the general practitioner in those numerous cases where the patient could not afford a specialist's consultation or expensive x-rays and laboratory tests. The dispensary could, that is, serve a vast urban constituency able perhaps to afford the services of a general practitioner but unable to manage the cost of more extended or elaborate medical care. And such occasions increased steadily as the profession's ability to understand and even cure increased. Yet even as they urged such prudent considerations, these advocates of social medicine were well aware of the threat posed to the independence and ultimately to the existence of the dispensary by rapid changes in medical ideas, techniques, and institutional forms.

These arguments were consistent as well with the motivations and social assumptions of the contemporary settlement-house movement and other pioneer social welfare advocates. The settlement-houses were often involved in dispensary-like programs themselves. But in a precisely timed irony, the dispensary as a viable independent institution was dying just as its most self-conscious advocates were formulating these brave contentions.

How did this come about? The dispensaries could hardly be said to have lost their social function; we have become quite conscious in recent years that their function is still not being adequately fulfilled. In retrospect, however, their dissolution was inevitable. By the 1920s, most significantly, the dispensary had become as marginal to the needs of the medical profession as it had been central in the first two-thirds of the nineteenth century. A century of work in the city's slums, a growing—if always somewhat ambiguous—awareness of the relationship between health and environment,

---

32. For useful descriptions of the tuberculosis clinics, see, for example: F. Elisabeth Crowell, *The Work of New York's Tuberculosis Clinics*... (New York, 1910); Louis Hamman, 'A Brief Report of the First Two Years' Work in the Phipps Dispensary for Tuberculosis of the Johns Hopkins Hospital,' *Johns Hopkins Hosp. Bull.*, 1907, *18*, 293–97. For samples of the more positive defense of the dispensary and its appropriate role, see: S. S. Goldwater, 'Dispensary Ideals: With a Plan for Dispensary Reform ...,' *Am. J. med. Sci.*, 1907, n.s. *134*, 313–335; Richard Cabot, 'Why Should Hospitals Neglect the Care of Chronic Curable Disease in Out-Patients?' *St. Paul med. J.*, 1908, *10*, 110–20; Cabot, 'Out-Patient Work. The Most Important and Most Neglected Part of Medical Service,' *J. Am. med. Ass.*, 1912, *59*, 1688–89; Good Samaritan Dispensary (New York), *29th Annual Report, 1919* (New York, 1920), p. 8. The most complete statement of a positive dispensary program is to be found in Davis and Warner, *Dispensaries* (n. 1).

the conscious commitment of a small leadership group to the need for working in that human environment—all proved ultimately of little importance.

As hospital-centered interne and residency programs became a normal part of medical education—following inclusion of clinical training in the undergraduate years—it was inevitable that those elite physicians who would in earlier generations have been anxious to receive a dispensary appointment would now prefer hospital posts. Not only had hospitals increased greatly in number, but they contained beds, laboratory and x-ray facilities, and a cluster of appropriately trained specialists. The hospital's increasingly exclusive claims to practice the best, indeed the only adequate medicine seemed to grow more and more plausible. When, for example, in 1922 the Managers of the Philadelphia Dispensary decided to merge with the Pennsylvania Hospital, they explained that they had 'found it practically impossible for an independent dispensary, unassociated with the facilities and specialists of a large modern hospital, to render the public adequate service.'[33]

As the intellectual and institutional aspects of medicine changed, economic pressures also pointed toward the centralized and capital-intensive logic of the hospital. Expensive laboratory facilities, x-rays, modern operating rooms all demanded the investment of unprecedently large sums of money. The routine low-budget dosing which characterized the independent nineteenth-century dispensary seemed no longer a real option; dispensary boards had to face a growing and embarrassing asymmetry between their limited resources and the demands of high quality medical care. The hospital out-patient department seemed to many medical men a substantial and inevitable improvement over its predecessor institution. The growing tendency in the twentieth century for medical schools to forge strong hospital ties only increased the centrality of the hospital.

Shorn of its relevance to the career needs of aspiring physicians, the dispensary was left with the clearly residual function of providing public health—charity—medical care, in itself a low-status occupation throughout the nineteenth century. Dispensary appointments had brought pres-

---

33. Philadelphia Dispensary, Minutes, 8 January 1923, APH. At the end of the nineteenth century, for example, the Boston Dispensary began a search for beds; it seemed a necessity if bright young men were to be kept on the staff. *Report of the Dinner given to the Board of Managers of the Boston Dispensary by the Staff of Physicians . . . January 25th, 1909* [Boston, 1909], p. 13. Once allied with a hospital, the dispensary had invariably a lower status. Francis R. Packard charged in 1903 that hospitals would casually spend two or three hundred dollars for new surgical instruments yet balk at ten or fifteen for the dispensary. F. B. Kirkbride, *Dispensary Problem in Philadelphia*, p. 21.

tige and clinical opportunities in generations during which there were few other badges of status or roads to the acquisition of clinical skills; by the end of the century, there were other, more prestigious options for the ambitious young physician. Positions as municipal 'out-door physicians' had a comparatively low status throughout the nineteenth century. The dominion of fee for service medicine remained essentially unchallenged by the liberal critics of the Progressive generation. Those ambitious young men incapable of remaining content with the mere accumulation of fees were—as the twentieth century advanced—ordinarily attracted not by social medicine but increasingly by the 'higher' and certainly less ambiguous demands of research; and even clinical investigation seemed in its most demanding forms to have little place in the dispensary.

If the dispensary had lost much of its appeal for the medical elite by the end of the nineteenth century, it had lost whatever goodwill it had had in the mind of the average practitioner decades earlier. There had always been occasional complaints in regard to the dispensaries intervening unfairly to compete with private physicians for a limited supply of paying patients. From the earliest years of their operation, American dispensaries had warned that their services were only for 'such as are really necessitous.' None however chose to investigate systematically the means of their patients until after the Civil War. Until the 1870s, criticism was comparatively muted; throughout the last third of the century, however, and into the twentieth, the dispensaries were widely attacked as purveyors of ill-considered charity to the unworthy. The more constructive critics sought to find alternatives, the most popular—in addition to simply demanding a small fee—being the provident dispensary, a species of pre-paid health plan which had proven workable in some areas in England. In city after city, local practitioners called meetings and commissioned reports predictably concluding that a goodly portion of those using dispensary services were quite capable of paying a private physician's fees.[34] Americans found it difficult to understand the social configuration of the society in which they lived; only abuse by those in fact capable of paying medical bills could

---

34. Probably most significant is the tone of this debate. It was the ordinary practitioner who generally resented the way in which dispensaries with their elite house staffs attracted cases which might otherwise have remained in the hands of private practitioners. Discussions of 'dispensary abuse' also served to express the resentment of many practitioners against the monopolization of hospital and dispensary posts by a minority of well-connected physicians. In its report on charity abuse, for example, the Medical Association of the District of Columbia also urged limited tenure in hospital staff appointments and access to hospital privileges for all 'reputable members of the profession.' *Report of the Special Committee . . . on the Hospital and Dispensary Abuse in the City of Washington* (Washington, 1896), pp. 15–16.

possibly explain the vast numbers who utilized dispensary services. To doubt this was to assume that large numbers of worthy and hard-working Americans were indeed too poor to pay for even minimally adequate medical care.[35]

Physicians were often unwilling to refer their paying patients—even if the payment were only twenty-five or fifty cents—to the more specialized facilities of neighboring dispensaries. As late as 1914 the director of Pennsylvania's tuberculosis program charged that local practitioners refused to refer patients in the early stages of the disease, unwilling to relinquish treatment until such working-people were too deteriorated to work—and pay. Attacks on the dispensary system were generally supported as well by the charity organization movement which, in city after city, attacked dispensary medicine as an excellent example of that undiscriminating alms-giving which served only to demoralize its recipients. (It should be noted that the majority of empirical studies of dispensary patients completed between the 1870s and the First World War indicated that most dispensary patients were not in fact able to pay for medical care.)[36]

By the last quarter of the nineteenth century the dispensary patient no longer fit into that same vision of an ordered social universe which had guided and inspired the efforts of those benevolent Americans who had founded the first dispensaries a century earlier. Those older views of community and stewardship implied in the contributor-sponsorship system had faded by mid-century, paralleling changes in the environmental reality of America's cities. Similarly, it would have been hardly plausible to argue that New York or Boston tenement-dwellers should be visited in their homes so as to spare them the indignity of hospitalization. The constituency of both hospital and dispensary had changed. By the closing years of the nineteenth century, the dispensary had very clearly become the provider of charity medicine for a class who—if indeed worthy of such charity—were sharply differentiated from paying patients and who ordinarily lived in a section of the city removed physically from that of contributors, physicians, and private patients. Before mid-century and especially in the first quarter of the nineteenth century, dispensary managers still sought to enforce requirements that visiting physicians actually reside in the district they served—a natural enough sentiment in the eighteenth

---

35. [William Lawrence], *Medical Relief to the Poor. September, 1877* (Boston, 1877), pp. 3-4; James Keiser, 'The Abuses in Hospital and Dispensary Practice in Reading,' *National Hospital Record*, 1899.

36. Albert P. Francine, 'The State Tuberculosis Dispensaries,' *Penn. med. J.*, 1914, *17*, 940. See Davis and Warner, *Dispensaries*, pp. 42-58 for a brief discussion of patient eligibility.

century but impracticable in post-bellum America.[37] The arguments employed by the end of the century to attract contributions had become almost exclusively prudential, appealing little either to explicitly religious convictions or to a feeling of identity with those at risk. Fund-raising circulars emphasized instead the need to avert crime, pauperism and prostitution.

Positive support for the dispensaries was, on the other hand, shaky indeed; aside from the support implicit in the inertia developed by all institutions, only a small group of socially-active physicians and proto-social-welfare activists defended the dispensaries as a positive good. Many social workers, as we have indicated, evinced little affection for an institution which seemed to embody so casual and unscientific an approach to philanthropy. Even the oldest dispensaries did not survive as independent institutions past the early 1920s.

Historians have devoted little attention to the dispensary. Yet as our contemporaries begin to concern themselves with the delivery of medical care this neglect may end; for the dispensary provides such would-be reformers with a potentially usable past. The dispensary did at first provide a flexible, informal, and locally-oriented framework for the delivery of public medicine. But the analogy to contemporary problems is limited; the flexibility and informality of the dispensary were a result of medicine's still primitive tools, its local orientation a consequence of the contributors being in some sense—or assuming themselves to be—part of the community served by the dispensary. Such conditions ceased to exist well before the end of the nineteenth century. And even within its own frame of reference, the nineteenth-century dispensary provided second-class, routine, episodic medicine, was a victim of shabby budgets, and even in its earliest decades marked by unquestioned distance between physician and patient. (A distance *perhaps* made tolerable by traditional attitudes of hierarchy and deference.)

Yet despite these imperfections, the death of the dispensary and the transfer of its functions and client constituency to general hospitals has not been an unqualified success. And though the history of the rise and fall of the dispensary provides no explicit program for contemporary medicine, it does underline a simple moral: any plan for the reordering of medical care must be based on the accommodation of at least three different factors. One is felt social need, felt that is by those with power to change social

---

37. G. F. Thayer to William Gray, 12 April 1838, BDA.

policy. A second factor is general social values and assumptions as they shape the world-view and thus help define the options available to such decision-makers. Third, there are the needs of the medical profession, needs expressed in the career decisions of particular physicians and needs defined by medicine's intellectual tools and institutional forms. Without a strong commitment to government intervention in health matters—a commitment impossible without an appropriate change in general social values —factors internal to the world of medicine have determined most forcefully the specific forms in которой medical care has been provided for the American people. Thus the rise and fall of the dispensary; it was doomed neither by policy nor conspiracy but by a steadily shifting configuration of medical perceptions and priorities.

Department of History
University of Pennsylvania